NURSING LEADERSHIP FROM A CANADIAN PERSPECTIVE

Verna C. Pangman, RN, BA, MEd, MN
Senior Instructor, Faculty of Nursing
University of Manitoba
Winnipeg, Manitoba

Clare H. Pangman, BSc, BEd, MA, PhD
Associate Professor (Retired), Faculty of Education
University of Manitoba
Winnipeg, Manitoba

Wolters Kluwer | Lippincott Williams & Wilkins
Health
Philadelphia · Baltimore · New York · London
Buenos Aires · Hong Kong · Sydney · Tokyo

Acquisitions Editor: Elizabeth Nieginski
Developmental Editor: Melanie G. Cann
Project Manager: Cindy Oberle
Manufacturing Manager: Karin Duffield
Marketing Manager: Jodi Bukowski
Design Coordinator: Joan Wendt
Production Service: Maryland Composition/ASI

© 2010 by **LIPPINCOTT WILLIAMS & WILKINS, a WOLTERS KLUWER business**
530 Walnut Street
Philadelphia, PA 19106 USA
LWW.com

Printed in China

Library of Congress Cataloging-in-Publication Data

Pangman, Verna C.
  Nursing leadership from a Canadian perspective / Verna C. Pangman, Clare H. Pangman.
    p. ; cm.
  Includes bibliographical references and index.
  ISBN 978-0-7817-7794-0
  ISBN 0-7817-7794-1
  1. Nursing services—Canada—Personnel management. 2. Nurse administrators—Canada. 3. Leadership—Canada.
I. Pangman, Clare H. II. Title.
  [DNLM: 1. Leadership—Canada. 2. Nursing, Supervisory—trends—Canada. 3. Clinical Competence—Canada.
4. Nurse Administrators—trends—Canada. WY 105 P191n 2009]
  RT89.3.P36 2009
  362.17'30680971—dc22
                                                                                          2008042712

About the Authors

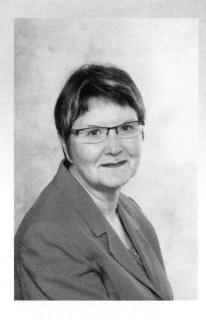

Verna C. Pangman is a Senior Instructor in the Faculty of Nursing, University of Manitoba. Verna has been course leader for many courses at the undergraduate level. Her nursing practice has been primarily with adults in mental health, palliative care, and long-term care settings. Her research interest lies in the field of gerontology, with a focus on family care. She is a Research Affiliate at a long-term care facility and at the Centre of Aging, University of Manitoba. She has published articles on older adults, both as a primary and secondary author, in peer-reviewed scholarly journals. She has presented papers provincially and nationally in the field of gerontology. Verna is involved in Faculty Practice, which helps to enhance her leadership and clinical skills.

Verna is a member of the College of Registered Nurses of Manitoba and a member of Sigma Theta Tau Nursing Honour Society, XI Lambda Chapter. Most recently, Verna received the Excellence in Professional Nursing Award from the College of Registered Nurses of Manitoba.

In the community, she volunteers for the Speakers Bureau, Alzheimer Society, Province of Manitoba. She is a member of the Senior Transport Institute, a committee that advocates for improved transportation facilities for seniors. Verna enjoys golfing and travelling with her husband, Clare. During the summer, they relax and enjoy their summer home on Lake Winnipeg near Gimli, Manitoba. During the winter, Verna enjoys teaching, researching current nursing publications, and writing manuscripts.

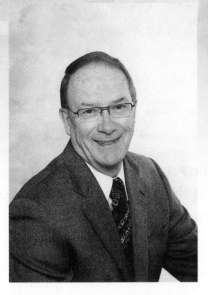

Clare H. Pangman is a retired professor from the Faculty of Education, University of Manitoba. Clare began his career teaching mathematics and science at the junior high and high school levels. Later in his career, Clare taught undergraduate psychology at Brandon University. While at the University of Manitoba, he taught at both the graduate and undergraduate levels in Education. At the undergraduate level, Clare taught courses on teaching and learning to pre-service undergraduate student teachers. At the graduate level, his emphasis was on teaching and learning in postsecondary institutions.

For more than 15 years at the University of Manitoba, Clare was a member of The University of Manitoba Teaching Services Unit, where teaching development workshops and seminars for university teachers were created and delivered to professors as well as to graduate students with university teaching assignments. These courses and seminars have since become part of the requirements University of Manitoba teachers can complete to qualify for the Certificate in University Teaching. Over the final 12 years of his career at the University of Manitoba, Clare served as Director of the Teaching Services Unit, which served more than 1,500 professors from all faculties and schools, both at the main campus and at the Health Sciences Campus.

Clare enjoys co-authoring with his wife, Verna. In addition, he is an avid gardener and golfer in summer and a curler in winter, and throughout the year, the Pangmans enjoy good movies, theatre, friends, and travelling.

To all student nurses who are on a quest to increase the visibility of the role of the nurse leader in order to meet the health care challenges of tomorrow.

Go gently.

Verna and Clare Pangman

Preface

The Canadian Nurses Association Position Statement on Nursing Leadership (2002) emphasized that the field of nursing requires visionary leaders who are visible and inspire others and who support professional practice. Significant changes in the health care delivery system require leaders to understand the structure and process of change in organizations. Leaders must assist others to develop the competencies of teamwork and collaboration. To provide the leadership required in this fast-paced and challenging health care environment, nurses need a current, effective, and established knowledge base from which they can draw evidence to develop their understanding of the leadership roles, relationships, and competencies needed to provide support and opportunities to a culturally diverse health care team.

This textbook presents to Canadian nursing students a current, research-based understanding of theory and development aimed at professional nursing competencies. It provides leadership insights rich in self-reflection to serve as the foundation for the development of the knowledge, competencies, and positive attitudes required for leadership. Related to the *business* of health care, the textbook provides an overview of the knowledge base and the set of competencies required of a nurse manager to deliver effective clinical health services. New nurse graduates will continually experience challenges resulting from dramatic technological development and rapid restructuring of the health care delivery system. This textbook helps to ensure that future nurse leaders are both knowledgeable about, and proficient in, the effective leadership practices they will need to meet these challenges. In addition, this textbook helps to prepare the nursing student to challenge the Canadian Registered Nurse Examination (CRNE).

Organization

The textbook comprises 15 chapters that are organized into four sections, as follows:

Section 1 (Chapters 1 through 5). Restructuring the Canadian Health Care System: Role of the Nurse Leader. This section begins with an overview of the Canadian health care system. The primary health care model is reviewed, the population health approach is described, and the dynamics of health care organizations are outlined to provide an understanding of organizations and the process of change. Featured throughout the chapters is the role of the nurse leader in relation to the continuum of health care services in various settings.

Section 2 (Chapters 6 through 9). Refocusing on the Leadership Role. This section introduces the current role of nursing leadership. The role of the nurse manager is described, and various financial and staffing issues are considered. The new Code of Ethics (2008) is described, along with its effect on nurse leaders. Emphasis is placed on the value of interdisciplinary teams for improving the health outcomes of clients.

Section 3 (Chapters 10 through 12). Reassessing Leadership Competencies. This section extensively reviews the competencies of decision making, conflict resolution, and time management and delegation, all of which are critical for nurse leaders.

Section 4 (Chapters 13 through 15). Reframing Leadership. This section begins with a chapter on role transition into career development. Current issues are discussed, including the aging population, sexuality, the environment and genetics, and the role of the nurse leader. The final chapter promotes thinking about the importance of connecting with others in the organization to promote change. The importance of spiritual issues in achieving improved levels of functioning and health within organizations is addressed.

Approach and Features

The material is presented through a narrative and pragmatic approach that invites both the student and the instructor to consider the topic from the position of their knowledge of the matter, along with their related personal experiences. A constructivist approach is used, whereby learners build new knowledge based on their previous knowledge. The learning process is intended to be active in nature. This means that by challenging existing knowledge and comprehension, new learning results.

The goal of each chapter is that the student feels increasingly more confident and sufficiently empowered to step into leadership roles. It is expected that the student will read and understand the material, reflect on ways the material relates to the student's own professional and life experiences, discuss alternative points of view in class, and be prepared to implement the skills of leadership as appropriate in different cultural contexts.

The methods and tools used in the textbook are intended to engage the student nurse actively in the learning process. Cartoons provide visual, and sometimes humorous, reinforcement of selected concepts. Figures, boxes, and tables are used to support the content provided in the text. The purpose of all the features incorporated throughout the text is to encourage students to reflect and to think critically about the many different leadership approaches to health care situations.

Quotes. Each chapter begins with a quote from a Canadian leader related to the chapter topic. A brief biography of the person quoted assists the reader to increase his or her knowledge and appreciation of that particular leader.

Chapter Overviews. Each chapter opens with an overview to help the reader focus his or her learning.

Learner-Centred Objectives. The objectives follow the Revised Bloom's Taxonomy, which places emphasis on instructional delivery and assessment. The objectives enable the reader to proceed into the chapter with a personal road map. It is intended that the reader will actually visualize himself or herself succeeding at the leadership skills presented in the text.

Reflective Thinking. Questions designed to encourage the reader to pause, think about what he or she has just read, and apply the material to his or her own development appear at appropriate points throughout the text.

Reflections on Leadership Practice boxes. Hypothetical situations and related questions prompt the reader to think in detail about particular clinical experiences, enabling the reader to gain additional insights into leadership situations.

Current Leadership Issues. Issues are presented with related questions to guide the reader to think critically and to apply the theoretical knowledge gained in the chapter. This feature promotes discussion with the instructor and colleagues about alternatives and options surrounding the issue.

Websites. Each chapter concludes with a list of useful and related Websites that the reader can visit for more information.

References. Each chapter concludes with a reference list that provides updated sources of information to support the chapter content and evidence-based practice.

Ancillaries

To further facilitate teaching and learning, ancillary materials are available on thePoint (http://thepoint.lww.com). The Point is a Web-based course and content management system that provides every resource instructors and students need in one easy-to-use site.

PowerPoint Presentations. A slide presentation to accompany each chapter in the book is available on ThePoint.

Test Generator. More than 300 multiple-choice questions and the Diploma test generator are provided to instructors on ThePoint. Each of the questions focuses on one of the four competency framework levels as reflected by the Canadian Registered Nurse Exam (CRNE). With the Diploma test generator, instructors can add their own questions, modify existing questions, and create chapter quizzes, section quizzes, and comprehensive exams at the push of a button.

Reviewers

Many thanks are extended to the instructors who read the manuscript during its various stages of development and provided us with valuable suggestions for improving it:

Donna Daines, RN BScN MEd EdD(c)
Year 3 / 4 Coordinator
Assistant Professor
School of Nursing
Thompson Rivers University
Kamloops, British Columbia

Lenore Duquette, BScN, MEd, EdD
Professor, Nursing
Humber College
Toronto, Ontario

Kathy Fukuyama, RN, BSN, MEd
Department Head, BSN Program
Vancouver Community College
Vancouver, British Columbia

Sandra Gessler, RN, BA, MPA
Program Coordinator and Instructor,
    Faculty of Nursing
University of Manitoba
Winnipeg, Manitoba

Angela Gillis, PhD, RN
Professor and Former Chair
St. Francis Xavier University School of
    Nursing
Antigonish, Nova Scotia

Mary Haase, RPN, RN, BScN, PhD
Instructor
Grant MacEwan Community College
Edmonton, Alberta

Lisa High RN, BScN, MScN
Director of Emergency and Critical Care
    Services
Metropolitan Hospital
Windsor Ontario

Linda Hughes, RN, BScN, MPA
Instructor, Faculty of Nursing
University of Manitoba
Winnipeg, Manitoba

Carole-Lynne Le Navenec, RN, PhD
Associate Professor, Faculty of Nursing
University of Calgary
Calgary, Alberta

Sheila McKay, RN, MN
Nursing Instructor
Red Deer College
Red Deer, Alberta

Mitzi Mitchell, RN, GNC (C), BScN, BA,
    MHSc, MN, DNS, PhD(c)
Lecturer, School of Nursing
York University
Toronto, Ontario

Tracy Oosterbroek, RN, BSN, MSc(c)
Nursing Faculty
University of Lethbridge
Lethbridge, Alberta

Aroha Page, RN, BA, BScN, Grad.Dip
   Health Sci, M.Phil(N), PhD(UCSF), FRCNA
Assistant Professor (Tenured)
Nipissing University
North Bay, Ontario

Beth Perry, RN, PhD
Associate Professor, Center for Nursing
   and Health Studies
Athabasca University
Athabasca, Alberta

Wanda Pierson, RN, MSN, MA, PhD
Chair, Nursing Department
Langara College
Vancouver, British Columbia

Donna Romyn, RN, PhD
Director and Associate Professor
Centre for Nursing and Health Studies
Athabasca University
Athabasca, Alberta

Lynn Theriault, RPN, RN, BScN, MHSA
Nursing Instructor
Grant MacEwan Community College
Edmonton, Alberta

Susan Wynne, RN, BsCN, ENC (C),
   CNCC(C)
Clinical Instructor
Trent/Fleming School of Nursing
Peterborough, Ontario

Acknowledgements

We wish to acknowledge and graciously thank all of the dedicated individuals who gave so freely of their time and who made available to us the use of facilities in the Faculty of Nursing at The University of Manitoba:

Dean Dauna Crooks, Faculty of Nursing, University of Manitoba

Jacqueline Dewar, Executive Assistant, Faculty of Nursing, University of Manitoba

The Research Assistants, in particular, Shauna Nelson, Payal Bhatt, Jennifer Gourlay, and Lindsey Kaminiski, for their dedication, enthusiasm, and unending work in assisting us to collect data from various scholarly books and journals.

We would also like to acknowledge and express our thanks to the staff members at Lippincott Williams & Wilkins who have been especially helpful and supportive to us throughout the preparation of this textbook:

Jean Rodenberger, Executive Editor, who believed in our capabilities to write this textbook and encouraged us to do so.

Deedie McMahon, Editor, and Melanie Cann, Senior Developmental Editor, Nursing Education, both of whom worked so tirelessly and supportively with us to complete the work.

Audrey Alt, Ancillary Editor, for her openness, supportive critiques of our work, and being constantly available to us.

Bob Galindo, Illustration Coordinator, and Carmen DiBartolomeo, Art Director, for their management of the art program.

Joan Wendt, Design Coordinator, for her assistance with the interior and cover designs.

Contents

RESTRUCTURING THE CANADIAN HEALTH CARE SYSTEM: ROLE OF THE NURSE LEADER

CANADIAN HEALTH CARE SYSTEM: NURSE LEADERS' JOURNEY DURING THE TRANSITION TO PRIMARY HEALTH CARE

The term primary health care is now entrenched in our minds and our actions. . . . Nursing has been involved in the development of primary health care from the beginning.

—Helen Glass

Dr. Helen Glass, OC, BSc (N), MA (N), MEd (N), Ed D (N), LLD (Hon), DSc (Hon), has received five honourary doctorates and the Jeanne Mance Award (1992), the most prestigious award of the Canadian Nurses Association. She is Professor Emerita, Faculty of Nursing, University of Manitoba, and the former Director of the (then) School of Nursing, University of Manitoba, Winnipeg.

Overview

The current structure of the Canadian health care system has undergone a gradual process of restructuring and revitalizing in its shift toward the primary health care (PHC) paradigm. Continued work is needed, however, by all sectors to enhance health promotion and disease prevention. Nurses have been highly instrumental and involved in PHC, and they believe that the necessary strategies exist to enhance the quality of care. Nurse leaders, more than ever before, are called upon to play a pivotal role to facilitate partnerships with members of other health care disciplines to integrate all health care services to best serve the health of all Canadians.

Objectives

By critically reflecting upon and processing knowledge throughout this chapter, you will be able to respond effectively to the following objectives:

1. Summarize the historical events of the health care system and the role of nurses within that journey.
2. Interpret the division of health care responsibilities among the federal, provincial, and territorial governments.
3. As a nurse leader, design a health care system utilizing the five principles of the Canada Health Act.
4. Critique the politically active role that the Canadian Nurses Association (CNA) has played toward endorsing PHC.
5. Compare and contrast themes between Kirby's Panel Report and the Romanow Commission Report.
6. Differentiate between public funding and privatization.
7. List activities of First Ministers during their meetings to promote health care reform
8. Create a table to summarize the political involvement of the CNA to promote leadership in nursing towards the transition to primary care.
9. Critique the increasing total health care expenditures in Canada.
10. Infer how PHC can reduce total health care expenditures.
11. Analyze how social trends will affect the Canadian health care system and the role of the nurse leader.

Perspectives on the Canadian Health System

Canada is a federation comprising 10 provinces and three territories where bilingualism and multiculturalism are not only encouraged, but also strongly supported (Vollman, Anderson, & McFarlane, 2004). Canada's well-established health care system is an important reflection of its principles, values, and overall national character (Vaillancourt Rosenau, 2006). The system serves a diversity of needs, and it has achieved, for the Canadian people, a level of health and wellness reflecting the notable progress of measures taken toward promoting health and preventing disease. Medicare is a distinctive feature of Canadian culture that expresses its unique value system in the Canadian health care system (Falk-Rafael & Coffey, 2005).

Nevertheless, major challenges that remain are characterized by an aging population, shifting family structures, rapid and irreversible social change, current finance and funding matters, and complex health care practices, as well as public expectations of care (Villeneuve & MacDonald, 2006). On a daily basis, nurses and other health care professionals witness the need to develop innovative approaches and integrate health care services to deal effectively with complicated health concerns of Canadians.

A sustainable and effective health care system is an important component of Canada's current and future success (Strelioff, Lavoie-Tremblay, & Barton, 2007). The Canadian Nurses Association (CNA) states that the principles of PHC coupled with the national conditions listed in the Canada Health Act provide the conditions that provincial/territorial health insurance plans must respect in order to receive federal cash contributions. CNA contends that these conditions provide the framework for Canada's health system of the 21st century (CNA 2000a, CNA 2000b).

To comprehend and appreciate fully the Canadian health care system and its transition to PHC, it is important to focus on the historical, political, economic, and social perspectives, as well as the roles of the nurse leader that have shaped, and are shaping, the system. Figure 1.1 represents four perspectives on Canadian health care. The figure also depicts the commitment, courage, cooperation, and collaboration of the nurse leaders who strive for quality health for Canadians.

Historical Perspective

Many significant events have occurred in the history of the Canadian health care system. Several milestones involve the nursing profession.

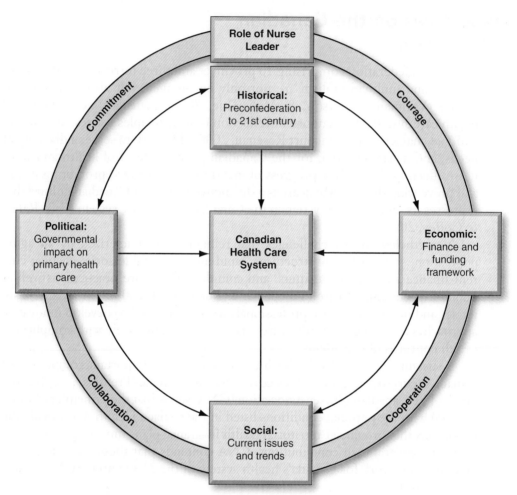

FIGURE 1.1 Perspectives in process on the Canadian health care system and role of nurse leaders.

Canada's First Nurse

Jeanne Mance, one of the most celebrated nurses in Canadian history, was the first nurse to arrive in the colony soon to be known as Canada. She took a leadership role, built the first hospital in Montreal, and ministered to Aboriginals and settlers alike (Ross-Kerr, 2003). Jeanne Mance negotiated with benefactors in France to bring more nurses to Canada (Storch, 2006). At present, the highest award given by the CNA to a nurse for contribution to the profession is the Jeanne Mance Award (Ross-Kerr, 2003).

Fathers of Confederation

As the fathers of confederation were developing the British North America Act of 1867, which continues to form a part of the current Constitution Act, they had little comprehension of how issues and trends would affect health care needs (Storch, 2006). They outlined basic responsibilities of the federal government but left much room and responsibility for the provincial governments to be key players in providing health care. As health care costs increased over time, provincial governments turned increasingly to the federal government for financial support (Birch & Gafni, 2005). The organization of Canada's health care system is largely determined by the Canadian constitution, whereby the federal, provincial, and territorial governments have been involved in ensuring both the availability and the funding of health care and social services (Health Canada, 2005).

Conception of Medicare

In the province of Saskatchewan, in 1947, Tommy Douglas and the Cooperative Commonwealth Confederation party introduced legislation to institute Medicare. Tommy Douglas is still referred to as the father of Medicare as a result of his role in bringing about this historic change (Falk-Rafael & Coffey, 2005). In 1966, following the lead of Saskatchewan and the 1964 Royal Commission on Health Services, the federal government introduced Medicare known as Canada's national health insurance program (Dickinson & Bolaria, 2002).

Medicare has been designed to ensure that all Canadians have reasonable access to medical treatment, hospital, and physician services on a uniform prepaid basis (Health Canada, 2006). Canadians generally support the publicly funded health care system. Several years ago, Canadians continued to resist privatization, by which clients pay for health care services, and grasped for proposals to protect and improve the health care system (Mendelssohn, 2002). But Soroka (2007) claims that there has been a slow and steady trend in the consideration of private services. That is, an increasing proportion of Canadians are giving serious consideration to private health care possibilities. The CNA is on record as supporting a publicly funded health care system and opposing privatization. CNA has advocated, through activities with the Health Action Lobby, to sustain Medicare in Canada (CNA, 2001).

reflective **THINKING**   As a nurse leader, what are your thoughts and feelings on privatization in regard to health care services? Compare and contrast the benefits and losses that a single-parent family might experience from privatization of health care services.

Significant Canadian Events

A highly significant Canadian event that occurred before the World Health Organization (WHO) conference at Alma Ata, USSR (1978), was the release of the federal government report (Lalonde, 1974). This report outlined a framework for health consisting of four determinants: lifestyle, environment, human biology, and health care organizations. The Lalonde Report, which continues to receive national and international acclaim, led to the development of successful health promotion programs associated with personal behaviours and lifestyles (Lemire Rodger & Gallagher, 2000).

The International Conference on Primary Health Care in Alma Ata, Kazakhstan, USSR, in 1978, established a goal to achieve "Health for All" by year 2000 (WHO, 2003). The basic aim of the conference was to address health care needs more effectively and equitably. Member states of the WHO, including Canada, decided to act toward the principles of "Health for All' (Lemire Rodger & Gallagher, 2006). A detailed discussion of the principles of PHC is found in chapter 2, Box 2.1.

The International Council of Nurses (ICN) urged nurses to become involved in the PHC movement. Furthermore, the ICN prepared and distributed extensive and valuable information to assist its members first to understand the primary health care concept and then encouraged nursing organizations to assume the much-needed leadership role (Glass, 2000).

These two key events—the Lalonde Report (1974) and the WHO conference (1978)—along with the Canadian federal government review of the national provincial health programs (Hall, 1980), provided the motivation for the Canadian nursing profession to take the leadership role to articulate and disseminate its vision of a future health care system. In 1980, the CNA submitted the document *Putting Health into Health Care* to the federal government's commission. The document served as a basis for major lobbying efforts by the nurses (Lemire Rodger & Gallagher, 2000).

Ottawa Charter

In 1986, Canada hosted the first International Conference on Health Promotion (Murray, Zentner, Pangman, & Pangman, 2006). Two key documents released at that conference were *Achieving Health for All: A Framework for Health Promotion* (Epp, 1986) and the *Ottawa Charter for Health Promotion* (Public Health Agency of Canada [PHAC], 2002). Conservative Health Minister Epp was emphatic that community participation was an essential strategy for enabling people to control factors affecting their health and to enhance their individual coping abilities (Epp, 1986). The *Ottawa Charter*, fundamental to health system reform, acknowledged that health promotion is the process of enabling individuals to increase control over and to improve their health.

The Charter outlines five strategies of health promotion:

1. Building healthy public policy
2. Creating supportive environments
3. Strengthening community actions
4. Developing personal skills
5. Reorienting health services (PHAC, 2002)

In essence, PHC ideology stems from the *Ottawa Charter*. PHC represents a shift in emphasis toward a social structure perspective of health, which remains mindful that biomedical and lifestyle considerations are not completely discarded (Boyce, 2002). The ICN and WHO held a conference in Tokyo (WHO, 1986) that enabled nurses to prepare themselves for leadership roles. Canada was specifically involved, assisting several countries that wished to educate their nurses in PHC (Glass, 2000). The CNA views PHC as the underlying foundation for the entire health system and as a specific model for improving health care (CNA, 2003).

> *reflective* **THINKING** Select a health problem likely to be prevalent in a rural community. As a nurse leader using the ideology of PHC reflected in the Ottawa Charter, what strategies can you implement to begin to resolve the problem?

Canada Health Act

According to Falk-Rafael and Coffey (2005), the introduction of the Canada Health Act (CHA) in 1984 was a proud moment in Canadian nursing history. The CHA consolidated previous legislation passed by the federal government to provide financial incentives to the provincial governments to establish universal hospital insurance. The Act also imposed financial penalties that endeavoured to prevent physicians from charging clients more than the amount listed in the negotiated provincial schedule of fees. This penalty led all provinces to ban the practice known as "extra billing" (Detsky & Naylor, 2003). The Act established principles and criteria for health insurance plans with the provinces. Territories must comply to receive full federal cash transfers in support of health. Figure 1.2 identifies these principles that affirm the beliefs and conditions on which Medicare was founded (Dickinson & Bolaria, 2002).

Intense lobbying and support by the CNA were instrumental in ensuring the passage of the bill, which resulted in the CHA. Nurses were not only instrumental in bringing the CHA into law, they were also influential in amending the CHA. Nurses and other health care workers, in addition to physicians, were recognized as potential providers of insurable services. This example of

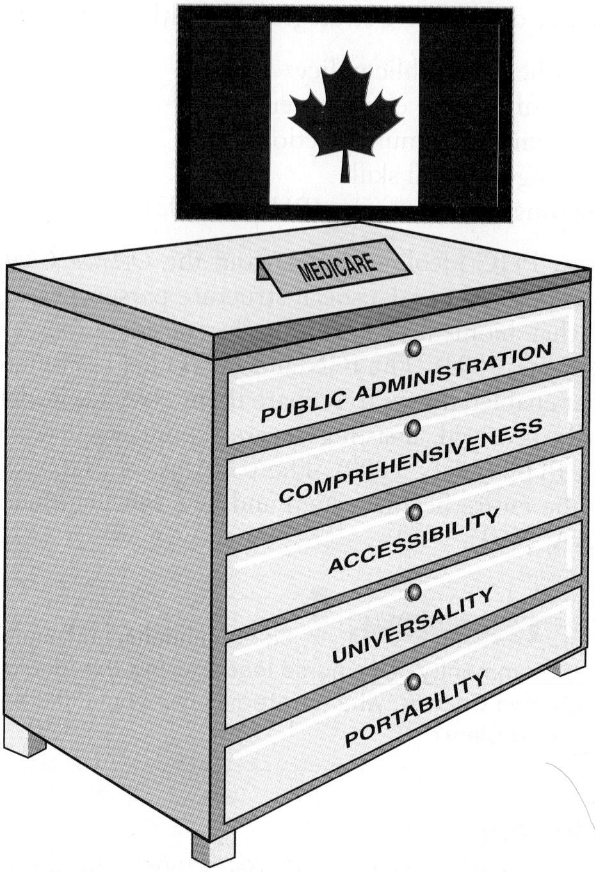

FIGURE 1.2 Basic principles of the Canada Health Act of 1984 sustaining Medicare. (Adapted with permission from Health Canada [2006].) (Source: Health Canada 2006. Canada's health care system. The role of government. Retrieved November 2008 from http://www.hc-sc.gc.ca/hcs-sss/pubs/system-regime/2005-hcs-sss/role-eng.php.)

assertive lobbying demonstrated by nurses showed the potential power of nurses when they remain unified (Wood, 2003). As a result of this change, the CNA is now seen as a viable professional organization promoting timely reform of the health care system. Such sustained professional activity has enabled nurses to assume a leadership role and to function more effectively in the health care system.

reflective **THINKING**   What types of political action can nurses take to influence change in health care reform?

Regionalization

Over the years, the health care system has expanded considerably to respond to the changing nature of health care, technology, genetics, and research findings in nursing and medical science. The roles and responsibilities of all governmental levels have changed over the decades. A related change that came into prominence in the late 1980s and 1990s was *regionalization*. Marchildon (2005) stated that regionalization was undertaken to save on public health care costs and to reallocate scarce resources from downstream illness care to upstream illness prevention and health promotion by transferring budgetary authority to geographically based regional health authorities. Generally, it is agreed that regionalization marks an important shift in health care governance and service delivery (Dickinson & Bolaria, 2002).

All provincial governments in Canada, except Ontario, which has only a consultative role, have accepted regionalization of health care services (Society of Rural Physicians of Canada, 2004; Romanow, 2004). The provinces created Regional Health Authorities (RHAs). RHAs are responsible for controlling costs; improving health outcomes; increasing responsiveness to health care needs; promoting greater citizen awareness of, and participation in, health care planning; and improving and integrating service delivery within a particular region of the province (Denis, Contandriopoulos, & Beaulieu, 2004; Romanow, 2004). All these responsibilities led to the continued transition toward the PHC paradigm.

Recently, governments across the Americas (including Canada) reaffirmed their commitment to the principles and strategies of PHC by signing, in 2005, the *Declaration of Montevideo*. The main thrust of this declaration is illness prevention and health promotion. This adjustment to health care services can be accomplished by:

- Assigning appropriate functions to each level of government.
- Integrating public and personal health services.
- Focusing on families and communities.
- Using accurate data in planning and decision making.
- Creating an institutional framework with incentives to improve quality of services (Martin, 2006).

reflective **THINKING** In examining Martin's plan (available at http://www.cachca.ca/) to adjust health care services, what individual and collective strategies can nursing leaders implement to promote PHC in the health care system?

CNA: Nursing Leadership

The CNA believes strongly that Canada's health system affects the well-being of Canadians. In addition, the CNA endorses the PHC approach to providing health care services (CNA, 2000; Villeneuve & MacDonald, 2006). If nurses are to be effective leaders in influencing the transition process toward PHC, they need to understand not only the history of structures of the health care system, but also the related political, social, and global trends within society. Nurses need to assess the needs of clients and their families, set goals, and collaborate with other health care professionals to achieve those goals for quality care (Storch, 2006). The CNA believes that through effective collaboration among health professionals, the responsiveness of the health care system can be strengthened (CNA, 2005).

The foundation of PHC reform is interdisciplinary team work (Villeneuve & MacDonald, 2006). In 2004, the New Health Professionals Network (NHPN) was founded by a group of students in nursing and pharmacy together with interns and residents in medicine to advocate for strengthening Medicare and interdisciplinary, team-based health care (NHPN, 2004). Presently, NHPN represents more than 20,000 new health professionals from across Canada in seven different health professions: nursing, medicine, pharmacy, social work, occupational therapy, physiotherapy, and chiropracty (Diamond, Somers, Garreau, & Martin, 2005). These upcoming graduates of various health care disciplines are developing innovative ways of working together to improve access to the health care system (Villeneuve & MacDonald, 2006).

The members of the new generation of health professionals have progressive expectations. They expect to work in teams where responsibility and accountability are shared. They intend to dismantle certain traditional hierarchies and give clients leadership in care. These new health care professionals support the principles that are consistent with the CHA and the vision that Tommy Douglas had for Medicare (Diamond et al., 2005).

---

reflective **THINKING**   After reading the article by Diamond et al. (2005) and the NHPN ("Strengthening Medicare: The Perspective of New Health Professionals," 2004), what strategies would you implement with other health care team members to continue the transition toward PHC?

Leadership Issue

*Y*ou are aware that a strong health care system begins with committed health care professionals. The current shortage of health care professionals—nurses, physicians, pharmacists, and many others—is well documented. As a nurse and a new health professional, what set of long-term solutions do you propose to "fix" the health/human resource problem?

POLITICAL PERSPECTIVES

The involvement of the federal government in Canada's health care plan has had an impact on the delivery system. A number of important reform initiatives have been considered and welcomed by the public and health care providers.

Romanow and Kirby Reports

Due in part to mounting tensions among the levels of government, the federal House of Commons commissioned former Saskatchewan Premier Roy Romanow to review the entire health care system and make specific recommendations. At the same time, the federal senate (a nonelected upper house) commissioned its own report to the Standing Senate Committee on Social Affairs, Science and Technology, chaired by Senator Michael Kirby (Detsky & Naylor, 2003).

In the fall of 2002, these two significant reports were released—the *Romanow Commission Report* and the *Kirby Panel Report* (Nagarajan, 2004). Romanow recommended sweeping changes to ensure the long-term sustainability of Canada's health care system (Commission on the Future of Health Care in Canada, 2002). Specifically, Romanow recommended establishing accountability as the sixth principle under the CHA and promoted the concept of a Health Council of Canada. The Health Council of Canada was intended to help foster cooperation and collaboration among provinces, territories, and the federal government (Storch & Meilicke, 2006). The council would play a significant role in establishing common indicators to measure the performance of the health care system and in reporting the results to Canadians on a regular basis (Murray, Zentner, Pangman, & Pangman, 2006). Other key themes in the Romanow Commission Report centred on:

- Maintenance and expansion of universal public funding and health care delivery.
- Improvement of Canada's health information technology.
- Provision of better access to care for rural and remote communities.
- Strategies for promoting the health of Aboriginal populations.
- Expansion of coverage by the provincial health insurance plans into home-based health care services and prescription drugs.
- Reform of primary care.
- Targeting of federal funds, with increased accountability for their use (Detsky & Naylor, 2003).

The Kirby Panel, on the other hand, suggested a more bureaucratically appointed council with fewer members and with limited advisory capacity. Kirby presented a controversial position when he supported the expansion of the private sector within a single-tier, publicly funded system, allowing for more outsourcing of services to investor-owned agencies and institutions, including private hospitals and clinics (Detsky & Naylor, 2003). Meanwhile, Romanow recommended that Medicare be maintained as a national asset, designed to preserve Canada's universally accessible, publicly funded health care system (Romanow, 2004). Both the Kirby Panel and Romanow Commission reports recognize the special health care problems faced by rural and remote communities (Nagarajan, 2004).

First Ministers' Accords

In September 2000, the First Ministers (provincial and territorial premiers) agreed that improvements to PHC were critical to the renewal of health services for Canadians. They agreed upon a vision, principles, and action plan for health system renewal (Health Canada, 2006). The government of Canada announced $23.4 billion of new federal investments over 5 years to support this agreement. This is one of the largest single expenditures by the Canadian government in Canadian history (Department of Finance, Canada, 2004). The First Ministers agreed specifically that improvements to PHC were critical to the renewal of health services highlighting the importance of multidisciplinary teams. The federal government established the $800 million Primary Health Care Transition Fund (PHCTF) to support the efforts of the provinces and territories to develop and implement transitional PHC reform initiatives (Department of Finance, Canada, 2006).

Collaboration among federal, provincial, and territorial governments is a critical element of the PHCTF. The PHCTF consisted of five funding envelopes (Provincial/Territorial, Multi-Jurisdictional, National, Aboriginal, and Official Languages Minority Communities). This funding was intended to support the transitional costs of fundamental changes to PHC delivery. For example, the Aboriginal funding envelope, accounting for $35.2 million, was to respond to the health needs of Aboriginal communities. One main thrust of the fund was to improve the quality of services delivered to the Aboriginal peoples, including cultural appropriateness (Health Canada, 2006).

> reflective **THINKING**   Given your general knowledge of Aboriginal people in your province or territory, which health needs do these people present that should be addressed? As a nurse leader, what strategies do you propose to address these needs?

In 2003, the First Ministers signed the Accord on Health Care Renewal to accelerate PHC renewal. The Accord outlines an action plan for reform reflecting renewed commitment by governments to work in partnership with each other, health care providers, and Canadians in shaping the future of the health care system. The First Ministers agreed to establish the Health Council of Canada (Health Council of Canada, 2007). Box 1.1 outlines the purpose of this Accord.

BOX 1.1 FIRST MINISTERS' ACCORD ON HEALTH CARE RENEWAL, 2003

First Ministers' Vision
- All Canadians have timely access to health services on the basis of need, not ability to pay—regardless of where they live or move in Canada.
- The health care services available to Canadians are of high quality, effective, patient-centered, and safe.
- Canada's health care system is sustainable and affordable and will exist for Canadians and their children in the future.

Purpose
The ultimate purpose of this Accord is to ensure that Canadians:
- Have access to a health care provider 24 hours a day, 7 days a week.
- Have timely access to diagnostic procedures and treatments.
- Do not have to repeat their health histories or undergo the same tests for every provider they see.
- Have access to quality home and community care services.
- Have access to the drugs they need without undue financial hardship.
- Are able to access quality care, no matter where they live.
- See their health care system as efficient, responsive, and adapting to their changing needs, and those of their families and communities, now and in the future.

Adapted from Health Canada (2006). 2003 First Ministers' Accord on Health Care Renewal. Author. Used with permission.

Further reforms were announced in 2004 by the First Ministers in the 10-Year Plan to Strengthen Health Care. The prime minister and premiers signed a second health care agreement. The Plan focused on improving access to quality care and reducing wait times because these were Canadians' largest concerns, and they constituted a national priority (Health Canada, 2006). Box 1.2 outlines the principles of the action plan to which the First Ministers agreed to adhere. The Health Council was given additional responsibilities to report on the health status of Canadians and health outcomes. Table 1.1 describes the reporting and accountability of the First Ministers' Accords from 2000 to 2004. The data provide transparency of governmental activities for Canadians.

Governmental Events

Since the year 2000, many governmental events have occurred to advance PHC. For example, a special meeting of First Ministers and National Aboriginal leaders, in September 2004, announced that a $200 million Aboriginal Health Transition Fund would be created over 5 years. The fund was designed to

(text continues on page 18)

BOX 1.2   FIRST MINISTERS' 10-YEAR PLAN

In 2004, the First Ministers met to develop a plan to ensure access to health care for all Canadians when they need it. Foremost on the agenda was the need to make timely access to quality care a reality for Canadians.

Dual Objectives of First Ministers' Commitment:
1. Better management of wait times.
2. Measurable reduction of wait times.

Strategies for Meeting Objectives
1. Cooperation among governments.
2. Participation of health care providers and patients.
3. Strategic investments in particular areas:
   a. Increasing the supply of health professionals (doctors, nurses, and pharmacists)
   b. Effective community-based services (including home care)
4. A pharmaceuticals strategy.
5. Effective health promotion and disease prevention.
6. Adequate financial resources.

Principles of the Action Plan
1. Universality, accessibility, portability, comprehensiveness, and public administration.
2. Access to medically necessary health services based on need, not ability to pay.
3. Reforms focused on the needs of patients to ensure that all Canadians have access to the health care services they need, when they need them.
4. Collaboration between governments, working together in common purpose to meet the evolving health care needs of Canadians.
5. Advancement through the sharing of best practices.
6. Continued accountability and provision of information to make progress transparent to citizens.
7. Jurisdictional flexibility.

Adapted from Health Canada (2006). First Ministers' Meeting on the Future of Health Care 2004: A 10-Year Plan to Strengthen Health Care. Author. Used with permission.

TABLE 1.1	REPORTING AND ACCOUNTABILITY OF CANADA'S FIRST MINISTERS

Reporting and Accountability

2000 Health Accord (September 2000)	2003 Health Accord (February 2003)	2004 10-Year Plan (September 2004)
First Minister Accord on Health Renewal and Early Childhood Development	First Minister Accord on Health Renewal	10-Year Plan to Strengthen Health Care
First Ministers committed their governments to report regularly to Canadians on: • Health status. • Health outcomes. • Performance of publicly funded health services. • Actions taken to improve these services.	First Ministers established an enhanced accountability framework. All governments committed to: • Provide comprehensive and regular reports to Canadians based on comparable indicators regarding health status, health outcomes, and quality of service. • Establish a health council to monitor and make annual public reports on the implementation of the Accord.	First Ministers agreed to collect and provide meaningful information to Canadians on progress made in: • Reducing wait times. • Establishing comparable indicators of access to health care services. • Establishing evidence-based benchmarks for medically acceptable wait times.

Source: Department of Finance Canada (2006). Federal transfer in support of the 2000/2003/2004 first ministers accords. Retrieved November 2008 from http://www.fin.gc.ca/FEDPROV/finAcce.html.

Reflections on Leadership Practice

As a nurse unit manager, you are in an interprofessional meeting on a unit in a hospital. One team member proposes that either the elderly spouse or the family members pay for a test that may produce a positive diagnosis for their loved one who has modest financial means. You recall the action plan for health care renewal agreed to by the First Ministers of the 2004 Accord and the principles that the ministers agreed would be followed. You agree with these principles.

How would you respond to this team member?

How can you influence the extent of the implementation of the principles of the First Ministers Accord?

improve the integration and delivery of services that better suited the Aboriginal people. One particularly important aspect of this action is that it increased the participation of Aboriginal people in the design, delivery, and evaluation of health programs and services (Health Council of Canada, 2007). Another example is that in the July 2006 First Ministers' conference, the premiers accepted a task force report on the national pharmaceutical strategy (NPS) and directed provincial and territorial ministers to release a report in September on the status of NPS and to continue working on key elements of the strategy, with a special focus on the Catastrophic Drug Program.

The establishment of the new Public Health Agency of Canada (PHAC) is one component of the Canadian government's broader strategy to strengthen the national public health system. The PHAC will be mandated specifically to build on strengths and capacities that exist across the country and facilitate collaboration with all levels of government on issues of public health (Bennett, 2004).

To date, achievements and shortcomings exist in the implementation of PHC in Canada. For example, Table 1.2 outlines the composition of PHC teams in selected Canadian jurisdictions. The data in the table indicate that continued progress is warranted to solidify the development of PHC teams. Most importantly, a need exists to improve the PHC data collection infrastructure in order to report on progress in a systematic fashion (Health Council of Canada, 2007).

reflective **THINKING**   In regard to nurse leaders in particular, what are the benefits of the PHAC?

CNA Nursing Leadership

The CNA has been a consistent influence in promoting PHC as a significant strategy to guide the reform of the health care system (Lemire Rodger, 2006). Many notable events have promoted reform of the health care system, including the following:

2000: Nursing Strategy for Canada

In 2000, the *Nursing Strategy for Canada* was made public by the federal, provincial, and territorial health ministers after significant consultations with nurses and other health care professionals (Health Canada, 2003). The goal was to describe strategic plans to achieve and maintain an adequate supply of nursing personnel who were well educated, well distributed, and deployed to meet the health needs of Canadian citizens (Health Canada, 2003).

TABLE 1.2	COMPOSITION AND DEVELOPMENT OF PRIMARY HEALTH CARE TEAMS: SELECTED JURISDICTIONS
Jurisdiction	**Multidisciplinary Teams**
British Columbia (BC)	BC measures gaps in care and monitors and reports on patient health outcomes. Interdisciplinary teams and/or networks are one component needed to close the gaps in care.
Saskatchewan (SK)	SK is working to increase the number of primary health care (PHC) teams across the province. Initial targets have been lowered to manageable targets of 2 to 3 new teams per quarter and about 10 per year. Currently 41 teams are in place, serving about 20% of the population.
Manitoba (MB)	Regional Health Authorities (RHAs) have made substantial progress in developing multidisciplinary teams. The Winnipeg RHA has developed access centres that integrate health and social services within specific neighbourhoods, and Brandon has developed an access centre based on a similar concept. Northern and rural RHAs have developed PHC centres where multidisciplinary teams provide integrated health care services that serve community and regional needs.
Ontario (ON)	As of November 2006, a total of 6,546 Ontario doctors were participating in PHC models, serving 6.9 million enrolled patients, out of a total population of 12.7 million. In April 2006, the government reached its goal and announced the creation of 150 Family Health Teams throughout Ontario. Family Health Teams include doctors, nurses, nurse practitioners, pharmacists, dieticians, physician specialists, social workers, health educators, mental health workers, and other health care providers.
New Brunswick (NB)	Community Health Centres (CHCs) in seven rural and urban communities offer access to a wide spectrum of PHC services, to approximately 51,000 residents during the fiscal year of 2005–2006. CHCs offer a wide spectrum of health services. As well as physicians and nurse/nurse practitioners (NPs), the CHCs include occupational therapists, physical therapists, respiratory therapists, speech therapists, psychiatrists, health promoters, social workers, pharmacists, and dieticians. NB has committed to improve services at CHCs and enhance the role of nurses, NPs, and other health care providers to increase patient access to PHC.

(table continues on page 20)

TABLE 1.2	COMPOSITION AND DEVELOPMENT OF PRIMARY HEALTH CARE TEAMS: SELECTED JURISDICTIONS (continued)
Jurisdiction	**Multidisciplinary Teams**
Nova Scotia (NS)	The composition of interdisciplinary, collaborative teams tends to be family physicians, family practice nurses, nurse practitioners, and pharmacists. These core team members are usually in place, though other team members and extended providers and contributors work interdependently in many areas. Some patients have access to teams including social workers, dieticians, and mental health workers.
Prince Edward Island (PEI)	25,000 people (18% of residents) routinely receive primary care through multidisciplinary teams in family health centres.
Newfoundland (NF) and Labrador	22% of residents presently receive PHC through teams. All of the eight teams currently in existence include professionals other than doctors and NPs.
Nunavut	Nunavut supports an integrated service approach at the community level for all health services. Departmental mandate includes both health and social services. PHC teams comprise nurses, community mental health workers, social workers, and visiting physicians.
Northwest Territories (NWT)	NWT has developed an integrated service delivery model as the theoretical base for health care delivery. Teams provide core services as set out in the delivery model. Six core services and protocols to access them have been established. Services are provided by health practitioners, social workers, nutritionists, occupational therapists, physicians, speech/ language therapists, community health workers, and mental health and addictions counsellors.
Yukon (YK)	Service in YK may be delivered by collaboration as opposed to co-located teams, especially in the communities. For diabetic patients, a chronic disease management program has been established as a collaborative practice. Two communities have contracted physicians. NPs are the front-line service providers in most communities outside Whitehorse. Other professionals may include dieticians, physiotherapists, and home care workers.

Adapted from Health Council of Canada (2007). *Health care renewal in Canada: Measuring up? 2007 Annual Report.* Toronto: Author. Used with permission.

2002: Our Health, Our Future—Creating Quality Workplaces for Canadian Nurses

Nurses make up approximately two thirds of all health professionals in Canada, and they play a pivotal role in maintaining a high-quality health care system, as well as meeting the health needs of Canadians. The recently created Canadian Nursing Advisory Committee presented its landmark report in August 2002, titled *Our Health, Our Future: Creating Quality Workplaces for Canadian Nurses*. The report contained 51 recommendations designed to implement conditions that would resolve workplace management issues and maximize the use of available resources.

2003: Report on the Nursing Strategy for Canada

The *Report on the Nursing Strategy for Canada*, released in September 2003, indicated that a collaborative approach resulted in significant progress in assuring that Canadians have access to quality nursing services. As well as summarizing the progress, this document outlines the challenges that still lie ahead. One such challenge is to continue support for provincial/territorial nursing advisory committees and/or other means of continuing a dialogue on nursing issues in each jurisdiction and to monitor the need for further action (Health Canada, 2003).

2004: CNA Role in First Ministers' 10-Year Plan

The CNA was an active participant in 2004, at the meeting with the First Ministers, for the 10-Year Plan to Strengthen Health Care. In preparation for this meeting, CNA collaborated with the Canadian Health Care Association, Canadian Medical Association, and the Canadian Pharmacists Association on joint policy and media relations initiatives. A common vision statement was prepared and delivered through media interviews, media statements, and media releases (CNA, 2006b).

2006: Nursing Matters!

The anticipated federal election of 2006 provided a valuable opportunity for CNA to be involved in developing an electronic, as well as print, election handbook and the e-newsletter *Nursing Matters!* This newsletter provided analyses of party platforms, background information, and evidence on issues. It also posed suggestions for strategies. CNA engaged the media on important issues affecting Canadians and the health system (CNA, 2006b).

Toward 2020: Visions for Nursing

The project *Toward 2020: Visions for Nursing* was released in the spring of 2006. Michael Villeneuve and Jane MacDonald, both nurses, were the principal investigators of this report based on interviews with Canadians within and beyond nursing. The authors provide an extensive literature review and a rich input from nursing practitioners. The report is intended to be provocative in nature, mainly to stimulate discussion and critical thinking among nurses about the future health and well-being of all Canadians.

Nursing Leadership: Unleashing the Power

The CNA believes that nursing leadership must be viewed as a strategic element that will gain momentum as nurses continue collectively to set the course for their own future. The document titled *Nursing Leadership: Unleashing the Power* (Broughton, 2001) strongly indicates that the area of leadership, both at the individual and organizational levels, is a priority for the CNA. The challenge is for nurses to have their collective voice heard, be proactive, and claim their leadership roles as the largest group of health care providers in the country. The report, *Nursing Leadership Development in Canada* (Kilty, 2005), presents several timely areas and approaches relevant to nursing leadership. One such area is the set of domains and competencies required by nursing leaders. Another area is the wide array of approaches available to leadership development. The CNA has a rich legacy of first advocating for and then providing strong professional support for nursing leadership. The CNA continues to organize national nursing leadership conferences, where far-reaching policy discussions result in clear and decisive reports related to nursing leadership.

CNA has taken the leadership role to advance the nursing profession and the publicly funded health care system. All nurses contribute to strengthen CNA as the national and credible voice of registered nurses, but most importantly, CNA has been paving a destiny, built on memorable past and insightful innovations, for a strong and vibrant future. Figure 1.3 represents the leadership visibility of CNA as it continues to shine in its involvement, support, and dedication to the PHC approach for health care services.

reflective **THINKING**   In what ways can leadership development be reflected in educational curricula, committee work, and the workplace?

Economic Perspective

The health care system requires an extensive array of resources to deliver health care services adequately and to meet the health needs of the Canadian population. Besides being financial in nature, these resources include human and physical resources (Romanow, 2004). Canada's health care system is financed by both the public and private sectors.

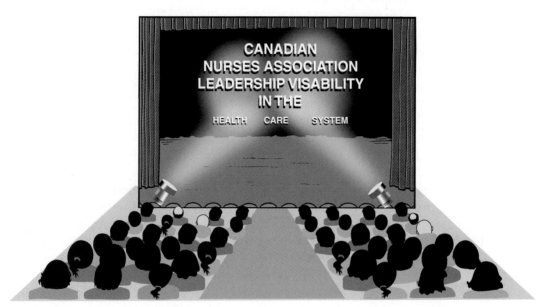

FIGURE 1.3 Lighting up leadership visibility in Canadian Nurses Association.

Public and Private Sectors

Public sector funding includes payments by governments at the federal, provincial/territorial, and municipal levels, and also by workers' compensation boards and other social security plans. The CHA established the principles and criteria for health insurance plans that the provinces and territories must meet in order to receive federal cash transfers in support of health. The federal government provides the provinces and territories with cash and tax transfers to be used in support of health. The financial package, including cash and tax transfers, is called the Canada Health Transfer. To support the costs of publicly funded services through the Canada Health Transfer, the federal government also provides equalization payments to less prosperous provinces and territories (Health Canada, 2006). Increases in federal transfers will be reflected primarily in increased expenditures by the provincial and territorial governments in the next several years (Canadian Institute for Health Information [CIHI], 2006). The public share has varied over the last 20 years as a result of the restructuring of the health care system. Meanwhile, private-sector funding consists primarily of health expenditures by households and private insurance firms (CIHI, 2006).

National Health Expenditures

The Canadian Institute for Health Information (CIHI) tracks health spending by each source of finance in the National Health Expenditure Data Base. The *National Health Expenditure Trends, 1975–2006*, is CIHI's tenth annual health expenditure trends publication, and it provides detailed and updated information on estimated health expenditures in Canada (CIHI, 2006). This publication reveals that the total health expenditures were estimated to be $139.8 billion in 2005 and $148 billion in 2006. Private-sector (households and insurance firms) spending on health care was close to 30% of the total expenditure.

Figure 1.4 shows how the total health expenditure forecasted for 2006 was apportioned. The category of drugs ranks second after hospitals in terms of its share of total health expenditure. Physicians are the third largest cost, followed by the category of other professionals. Other nonhospital institutions, such as personal care homes, make up the fifth largest cost in Canada's health care system. Twenty-five years ago, a much larger share went to the hospital, while payments to physicians came in second. Both shares of spending have since been overtaken by drug costs. Trends in health care costs have changed as well, and they are changing as a result of patterns of care, technology, advances in genomics, and the scope of how health professionals work together. All of these trends, and others, have an impact on how the Canadian health care system is organized and how health care is delivered.

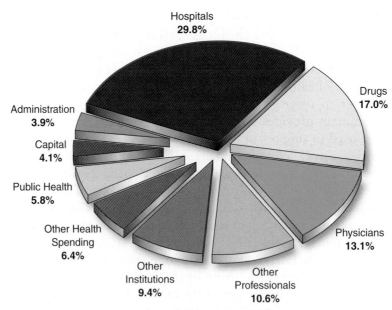

FIGURE 1.4   Health expenditure for 2006 was about $148 billion (Source: Canadian Institute for Health Information).

reflective **THINKING** What impact do you anticipate that health care spending trends will exert on the future costs of the health care system for clients and their families? In what ways can nurse leaders help to achieve cost-saving measures in various health care settings?

Questions and debates about the increasing costs of health care, who pays for what aspects of the health care system, and whether the health care system is sustainable in the future play significant roles in discussions about health care expenditures (Romanow, 2004). Overwhelming evidence concludes that direct charges, such as user fees, place the heaviest burden on the poor. User fees actually impede the access of Canada's poor to the health care they require (Romanow, 2004). Meanwhile, studies indicate that a publicly funded system provides many economic benefits. One of the benefits is that public funding spreads the cost of health care services across the entire population (Health Canada, 2005).

CNA: Nursing Leadership

The CNA believes that health services should be accessible to all and that governments are responsible for providing funding for health services (CNA, 2001). Further, the organization recommends that federal governments must focus on identifying health needs of Canadians, both now and into the future (CNA, 2006). CNA also believes that the federal government has key responsibilities in maintaining and improving the health and health care of Canadians. A healthy population is vital to a vigorous and productive economy (CNA, 2006a).

reflective **THINKING** As a nurse leader, how are you able to advocate for a client who is unable to pay for his/her prescribed medication?

Social Perspective

Social trends in society are changing rapidly. The health system of today might not look the same in a few years. Technology, genetics, cultural diversity, and interdisciplinary care, as well as community and consumer involvement, will shape health priorities (Villeneuve & MacDonald, 2006).

Trends in Health Care

As the population ages, increases in chronic health diseases will take priority among health conditions (Health Council of Canada, 2007). An increase in the influence of cultural and social issues, including those related to poverty and immigration, will continue to be prevalent in our society.

Reflections on Leadership Practice

*A*s you admit a male client to the surgical unit for quadruple bypass surgery, his partner informs you that the client strongly believes in herbal remedies and has taken them for many years. How will you approach this client regarding his herbal therapy in preparation for his surgery?

Another social concern is the impact of the environment on health, which is a critical issue in most industrialized countries, including Canada. For example, the prevalence of asthma in children is escalating (Manfreda, Becklake, Chan-Yeung, et al., 2001). The impact of environmental changes that affect health, such as allergies and infectious diseases, are already being experienced by Canadians (Villeneuve & MacDonald, 2006).

In responding to cultural and social issues, the Health Council of Canada (2005) indicated that health disparities in the level of health care available to some Canadians are the number one problem. Without action, the equity gap in health care will likely widen. Complementary and alternative health care options are growing at a rapid pace, and consumers will soon have the ability to make informed choices about their health care (Smith & Simpson, 2003).

What the Future Holds

Adequate support and services will be needed for families (informal caregivers) who are taking care of their loved ones at home. Informal care is a crucial element of home care. In fact, home care and family caregiving become "women's issues." Women make up the vast majority of home care workers, and they provide a high percentage of unpaid care to relatives (Prince, 2003). In many cases, the financial burden of home care is substantial to families. In many Canadian provinces and territories, drugs, supplies, and nursing hours or care hours, in excess of those provided by the health care system, must be paid for by the family (McDaniel & Tepperman, 2002).

Today, Canadian consumers want more health information and are actively looking for it. The internet has become a frequently used source of health information, despite the fact that many health professionals express concerns about the validity of the information. Currently, nurses use informatics for many kinds of health system initiatives—education being one of them. Systems of informing individuals include Telehealth and nurse-led client advice lines (CNA, 2006c). Roberts, Tayler, MacCormack, and Barwich (2007) outline in their article, "Telenursing in Hospice Palliative Care," how information and communication technology in palliative care achieve improved client outcomes. Nursing leaders need to be aware of technological advances and developments to sustain effective health care.

The disease trends related to obesity, inadequate exercise, and poor nutrition will improve because of health promotion efforts now underway (Villeneuve & MacDonald, 2006). Interdisciplinary care, collaboration, cooperation, and coordination among health care practitioners will be the norm. Tertiary care will still be required, but as technology improves, health care costs will diminish. Leeb, Jokovic, Sanhu, and Zinck (2006) explain that, currently, intensive care makes up about 16% of hospital costs, but only 8% of hospital days. Therefore, reducing stays in high-cost intensive care units is an important strategy to reduce overall costs.

To move forward in primary health care, a leadership structure remains prevalent for nurses so that nursing can flourish and function in both an autonomous and interdependent way as trends in health care delivery change. Nurses will need to continue to create partnerships with clients, physicians, and health care workers from other disciplines. However, it will become even more necessary to discover ways and means to promote an empowered nursing workforce whose potential can be realized as part of the interdisciplinary team (Shannon & French, 2005).

WEBSITES

▦ Tommy Douglas Research Institute

http://www.tommydouglas.ca/
The Tommy Douglas Research Institute is an independent, nonprofit Canadian economic and social research and educational organization. Named after T. C. Douglas, the former premier of Saskatchewan and acknowledged father of Medicare in Canada, the Institute's main goal is to raise public awareness of the respective role of both the large business sector and governments in providing for the well-being of Canadians. Visit this site to learn more about "the Greatest Canadian of all time."

▦ Health Council of Canada

http://www.healthcouncilcanada.ca/
The Health Council of Canada fosters accountability and transparency by assessing progress in improving the quality, effectiveness, and sustainability of the health care system. Through insightful monitoring, public reporting, and facilitating informed discussion, the Council shines a light on what helps or hinders health care renewal and the well-being of Canadians.

▦ Canadian Nurses Association (CNA)

http://www.cna-nurses.ca/
The CNA is the national professional voice of registered nurses, supporting them in their practice and advocating for healthy public policy and a quality, publicly funded, not-for-profit health system. The CNA has established a set of six important goals which, along with extensive professional current information, may be viewed at this valuable Website. The CNA is a federation of 11 provincial and territorial nursing associations representing more than 125,000 registered nurses.

▩ World Health Organization (WHO)

http://www.who.int/

The WHO is the United Nations' specialized agency for health. Established in 1948, WHO's objective is the attainment by all peoples of the highest possible level of health. Its constitution describes health as a state of complete physical, mental, and social well-being and not merely the absence of disease or infirmity. You will be amazed to realize the breadth and depth of WHO's involvement in world health, as shown on this Website.

REFERENCES

Bennett, C. (2004). Building a national public health system. *Canadian Medical Association Journal, 170*(9), 1425–1437.

Birch, S., & Gafni, A. (2005). Achievements and challenges of medicare in Canada: Are we there yet? Are we on course? *International Journal of Health Services, 35*(3), 443–463.

Boyce, W. F. (2002). Influence of health promotion bureaucracy on community participation: A Canadian case study. *Health Promotion International, 17*(1), 61–68.

Broughton, H. (2001). *Nursing leadership: Unleashing the power.* Ottawa: Canadian Nurses Association.

Canadian Institute for Health Information. (2006). *National health expenditure trends, 1975–2006.* Ottawa: CIHI.

Canadian Nurses Association. (2000a). *Position statement: Healthy public policy. Framework for Canada's health system.* Ottawa, ON: Author. Retrieved February 2007 from http://www.cna-nurses.ca/

Canadian Nurses Association. (2000b). *Fact sheet: The Canada Health Act.* Ottawa, ON: Author. Retrieved June 2007 from http://www.cna-nurses.ca/

Canadian Nurses Association. (2001). *Optimizing the health of the health system: Brief to the Commission on the future of health care in Canada.* Ottawa, ON: Author. Retrieved February 2007 from http://www.cna-nurses.ca/cna/documents/pdf/publications/romanow_brief_oct_31_e.pdf

Canadian Nurses Association. (2005). *Position statement: Primary health care. Interprofessional collaboration.* Ottawa, ON: Author. Retrieved February 2007 from http://www.cna-nurses.ca/

Canadian Nurses Association. (2001). *Position statement: Financing Canada's health system.* Ottawa: Author.

Canadian Nurses Association. (2003). *Primary health care: A summary of the issues.* Ottawa: Author.

Canadian Nurses Association. (2005, January). Nursing leadership in a changing world. *Nursing Now: Issues and Trends in Canadian Nursing, 18.*

Canadian Nurses Association. (2006a). *Online consultations on restoring fiscal balance in Canada: Submission to the federal-provincial relations and social policy branch, Department of Finance.* Ottawa, ON: Author.

Canadian Nurses Association. (2006b). *Operational report of the chief executive officer: June 2004 to June 2006.* Ottawa, ON: Author.

Canadian Nurses Association. (2006c). *Position statement: Nursing information and knowledge management.* Ottawa, ON: Author. Retrieved June 2007 from http://www.cna-aiic.ca/

Commission on the Future of Health Care in Canada. (2002). *Shape the future of health care.* Ottawa, ON: Author.

Denis, J.-L., Contandriopoulis, D., & Beaulieu, M.-D. (2004). Regionalization in Canada: A promising heritage to build on. *Healthcare Papers, 5*(1), 40–45.

Department of Finance. (2004). *Economic statement and budget update 2000. Key investments.* Author. Retrieved from http://www.fin.gc.ca/ec2000/ecch6e.htm

Department of Finance. (2006). *Transfer payments to provinces. Federal transfers to provinces and territories (October 2006). Federal transfer in support of the 2000/2003/2004 First Ministers' Accords.* Retrieved February 2007 from http://www.fin.gc.ca/

Detsky, A. S., & Naylor, C. D. (2003). Canada's health care system: Reform delayed. *The New England Journal of Medicine, 349*(8), 804–810.

Diamond, J., Somers, A., Garreau, M., & Martin, D. (2005). New health professionals' network: The future face of medicine. *Canadian Journal of Nursing Leadership, 18*(4), 44–6.

Dickinson, H., & Bolaria, S. (2002). The Canadian health care system: Evolution and current status. In B. Singh Bolaria, & H. D. Dickinson (Eds.), *Health, illness, and health care in Canada* (3rd ed., pp. 20–32). Toronto, ON: Nelson Thomson Learning.

Epp, J. (1986). Achieving health for all: A framework for health promotion. *Health Promotion International, 1*(4), 419–428.

Falk-Rafael, A., & Coffey, S. (2005). Financing, policy, and politics of health care delivery. In L. Leeseberg Stamler (Ed.), *Community health nursing: A Canadian perspective* (pp. 17–37). Toronto, ON: Pearson Education Canada.

Glass, H. (2000). Primary health care: Then and now. *Canadian Journal of Nursing Research, 32*(1), 9–16.

Hall, E. M. (1980). *Canada's national-provincial health program for the 1980s: A commitment for renewal.* Justice E. M. Hall, Special Commissioner. Ottawa, ON: Department of National Health and Welfare.

Health Canada. (2002). *Canada health act overview.* Retrieved February 2007 from http://www.hc-sc.gc.ca/hcs-sss/medi-assur/cha-lcs/overview-apercu-eng.php

Health Canada. (2003). *A report on the nursing strategy for Canada.* Ottawa: Advisory Committee Health Delivery and Human Resources.

Health Canada. (2005). *Canada's health care system.* Ottawa, ON: Author. Retrieved February 2007 from http://www.hc-sc.gc.ca/hcs-sss/pubs/system-regime/2005-hcs-sss/index-eng.php

Health Canada. (2006). *Health care system. Primary health care. Primary health care transition fund.* Retrieved February 2007 from http://www.hc-sc.gc.ca/

Health Council of Canada. (2005). *Health care renewal in Canada: Accelerating change.* Toronto, ON: Author.

Health Council of Canada. (2007). *Health care renewal in Canada: Measuring up? Annual report to Canadians 2006.* Toronto, ON: Author.

Kilty, H. L. (2005). *Nursing leadership development in Canada.* Ottawa, ON: Canadian Nurses Association.

Lalonde, M. (1974). *A new perspective on the health of Canadians.* Ottawa, ON: Information Canada.

Leeb, K., Jokovic, A., Sandhu, M., & Zinck, G. (2006). CIHI survey: Intensive care in Canada. *Health Care Quarterly, 9*(1), 32–33.

Lemire Rodger, G. (2006). Canadian nurses association. In M. McIntyre, E. Thomlinson, & C. McDonald (Eds.), *Realities of Canadian nursing: Professional, practice, and power issues* (pp. 134–151). Philadelphia: Lippincott Williams & Wilkins.

Lemire Rodger, G., & Gallagher, S. (2000). The move toward primary health care in Canada: Community health nursing from 1985 to 2000. In J. Stewart (Ed.), *Community nursing: Promoting Canadians' health* (2nd ed., pp. 33–56).

Manfreda, J., Becklake, M. R., Sears, M. R., Chan-Yeung, M., Dimich-Ward, H., Siersted, H. C., et al. (2001). Prevalence of asthma symptoms among adults aged 20–40 years in Canada. *Canadian Medical Association Journal, 164*(7), 995–1001.

Marchildon, G. P. (2005, November 17). *Regionalization and health services: Restructuring in Saskatchewan.* Conference paper, Queen's University, Kingston, ON.

Martin, C. M. (2006). *Towards a framework for primary health care transition in Canada.* Canadian Alliance of Community Health Centre Associations. Discussion document. Retrieved February 2007 from http://www.cachca.ca/local/files/Martin%20Discussion%20Document.pdf

McDaniel, S. A., & Tepperman, L. (2002). *Close relations: An introduction to the sociology of families* (Brief ed.). Toronto, ON: Prentice Hall.

Mendelssohn, M. (2002). *Canadians' thoughts on their health care system: Preserving the Canadian model through innovation.* Ottawa, ON: Commission on the Future of Health Care in Canada.

Murray, R. B., Zentner, J. P., Pangman, V., & Pangman, C. (2006). *Health promotion strategies through the lifespan.* Toronto, ON: Pearson Education Canada.

Nagarajan, K. V. (2004). Rural and remote community health care in Canada: Beyond the Kirby Panel Report, the Romanow Report and the federal budget of 2003. *Canadian Journal of Rural Medicine, 9*(4), 245–251.

New Health Professionals Network. (2004). *Strengthening Medicare: The perspective of new health professionals.* Retrieved February 2007 from http://pairo.rtihosting.com/Content/Files/Strengtheningmedicare.pdf

Prince, M. J. (2003, September). *Respecting family caregivers: What's been happening recently?* Paper presented at the Family Caregiver Network Society Annual General Meeting, Victoria Health Unit, Victoria, BC.

Public Health Agency of Canada. (2002). *Population health approach – Ottawa charter for health promotion: An international conference on health promotion.* Ottawa, ON: Author.

Roberts, D., Tayler, C., MacCormack, D., & Barwich, D. (2007). Telenursing in hospice palliative care. *Canadian Nurse, 103*(5), 24–27.

Romanow, R. (2004). Sustaining Medicare: The Commission on the Future of Health Care in Canada. In F. Baylis, J. Downie, B. Hoffmaster, & S. Sherwin (Eds.), *Health care ethics in Canada* (3rd ed., pp. 79–98). Toronto, ON: Thomson Nelson.

Ross-Kerr, J. C. (2003). Early nursing in Canada, 1600 to 1760: A legacy for the future. In J. Ross-Kerr, & M. J. Wood (Eds.), *Canadian nursing: Issues and perspectives.* (4th ed., pp. 3–13). Toronto, ON: Mosby.

Shannon, V., & French, S. (2005). The impact of the re-engineered world of health-care in Canada on nursing and patient outcomes. *Nursing Inquiry, 12*(3), 231–239.

Smith, M., & Simpson, J. (2003, November). Alternative practices and products: A survival guide. *Health Policy Research Bulletin, 7*, 3–5.

Society of Rural Physicians of Canada. (2004). *Policy paper on regionalization: Recommended strategies.* Shawville QC: Author. Retrieved February 2007 from http://www.srpc.ca/librarydocs/Regionalization_SRPC.PDF

Soroka, S. N. (2007). *Canadian perceptions of the health care system: A report to the Health Council of Canada,* Toronto, ON: Health Council of Canada.

Storch, J. (2006). Canadian health care system. In M. McIntyre, E. Thomlinson, & C. McDonald (Eds.), *Realities of Canadian nursing: Professional, practice, and power issues* (pp. 29–53). Philadelphia: Lippincott Williams & Wilkins.

Storch, J. L., & Meilicke, C. A. (2006). Political, social, and economic forces shaping the health care system. In J. M. Hibberd, & D. L. Smith (Eds.), *Nursing leadership and management in Canada* (3rd ed., pp. 5–28). Toronto, ON: Elsevier Mosby.

Strelioff, W., Lavoie-Tremblay, M., & Barton, M. (2007). Collaborating to embrace evidence-informed management practices within Canada's health system. *Healthcare Papers: New Models for the New Healthcare, 7* (special issue), 36–41.

Vaillancourt Rosenau, P. M. (2006). U.S. newspaper coverage of the Canadian health system: A case of seriously mistaken identity? *The American Review of Canadian Studies. 36*(1), 27–58.

Villeneuve, M., & MacDonald, J. (2006). *Toward 2020: Visions for nursing.* Ottawa, ON: Canadian Nurses Association.

Vollman, A. R., Anderson, E. T., & McFarlane, J. (2004). *Canadian community as partner: Theory and practice in nursing.* Philadelphia: Lippincott Williams & Wilkins.

Wood, M. L. (2003). The role of the Canadian Nurses Association in the development of nursing in Canada. In J. Ross-Kerr, & M. J. Wood (Eds.), *Canadian nursing: Issues and perspectives* (4th ed., pp. 39–64). Toronto, ON: Mosby.

World Health Organization. (2003). *International Conference on Primary Health Care, Alma-Ata: Twenty-fifth Anniversary.* Geneva: Author. A56/27 Provisional Agenda Item 14.18.

World Health Organization. (1986). *Why leadership for health for all? Leadership in Nursing for Health for All Conference.* Geneva: Author.

PRIMARY HEALTH CARE: ROLE OF THE NURSE LEADER

2

Primary health care is the most effective way to provide health care to a population. Primary health care places an emphasis on illness prevention and health promotion. And it focuses on the delivery of integrated health services where health care professionals work together to ensure that patients and their families receive the support and treatments they require.

—Robert Calnan

Rob Calnan has demonstrated outstanding professional leadership in British Columbia and in Canada. After beginning his career as an LPN, he obtained the BScN degree (1987) and the MEd degree (1990) and served as president of the Registered Nurses Association of British Columbia (1997–1999). He then served as President of the Canadian Nurses Association from 2002 to 2004, during which he received the Queen's Golden Jubilee Medal for his contributions to health care. More recently, he represented Canadian nurses at the International Council of Nurses (ICN) Council of Representative Nations and the Commonwealth Nurses Federation and was one of four nurses selected to participate in the ICN delegation to the World Health Assembly in Geneva.

Overview

Primary health care (PHC), proposed as the cornerstone of the Canadian health care system, is a critical element in providing high-quality care to clients and their families in various health care settings, as well as in communities. It is imperative that community health centres be recognized and regarded as an integrated and accessible PHC model suited to deliver health care services to Canadians. Interprofessional health care teams are the key to PHC. The emphasis on greater collaboration and integration among health care professionals is both challenging and rewarding. The roles of the nurse leaders require a definite way of being, knowing, and doing as they relate to clients, families, and other health care professionals to advance the principles of PHC.

Objectives

By critically reflecting upon and processing knowledge throughout this chapter, you will be able to respond effectively to the following objectives:

1. Compare and contrast PHC with primary care.
2. Review the movement of PHC in Canada beginning with the declaration of Alma Ata to the present in Canada.
3. Critically appraise the role of the Canadian Nurses Association in the endorsement of PHC.
4. Evaluate the paradigm shift from primary care to PHC in health care centres.
5. Examine your values as a nurse leader regarding PHC.
6. Evaluate the determinants of health.
7. Describe how social justice and equality can affect the role of the nurse leader in the practice of nursing.
8. Evaluate the significance of the principles of PHC on the quality of care delivered by health professionals.
9. Analyze community health centres as a model of PHC.
10. Formulate a research hypothesis to study the performance of community health centres.
11. Justify the role of the nurse leader in the process of collaboration.

Perspective on PHC

The basic premise of the PHC approach focuses on promoting health and preventing illness. Globally, the International Council of Nurses (ICN) believes that equity and access to PHC services, notably nursing services, are critical to improving the health and well-being of all people (ICN, 1999). In Canada, the Canadian Nurses Association (CNA) views PHC as a foundation for the health care system and as a model for improving health care delivery (CNA, 2005). In fact, the CNA lobbied the federal government to ensure that nurses are PHC providers (Orchard, Smille, & Meagher-Stewart, 2000). CNA believes that this approach is the most effective strategy for improving health care in an equitable and accessible way (CNA, 2005). To appreciate PHC fully, the nurse leader must have an in-depth understanding of the following:

- The difference between primary care and PHC
- The conception and development of PHC
- The philosophy and principles of PHC
- The importance of community health centres

The shift toward community health centres is occurring as one component of a broader health network. Consequently, nurse leaders must work in interdisciplinary teams and adapt to a more caring and empowering PHC model. Figure 2.1 depicts the four main elements that are considered to be necessary to promote the understanding of PHC by nurse leaders.

PHC Versus Primary Care

Muldoon, Hogg, and Levitt (2006) claim that PHC and primary care (PC) are similar terms that are often used interchangeably but denote different concepts. The World Health Organization's (WHO) 1978 Declaration of Alma Ata defines PHC in the following way:

- PHC is made accessible to individuals and families in the community through their full participation and at a cost that the community and country can afford.
- PHC forms an integral part of the country's health system, which is the central focus, and of the overall social and economic development of the community.
- PHC is the first level of contact of individuals, families, and the community with the national health care system, bringing health care as near as possible to where people live and work.
- PHC constitutes the first element of a continuing health care process (Declaration of Alma Ata, 1978).

Meanwhile, PC has been traditionally viewed as provider driven, focused on clinical diagnosis and treatment, institutionally oriented, individually focused, and

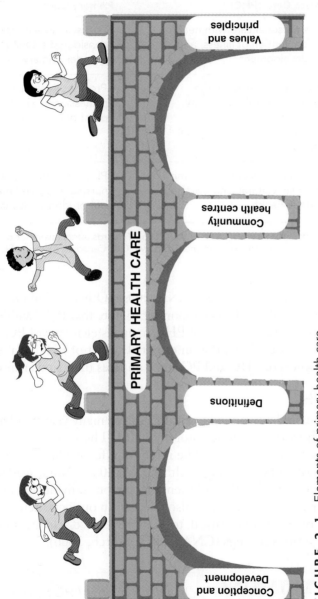

FIGURE 2.1 Elements of primary health care.

TABLE 2.1	COMPARING PRIMARY HEALTH CARE AND PRIMARY CARE	
Primary Health Care (PHC)		**Primary Care**
• Incorporates personal care with health promotion, prevention of illness, and community development		• Focuses more on clinical care—can be considered a subcomponent of the broader primary health care system
• Includes philosophy based on the interconnecting principles of equity, access, empowerment, community self-determination, and intersectorial collaboration		• Provides health care by a medical professional, which is a client's first point of entry into the health system
• Encompasses an understanding of the social, economic, cultural, and political determinants of health		• Places health care widely in area of nursing and allied health professionals, but predominantly in general practice

Reprinted with permission from Martin, C. M. (2006). *Towards a framework for primary health care transition in Canada: A discussion document.* Ottawa, ON: Canadian Alliance of Community Health Centre Associations.

emphasized by service delivery (CNA, 2003). Other definitions of PHC and PC are provided in Table 2.1. It is important to note that PHC and PC are not mutually exclusive; every definition of PHC includes elements of PC. In fact, PC does not disappear under PHC; it is an essential subset of PHC. Table 2.2 depicts the common features of PHC and PC and compares their similarities and differences.

Approach to PHC

Canadian nurses have strived toward PHC for many years, and it continues to be an approach worth pursuing (Storch, 2006). The goal of nursing practice is to improve the health of clients. The intent of effective health care delivery is preventing illness and promoting health (CNA, 2002). Nurse leaders must comprehend the concept of PHC and then take action individually and collectively on the PHC principles. They must also take action on social determinants of health, which are relevant and critical to comprehensive, client, and family-centred practice in various settings (CNA, 2005a; Storch, 2006).

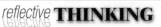 **THINKING**   In what way does PHC benefit clients and their families in a rural area?

Before the 1978 Declaration of Alma Ata, the federal and provincial governments in Canada had shifted in the direction of some of the main components of

TABLE 2.2	FEATURES OF PRIMARY CARE (PC) AND PRIMARY HEALTH CARE (PHC)

Features common to both forms of care
1. First-contact care (except IOM)
2. Accessibility
3. Comprehensiveness
4. Coordination of care

Features of PHC not found in PC	Features of PC not found in PHC

1. Offers essential services/universal accessibility
2. Forms nucleus of country's health care system. Constitutes integral part of overall social and economic development of the country (WHO)
  1. Provides care at a cost the community and country can afford; better use of resources
  2. Brings health care as close as possible to where people live and work
  3. Provides services to community as a whole
  4. Services are organized and adapted to needs of population served
  5. High-quality services
  6. Requires teamwork and interdisciplinary collaboration
  7. Decentralizes services to community-based organizations
  8. Provides services by health care professionals who have the right skills to meet the needs of individuals and the communities being served
	1. Is person-focused (not disease-oriented) care
	2. Involves care over time
	3. Includes sustained partnership with patients (IOM).

Adapted with the permission from Muldoon, L. K., Hogg, W. E., & Levitt, M. (2006). Primary care (PC) and primary health care (PHC). *Canadian Journal of Public Health, 97*(5), 409–411.

PHC (Ogilvie & Reutter, 2003). Examples include the introduction of universal health insurance in 1966 and the presentation of the Lalonde Report by the federal health minister in 1974 (Dickinson & Bolaria, 2000). In the Lalonde Report, Ogilvie and Reutter (2003) state, "The groundwork for building an accessible health-care system oriented to prevention, health promotion, and intersectorial collaboration was in place" (p. 445).

As noted above and in Chapter 1, the 1978 WHO global conference at Alma Ata resulted in a declaration. This key conference defined and granted international recognition to the concept of PHC as a strategy to achieve "Health for All by the Year 2000" (Smith, 2005). A landmark document, the Declaration of Alma Ata, marked a dramatic point by confirming that access to basic health services is a fundamental human right (Declaration of Alma Ata, 1978). The document challenged the health care system to move from the traditional biomedical model to a framework that promoted health (Vollman, Anderson, & McFarlane, 2004).

PHC involves a shift from traditional practices and power dynamics in health care to a paradigm model in which all health care professionals are used to their maximum potential to deliver effective client health care outcomes (Storch, 2006). PHC is both a philosophy of health care and an approach to providing services and emphasizes five basic principles. The five principles are explained, with examples, in Table 2.3. PHC is cost effective and has the capacity to benefit those people in greatest need (CNA, 2003).

Philosophy of PHC

The philosophy of PHC focuses on social justice and equality, whereas the approach embraces five types of essential care: promotive, preventive, curative, rehabilitative, and supportive/palliative (Vollman & Potter, 2006). In delivering each type of care, the focus is on preventing illness and promoting health for various client groups, from individuals and families to communities and populations (CNA, 2000).

> reflective **THINKING**   What is your understanding of basic health services? Describe four or five PHC strategies to promote health in a northern region of Saskatchewan.

Nursing Leadership in PHC

In 1985, the WHO statement entitled *Nurses Lead the Way* recognized officially the importance of the leadership role that nurses could provide in implementing primary health care. In the following year, 1986, a major WHO conference in Tokyo, "Leadership in Nursing for Health for All," marked the international recognition of the leadership role of nurses in primary health care (Lemire Rodger & Gallagher, 2000). In Canada, nursing leaders were positioned to take up the challenge to improve the quality of health in clients and their families by implementing the principles of PHC.

According to Lemire Rodger and Gallagher (2000), two key developments in 1986—the discussion paper "Achieving Health for All" and the Ottawa Charter for Health Promotion—manifested the political will for health care reform. The Ottawa Charter for Health Promotion presented fundamental strategies and approaches for health promotion that were considered vital for major progress

TABLE 2.3	CANADIAN NURSES ASSOCIATION: FIVE PRINCIPLES OF PRIMARY HEALTH CARE	
Principles	**Explanation**	**Example**
Accessibility	Effective health care is accessible and equitable to all individuals and communities. Whether the individuals, families, groups, or communities are seeking diagnosis, treatment, rehabilitation, and/or palliative care, as well as support and advice to prevent disease, the PHC approach ensures the right provider is offering the right care at the right time and the right place.	The North Shore Ambulatory Nursing Clinic in North Vancouver had noted a high number of home visit appointment cancellations by cancer patients. This was attributed to conflicting appointments with other health professionals. A program of centralized nursing clinics to replace home visits was developed. The results of the program include coordination of care for cancer patients, improved access to appropriate services by appropriate health professionals, and more efficient use of resources.
Public participation	Effective care means individuals, families, and communities actively participate in decisions affecting their health.	The *Better Beginnings, Better Futures* project, being implemented in eight disadvantaged communities in Ontario, found that the strong involvement of local residents in all aspects of program delivery and implementation are critical to the acceptance and appropriateness of the programs.
Health promotion	Effective health care encompasses more than physical and mental health—it takes into account social, economic, environmental, and spiritual factors. The goal of health promotion is to enable individuals, families and communities, to live healthy lives. It involves activities related to health education, advocacy, illness prevention, and strong community participation.	The Montreal Dietary Dispensary (MDD) Program is an award-winning program established to help disadvantaged women by providing nutritional counselling and support to expectant mothers at risk. A cost/benefit analysis revealed that for every $1 spent on an MDD client, $8 was saved in health care costs. It was estimated that the $6 million required to provide intervention for all low-income pregnant women at any one time in the Province of Quebec could be entirely recovered within 12 to 14 months through reduced health care costs.
Appropriate skills and technology	Effective health care uses appropriate technology based on health needs of communities. It involves consideration of alternatives to high-cost, high-tech services.	The University of Ottawa's Heart Institute provides cardiac consultations to clients in the North, especially in Aboriginal communities, via telehealth and telemedicine.

(table continues on page 40)

TABLE 2.3	CANADIAN NURSES ASSOCIATION: FIVE PRINCIPLES OF PRIMARY HEALTH CARE (continued)	
Principles	**Explanation**	**Example**
Intersectorial cooperation	Effective health care means working with other sectors that influence the health of communities and individuals, e.g., education, social services, environment, etc.	Dr. Gina Browne, from McMaster University, conducted a groundbreaking study looking at what financial and social implications happen when you provide comprehensive care for single mothers on welfare and their children instead of leaving them to fend for themselves in a fragmented system. They found that providing comprehensive services to families enabled them to leave income-maintenance programs.

From Canadian Nurses Association. (2002). *Fact sheet: Effective health care equals primary health care (PHC)*. Ottawa, ON: Author.

within the health care system (Vollman, Anderson, & McFarlane, 2004). Health promotion is the process of enabling individuals to improve and to increase control over their health (Public Health Agency of Canada, 2002, p. 37; see also Chapter 1).

Despite the evident political will, the barriers created by the medical model in most Western industrialized countries—which are frequently in opposition to the principles of a PHC model—remain a challenge for the Canadian nursing profession. However, considering the drawbacks presented by the medical model, the leadership role of the CNA has always been impressive. Many leadership development initiatives mounted by universities, unions, and professional nursing organizations are geared toward developing strategic actions needed to provide the quality of nursing leadership required to deal with Canadian as well as global health care (CNA, 2005b). In brief, all provincial and territorial nursing associations have been involved in PHC activities. Such activities include the development of public policies on health, political action for the reform of the health care system, and PHC projects.

For example, the College of Registered Nurses in Manitoba, in one of its leadership roles, was successful in the endeavour to launch a campaign in two phases to encourage Manitobans and their families to make frequent handwashing a habit. Hildebrand (2006) states that an evaluation of the campaign showed that the overall message was well received by the public. Those exposed to the message reported that they would likely change their personal behaviour and wash their hands more frequently as a result of the increased awareness of handwashing and its value in their life. This campaign had several objectives, the most significant being that it assisted the public to understand the value and importance of nurses and the critical role they play within the health care system.

reflective **THINKING**   As a nurse leader, what steps can you take to advocate implementing PHC strategies in your area of work?

In 2002, the CNA updated its fact sheet from "The PHC Approach" to "Effective Health Care Equals Primary Health Care (PHC)" (CNA, 2002). In doing so, the CNA emphasized the role of the nurse in effective PHC. Later, in 2005, the CNA developed an important and timely position statement on *interprofessional collaboration*. The association believes that the responsiveness of the health care system can be strengthened through effective collaboration among health professionals (CNA, 2006). Provincially speaking, the College of Registered Nurses of British Columbia (CRNBC) has a position statement entitled *Primary Health Care*. CRNBC endorses PHC as key to the sustainability of the Canadian health care system (CRNBC, 2005).

The *Romanow Commission Report* stated that primary health care offers tremendous benefits to Canadians and to the health care system (Romanow, 2002). In 2006, Health Canada stated that PHC is key to maintaining and improving the health of Canadians. All provinces and territories are implementing plans for PHC reform. Nationwide, these reforms are garnering financial support from the government of Canada through a special $800 million fund (discussed in Chapter 1), called the Primary Health Care Transition Fund (Health Canada, 2006). Specifically, the fund provides support for the transitional costs associated with introducing new approaches to primary health care delivery. It has funded the search for innovative ways to deliver effective and appropriate health care (Villeneuve & MacDonald, 2006). Although the Primary Health Care Transition Fund is time-limited, the changes that it supports are intended to have a lasting and sustainable impact on the health care system. At present, all funding allocations have been completed, and no further funding is available (Health Canada, 2006).

Lemire Rodger and Gallagher (2000) state that the increased focus on health promotion and illness and injury prevention has been integrated throughout all reported nursing activities. In 2004, the CNA collaborated with various partners for such projects as the Canadian Nurse Practitioner Initiative, the development of a national nursing portal, and the project "Toward 2020: Visions for Nursing" (Villeneuve & MacDonald, 2006). Interdisciplinary education and care are of particular interest and are being experimented with in various jurisdictions throughout Canada. Such experimentation seems fully warranted because the basis of PHC is interdisciplinary team work (Villeneuve & MacDonald, 2006). It is crucial that the nursing profession continues to assume leadership and to ensure the integration of these essential activities into the health system.

> *reflective* **THINKING** In what projects do you see nurse leaders taking the initiative to advocate for, and to increase knowledge about, primary health care in your community?

Determinants of Health

The philosophy of social justice and equity, found in the Alma Ata Declaration: Health for All by Year 2000, called for countries to provide essential health services for everyone. The essential health services were health education, safe water, adequate sanitation, maternal and child health care, adequate food, and immunization. Also addressed in the declaration were the prevention and control of endemic diseases, appropriate treatment of common diseases and injuries, and the provision of essential drugs (WHO, 1978). PHC is committed to promoting essential health services that lead to improved health outcomes for an entire population (Potter et al., 2006).

Economic and Social Determinants of Health

According to Smith (2005), social justice "refers to the degree of equality of opportunity for health made available by the political, social, and economic structures and values of a society" (p. 88). Extensive research indicates that economic and social conditions, rather than medical treatments and lifestyle choices, are the major factors in determining the health status of individuals. One of the critical important life conditions that determine whether individuals stay healthy or become ill is their income. For example, cardiovascular disease among Canadians is the disease most frequently associated with low income. It is estimated that among Canadians, income differences account for a 24% excess in premature deaths from cardiovascular disease before age 75 years. An estimate of the annual costs to Canada, of those income-related cardiovascular disease effects, is $4 billion (Raphael, 2002).

In 2002, at a conference at York University in Toronto, a special group of social and health policy experts, community representatives, and health researchers considered the state of 10 key social or societal determinants of health. This conference was held in response to the accumulating body of evidence that growing social and economic inequalities among Canadians were contributing to higher health care costs and other social burdens. The social determinants identified as relevant and important to the health of Canadians are as follows:

- Early childhood development
- Education

- Employment and working conditions
- Food security
- Health care services
- Housing
- Income and its equitable distribution
- Social exclusion
- Social safety nets
- Unemployment and employment security.

These social determinants reflected an increasing concern that social safety nets were eroding (Potter et al., 2006). As a result of the conference, the "Toronto Charter on the Social Determinants of Health" was developed to outline action for governments at all levels, the media, public health, and health care agencies and associations. This charter is, and will continue to be, a valuable tool for promoting health and social justice (Raphael, Bryant, & Curry-Stevens, 2004).

Social Justice and Equality

It is imperative that nurse leaders contemplate ways in which the concept of social justice is enacted in nursing practice. One way is for individual nurse leaders to reflect on their own personal and professional values. Nurse leaders must also consider how the management of various health care organizations, in the delivery of health care, will affect health outcomes. Nurses must play a pivotal role in becoming politically active to mobilize actions for change in individual, family, and organizational health behaviours.

reflective **THINKING** After thinking about the social health determinants, what health problems do you see in your community? As a nurse leader, what primary prevention strategies should you consider implementing?

Inequities as Determinants

According to Kawachi, Subramanian, and Almeida-Filho (2002), both equity and inequity are "political concepts, expressing a moral commitment to social justice" (p. 647). *Health inequality* is a term used to denote differences, variations, and disparities in the health attainments of individuals and groups. The Health Council of Canada (2007) states that a growing level of health inequality between different groups in Canada exists. The key factors in health inequalities are income, gender, and disability. For example, Aboriginal Canadians in particular have noticeably poor health status compared with the rest of the Canadian population. Children and youth who grow up in lower-income families tend to have declining health, and Aboriginal children and recent immigrants are more likely to become poor (Health Council of Canada, 2006).

In 2004, British Columbia, Newfoundland and Labrador, Saskatchewan, and Manitoba were the four provinces with the highest rates of child poverty (Campaign 2000, 2006a). The provincial rate tends to be higher than the national average (Campaign 2000, 2006b). Health Council of Canada (2006) claims that effective child development and parenting support programs can overcome some of the negative effects of poverty. Governments at all levels need to attack poverty and strive to reduce it by regularly re-evaluating their direct programs of income support and their indirect programs designed to address housing, food security, prescription drugs, and dental care.

Ill health among homeless people is also a huge and growing concern in Canada. Homelessness is associated with increased hospital costs, length of stay, and medical or surgical conditions complicated by secondary diagnoses of substance abuse or mental illness (Podymow, Turnbull, Tadic, & Muckle, 2006).

The Ottawa Inner City Health Project was developed as a pilot research project in partnership with city health and social agencies and the University of Ottawa. The project implemented a harm-reduction paradigm to deliver health services to homeless adults within the existing shelter system. Podymow et al. (2006) found that a shelter-based convalescence unit can provide health care to homeless persons, treat mental and medical illness, facilitate adherence to treatment regimens, decrease substance abuse, and assist with housing. The researchers indicate that those responsible for the homeless should consider implementing and evaluating such programs by integrating health services with shelters for the homeless.

Concerns about adequate food supply is a mounting problem in Canada. The food offered at the 650 food banks in Canada has become a critical part of the nutritional intake of more than 820,600 Canadians each month; approximately 40% of food bank users are children (Irwin et al., 2007). In their study of comparing food hamper contents with Canadian guidelines that intend to provide 3 days worth of food per person, Irwin et al. (2007) found that food hampers did not provide sufficient macro- or micronutrients, food-group servings, or energy per person for the intended 3 days. This is a serious concern because food banks have become a highly important source of nutrition for low-income and highly vulnerable subpopulations in Canada (Ledro & Gervais, 2005). This situation requires meaningful and immediate attention. In fact, the readers' attention is drawn to the work of Cathy Crowe, Toronto street nurse. (Visit her at http://www.trdc.net/cathycrowe.htm.)

reflective **THINKING**   After visiting Cathy Crowe's Website, what is your understanding of a street nurse? What leadership skills does the street nurse need?

The gap between low-income families and well-off families is widening in relation to their income (Campaign 2000, 2006c). The benefits of a strong Canadian economy have not been evenly distributed among Canadians, and the inequality results in devastating health effects for those in the lower income level (Campaign 2000, 2006c).

The health of individuals and their families is affected by the community environment and society in which they live. In fact, the societal context for living can either sustain and expand health potentials or inhibit health and well-being. Nurses frequently encounter unique opportunities to provide leadership to health professionals in various settings and to the government in the promotion of better health in society. Nurses, as the largest single group of health care providers, play a vital role in making health promotion and illness prevention strategies available to all population groups, including those who are underserved and vulnerable (Pender, Murdaugh, & Parson, 2006). In fact, nurse leaders are key players in planning and implementing health promotion interventions and measuring their effectiveness (Smith, 2005). This approach is fundamental to PHC.

Principles of PHC

In 1978, the WHO adopted the PHC approach, which is both a philosophy and a model, as the conceptual basis for the effective delivery of health care services (CNA, June 2002). CNA endorses the PHC approach as the most highly effective

Reflections on Leadership Practice

As you are preparing yourself for a leadership seminar group on primary health care (PHC), you decide to read this chapter. You reflect on the value "equity in health" and on the premise that income affects health and, furthermore, that living in poverty is a primary indicator of poor health. In your seminar group, you and the rest of the students begin to discuss how poverty throughout Canada continues to be a reality for the lives of many children, youth, and families. Someone in the group comments on the degree of health disparity that occurs across income levels.

Take the time in your group to compare and contrast the health problems that poor youth experience compared with more affluent youth.

As a nurse leader, what health promotion strategies could you implement for the health issues you identify for both groups?

Identify some actions that you as a group of nurse leaders can initiate to begin reducing poverty in your community?

way of preventing illness and promoting health care to a population (CNA, November 2002). The five principles associated with PHC are as follows:

1. Accessibility
2. Public participation
3. Health promotion
4. Appropriate skills and technology
5. Intersectorial cooperation.

Table 2.3 presents explanations and examples of each principle.

> reflective **THINKING**   Identify your own example for each of the principles. Choose examples from an area with which you are familiar. Conversely, you might create examples and bring them to class for discussion purposes.

Integrating Principles in Practice

It is important to be aware that nurses continually are integrating with increased effectiveness the principles of PHC in their practice. Such professional development is extremely valuable for nurses involved in direct care, whether in roles of education, research, administration, or policy (CNA, April 2002). These nurses are actively addressing the challenge of working productively as members of an interdisciplinary health care team (CNA, 2005c). Nurse leaders need to provide active support to all nurses who are conscientiously adopting the principles of PHC. Nurses, who make up the largest number of health care providers, must continue to work toward client, family, and societal wellness through disease prevention and health promotion strategies for all (Smith, 2005).

PHC Model

Over the last 15 years, the Canadian health care system has experienced major reform (Richard et al., 2005). In fact, one of the major challenges facing the Canadian health care system in the 21st century is the organization of PHC. Although PHC has been interpreted in many ways, six broad effects exist that a PHC model should deliver. The six effects are as follows:

- Effectiveness: the ability to produce the expected outcome—either maintain or improve health.
- Productivity: the relationship between the delivery of services and the use of resources to deliver them.

- Accessibility: the ability to visit a PHC physician promptly. It includes the ease of accessing specialized and diagnostic services.
- Continuity: the availability of services offered while keeping up with the health needs and personal contexts of clients.
- Quality: the appropriateness and effectiveness of care as perceived by clients and professionals. It includes compliance with guidelines, as well as the suitability of services.
- Responsiveness: respect and consideration extended in response to the expectations and preferences of service users and health care providers (Canadian Health Services Research Foundation, 2003).

Community Health Centres

The Canadian Alliance of Community Health Centre Associations (CACHCA) represents more than 250 community health centres in Canada. CACHCA advocates for the further development of community health centres as a comprehensive, integrated, and accessible PHC model that is well suited to the pan-Canadian health care system (Romanow, 2001). In the document *The Future of Canada's Public Health Care System* (Romanow, 2001), CACHCA reviews the community health centres as a model that incorporates many of the principles inherent in the practice of PHC as defined by the WHO and contends that the model should be accessible to all Canadians.

The main objective of CACHCA is to work for quality health care services for individuals and their families in communities across Canada. CACHCA advocates community health centres as a cost-effective and successful method for delivering PHC (CACHCA, n.d.). Box 2.1 outlines the characteristics of community health centres as promoted in the CACHCA (2007) document.

> *reflective* **THINKING**   After reading the characteristics of the Community Health Centres (Box 2.1), to what extent do the broad effects that a PHC model should deliver meet the given characteristics?

Canada and many other countries are indicating a renewed interest in PHC. In fact, many believe it to be the critical element in responding to the numerous challenges facing the health care system (Canadian Health Services Research Foundation, 2003). Although community health centres have been viewed as the ideal settings in implementing the PHC approach, more research is needed to evaluate the performance of Community Health Centres in the delivery of PHC. For example, the study by Richard et al. (2005) of *centres locaux de services communautaires*, local community health and social service centres in Quebec, is noteworthy. Being one of the very few such studies in Canada, the findings make a

> ## BOX 2.1   CHARACTERISTICS OF COMMUNITY HEALTH CENTRES (CHCS)
>
> A community health centre generally has the following characteristics:
> 1. Nonprofit or government-sponsored organization
>   - Governed by locally elected board of directors, OR by an advisory board.
>   - In either case, the board consists mostly of local residents and/or clients.
> 2. Defined by geographic area, OR by a group, or groups, of people who have experienced barriers in accessing primary health services.
> 3. A range of services
>   - Includes primary health, social, rehabilitation, and other institutional services
>   - Emphasizes prevention, health promotion, health education, and community development services
> 4. Partnership with organizations in other sectors
>   - Emphasizes education, justice, recreation, and economic development
>   - Promotes the health of the community
> 5. Interdisciplinary teams provide services.
> 6. Staff remuneration by salary and/or *capitation**
>
> ---
>
> **capitation*: A tax levied per head; a method of payment for health services in which an individual or institution is paid a fixed amount for each person served, without regard to the actual number or nature of services provided to each person.
>
> Adapted with permission from Canadian Alliance of Community Health Centre Associations (n.d.). *What is a CHC?* Author.

valuable contribution to building knowledge about the performance of community health centers.

Leadership Issue

*Y*ou are employed at a new Community Health Centre, which is beginning to provide a full range of health-related services focusing on health promotion and prevention of illness. As a nurse leader, you are asked to design a program on immunization. How will you begin? What resources will you need?

Role of the Nurse Leader

In recent years, the desire to shift the focus of the health care delivery system from illness to health has resulted in the growth of the PHC movement (Gottlieb & Feeley, 2006). A critical underlying premise of PHC is collaboration between health care practitioners and consumers of care (Villeneuve & MacDonald, 2006). Collaborative client-centred practice promotes the active participation of each discipline in client care by encouraging respect for the contributions of all health care professionals and by optimizing staff contribution and participation in decision making. The Canadian Nurses Association (CNA) published a position statement entitled *Interprofessional Collaboration* (CNA, 2006). CNA, as a partner in the Enhancing Interdisciplinary Collaboration Project, has contributed to the development of the document *The Principles and Framework for Interdisciplinary Collaboration in Primary Health Care.* This statement describes the effectiveness of health care service integration for all Canadians (CNA, 2005c). The six principles, found in Box 2.2, will facilitate collaboration among professions and professionals.

BOX 2.2 SIX PRINCIPLES TO FACILITATE COLLABORATION AMONG PROFESSIONS AND PROFESSIONALS*

Focus on the Patient/Client
- The needs of individual patients and clients must be the focus of health services.
- Health professionals work together to:
  1. Optimize the health and wellness of each individual
  2. Involve the individual in decision-making about his/her health.
- Individuals and their families are actively engaged in the prevention, promotion, and management of health problems.
- Health professionals respect that personal health information must be kept confidential.

Population Health Approach
- Assessments of the demographics and health status of a community are used to:
  1. Ensure the relevance of the health service.
  2. Identify appropriate health professionals.
- Trends in the health of the population are tracked to assess the impact of the services offered.

Quality Care and Services
- Health professionals work together to identify and assess research evidence:
  1. As a basis for identifying treatments.
  2. As a basis for management of health problems.
- Health outcomes are continuously evaluated:
  1. To track the effectiveness of services.
  2. To track the appropriateness of services.

Access
- The right service is provided at the right time, in the right place, and by the right care provider.
- Geographic barriers are minimized.
- Service delivery is respectful of age, gender, culture, language, religion, and lifestyle of patients/clients.

(box continues on page 50)

> **BOX 2.2**   SIX PRINCIPLES TO FACILITATE COLLABORATION AMONG
> PROFESSIONS AND PROFESSIONALS* (continued)
>
> **Trust and Respect**
> - Each profession brings its own set of knowledge and skills—the result of educa-
>   tion, training, and experience—to collaborative health services.
> - Each professional contributes to an individual's health.
> - Shared decision making, creativity, and innovation allow providers to learn from
>   one another and enhance the effectiveness of their collaborative efforts.
>
> **Communication**
> Active listening and effective communication skills facilitate both information shar-
> ing and decision making.
>
> ---
>
> *As outlined in *Principles and Framework for Interdisciplinary Collaboration in Primary Health Care.*
> From Canadian Nurses Association. (2006). *Position statement: Interprofessional collaboration.* Ottawa, ON:
> Author.

Interdisciplinary collaboration requires teamwork. For a team to function well, the team must be supported by a strong team leader and the health care organization involved (Enhancing Interdisciplinary Collaboration in Primary Health Care, 2005). Nurses constitute a major component of health care professionals and are the cornerstone of Canada's health care system (Buckland, Lawless, & Bowmer, 2007). Nurse leaders need to learn about collaboration as well as the roles of other nurse professionals to work effectively in the provision of PHC to clients and their families (Herbert, 2005). Nurses will be called to lead the collaborative process in teams involved in health care delivery as they play an integral role in the management and delivery of health care services.

WEBSITES

■ Primary Health Care Transition Fund (2000–2006)

http://www.hc-sc.gc.ca/hcs-sss/prim/phctf-fassp/index_e.html

On September 11, 2000, First Ministers agreed that "improvements to primary health care are crucial to the renewal of health services" and highlighted the importance of multi-disciplinary teams. In response to this agreement, the Government of Canada established the $800 million Primary Health Care Transition Fund (PHCTF). Over a 6-year period (2000–2006), the PHCTF supported provinces and territories in their efforts to reform the primary health care system. Specifically, it provided support for the transitional costs associated with introducing new approaches to primary health care delivery.

■ The Canadian Institute for Health Information (CIHI)

http://www.cihi.ca/

The CIHI is a not-for-profit organization that provides timely, accurate, and comparable health information and seeks to improve the health of Canadians and the health care system. CIHI data and reports inform about health policies, support the effective delivery of health services, and raise awareness among Canadians of the factors that contribute to good health.

■ The Canadian Alliance of Community Health Centre Associations (CACHCA)

http://www.cachca.ca/

The CACHCA was established in 1995 to provide support to Canada's provincially based community health centre organizations and to represent the interests of those organizations at the national level.

REFERENCES

Buckland, R., Lawless, V., & Bowmer, M. I. (2007, February). The power of collaboration. *Health Policy Research, 13,* 36–39.

Calnan, R. (2003). My opinion: Primary health care. *SRNA Newsbulletin, 5*(2), 11.

Campaign 2000. (2006a). *Manitoba child and family poverty report card 2006: Back to the future: Approaching 1989.* Toronto, ON: Campaign 2000 Continues Steering Committee of the Social Planning Council of Winnipeg. Retrieved March 2007 from http://www.campaign2000.ca/

Campaign 2000. (2006b). *Report card on child poverty in Saskatchewan.* Toronto, ON: The Social Policy Research Unit, Faculty of Social Work, University of Regina. Retrieved March 2007 from http://www.campaign2000.ca/

Campaign 2000. (2006c). *Oh Canada! Too many children in poverty for too long.* Toronto, ON: Family Service Association of Toronto. Retrieved March 2007 from http://www.campaign2000.ca/

Canadian Alliance of Community Health Centre Associations (CACHCA). (n.d.) *What is a CHC?* Ottawa, ON: Author. Retrieved June 2007 from http://www.cachca.ca/

Canadian Health Services Research Foundation. (2003). *Choices for change: The path for restructuring primary healthcare services in Canada.* Ottawa, ON: Author. Retrieved March 2007 from http://www.chsrf.ca/

Canadian Nurses Association. (2000). *Fact Sheet: The primary health care approach*. Ottawa, ON: Author.

Canadian Nurses Association. (2002). *Three stages for optimizing the health of the health system: Statement to the Commission on the Future of Health Care*. Ottawa, ON: Author.

Canadian Nurses Association. (2002, June). *Primary health care: A new approach to health care reform*. Ottawa, ON: Author.

Canadian Nurses Association. (2002, November). *Fact sheet: Effective health care equals primary health care (PHC)*. Ottawa, ON: Author.

Canadian Nurses Association. (2003). *Nursing Now: Primary health care—the time has come*. Ottawa, ON: Author.

Canadian Nurses Association. (2005a). *CNA backgrounder, Primary health care: A summary of the issues*. Ottawa, ON: Author.

Canadian Nurses Association. (2005b). *Nursing leadership development in Canada*. Ottawa, ON: Author.

Canadian Nurses Association. (2005c). *Position statement: Interpersonal collaboration*. Ottawa, ON: Author.

Canadian Nurses Association. (2006). *Position statement: Interprofessional collaboration*. Ottawa, ON: Author.

College of Registered Nurses of British Columbia. (2005). *Position statement: Primary health care*. Vancouver, BC: Author.

Dickinson, H., & Bolaria, S. (2002). The Canadian health care system: Evolution and current status. In B. Singh Bolaria, & H. D. Dickinson (Eds.), *Health, illness, and health care in Canada* (3rd ed., pp. 20–32). Toronto, ON: Nelson Thompson Learning.

Enhancing Interdisciplinary Collaboration in Primary Health Care Initiative. (2005). *Enhancing interdisciplinary collaboration in primary health care in Canada*. Ottawa, ON: The Conference Board of Canada.

Gottlieb, L. N., & Feeley, N., with Dalton, C. (2006). *The collaborative partnership approach to care: A delicate balance*. Toronto, ON: Elsevier Canada.

Health Canada. (2006, July). *Primary health care transition fund*. Retrieved March 2007 from http://www.hc-sc.gc.ca/hcs-sss/prim/phctf-fassp/index-eng.php

Health Council of Canada. (2006). *Their future is now: Healthy choices for Canada's children & youth June 2006*. Ottawa, ON: Author.

Health Council of Canada. (2007). *Health care renewal in Canada: Measuring up?* Ottawa, ON: Author.

Herbert, C. (2005). Changing the culture: Interprofessional education for collaborative patient-centred practice in Canada. *Journal of Interprofessional Care, Supplement 1*, 1–4.

Hildebrand, G. (2006). College's successful hand washing campaign expands, Second phase: Province-wide TV public service announcements. *Manitoba RN Journal, 31*(4), 31–32.

International Council of Nurses. (1999). *Position Statement: Nurses and primary health care*. Geneva, Switzerland: Author. Retrieved March 2007 from http://www.icn.ch/psprimarycare.htm

Irwin, J. D., Ng, V. K., Rush, T. J., Nguyen, C., & He, M. (2007). Can food banks sustain nutrient requirements? *Canadian Journal of Public Health, 98*(1), 17–20.

Kawachi, I., Subramanian, S., & Almeida-Filho, N. (2002). A glossary for health inequalities. *Journal of Epidemiology and Community Health, 56*(9), 647–652.

Ledrou, I., & Gervais, J. (2005). Food insecurity. *Health Reports, 16*(1), 47–51.

Lemire Rodger, G., & Gallagher, S. (2000). The move toward primary health care in Canada: Community health nursing from 1985 to 2000. In M. J. Stewart (Ed.), *Community nursing: Promoting Canadians' health* (2nd ed., pp. 33–55).

Martin, C. M. (2006). *Towards a framework for primary health care transition in Canada: A discussion document.* Ottawa, ON: Canadian Alliance of Community Health Centre Associations. Retrieved March 2007 from http://www.cachca.ca/english/useful%20resources/documents/default.asp?s=1

Muldoon, L. K., Hogg, W. E., & Levitt, M. (2006). Primary care (PC) and primary health care (PHC). *Canadian Journal of Public Health, 97*(5), 409–411.

Ogilvie, L., & Reutter, L. (2003). Primary health care: Complexities and possibilities from a nursing perspective. In J. C. Ross-Kerr, & M. J. Wood (Eds.), *Canadian Nursing: Issues and Perspectives* (4th ed., pp. 441–465). Toronto, ON: Mosby.

Orchard, C. A., Smille, C., & Meagher-Stewart, D. (2000). Community development and health in Canada. *Journal of Nursing Scholarship*, Second Quarter, 205–209.

Pender, N. J., Murdaugh, C. L., & Parsons, M. A. (2006). *Health promotion in nursing practice* (5th ed) Upper Saddle River, NJ: Prentice Hall.

Podymow, T., Turnbull, J., Tadic, V., & Muckle, W. (2006). Shelter-based convalescence for homeless adults. *Canadian Journal of Public Health, 97*(5), 379–383.

Public Health Agency of Canada. (2002). *Population health: Ottawa charter for health promotion: An international conference on health promotion, November 17–21, 1986.* Ottawa, ON: Author.

Raphael, D. (2002). *Social justice is good for our hearts: Why societal factors—not lifestyles—are major causes of heart disease in Canada and elsewhere.* Toronto, ON: Centre for Social Justice Foundation for Research and Education.

Raphael, D., Toba, B., & Curry-Stevens, A. (2004). Toronto charter outlines future health policy directions for Canada and elsewhere. *Health Promotion International, 19*(2), 269–273.

Richard, L., Pinneault, R., D'Amour, D., Brodeur, J.-M., Sequin, L., Latour, R., et al. (2005). The diversity of prevention and health promotion services offered by Quebec community health centres: A study of infant and toddler programmes. *Health and Social Care in the Community, 13*(5), 399–408.

Romanow, R. (2001, December). *The future of Canada's public health care system: Submission by the Canadian Alliance of Community Health Centre Associations.* Toronto, ON: Walter Weary and Associates.

Romanow, R. (2002). *Shape the future of health care.* Ottawa: Commission on the Future of Health Care in Canada.

Smith, D. (2005). Primary health care. In L. Leeseberg Stamler & L. Yiu (Eds.), *Community health nursing: A Canadian perspective.* Toronto, ON: Pearson Prentice Hall.

Storch, J. (2006). Canadian health care system. In M. McIntyre, E. Thomlinson, & C. McDonald (Eds.), *Realities of Canadian nursing: Professional, practice, and power issues.* Philadelphia: Lippincott Williams & Wilkins.

Villeneuve, M., & MacDonald, J. (2006). *Toward 2020: Visions for nursing.* Ottawa, ON: Canadian Nurses Association.

Vollman, A., Anderson, E. T., & McFarlane, J. (2004). *Canadian community as partner: Theory and practice in nursing.* Philadelphia: Lippincott Williams & Wilkins.

Vollman, A. R., & Potter, P. A. (2006). The Canadian health care delivery system. In P. A. Potter, A. G. Perry, J. C. Ross-Kerr, & M. J. Wood (Eds.), *The Canadian health care delivery system* (pp. 18–34). Toronto, ON: Elsevier Canada.

World Health Organization. (1978). *Declaration of Alma-Ata: International conference on primary health care, Alma-Ata, USSR, 6–12 September 1978.* Geneva, Switzerland: Author.

3

POPULATION HEALTH APPROACH: STRATEGIES FOR NURSE LEADERS

want to inspire and engage Canadians from all walks of life, to empathize and respond to the injustice of homelessness in their community and motivate them to become involved in calling for the solution—a national housing program.

—**Cathy Crowe,**
in receiving the Atkinson Economic Justice Award, January 2004

Cathy Crowe, RN, BA (Nursing), MEd, has worked as a Toronto street nurse for almost 20 years. She has been involved in numerous coalitions and extensive public education work regarding the homeless. In 1998, she cofounded the Toronto Disaster Relief Committee, an organization that dramatically increased public understanding of homelessness by calling it "a national disaster." Two Canadian universities have awarded her honourary doctoral degrees.

Overview

In Canada and globally, there is growing awareness of the broad range of multiple factors that influence health and well-being in populations. Population health is an approach that includes examining population growth and trends, focusing on the complex patterns of health determinants that affect health outcomes, and examining health inequities and disparities of various population groups. The population approach also includes implementing strategies and policies to improve the health of Canadians, evaluating the health outcomes and, finally, providing a framework for action that can be adapted by all sectors in society to enhance the health of the population as a whole. A population health approach involves a concerted effort by all health care practitioners, including nurse leaders, to pool their resources and expertise so everyone can reap the benefits of collaborating to promote health in populations.

Objectives

By critically reflecting upon and processing knowledge throughout this chapter, you will be able to respond effectively to the following objectives:

1. Summarize briefly the population health perspective.
2. Illustrate in your own manner the meaning of population health.
3. Design a case situation whereby all eight elements of the population health approach are implemented.
4. Propose a health care system that will address the current health status of the Baby Boomers.
5. Compare and contrast the effect of health status indicators and determinants on population health.
6. Evaluate the importance of social determinants of health and their effect on health status of the population.
7. Defend the role of the nurse in addressing the social determinants of health.
8. Emphasize the importance of the interdisciplinary health team to implement health promotion strategies.
9. Advocate verbally or on paper for nurse leaders to be politically active for clients and families in communities.
10. Assess the role of the nurse in implementing the population health promotion model.
11. Interpret to your classmates the integrated Pan-Canadian Healthy Living Strategy.
12. Paraphrase how the ecological approach affects the role of the nurse leader.
13. Construct a framework to evaluate the strategies you might use to implement, maintain, and improve the health status of the population and to decrease inequalities in health status between groups and subgroups.

Population Health Perspective

Health Canada has played a leading role in developing a thorough understanding of health for more than 20 years (Health Canada, 1998). The highly acclaimed *Lalonde Report: A New Perspective on the Health of Canadians* (1974) was a turning point in assisting Canadians to understand not only the factors that contribute to health, but also the role of the government in promoting the health of the Canadian population. The Lalonde Report identified human biology, lifestyle, environment, and health care organization as the four main elements affecting health (Vollman, Anderson, & McFarlane, 2004). The report indicated the first stage of health promotion in Canada (Glouberman & Millar, 2003). Health promotion is the process of enabling individuals to increase control over, and to improve, their health (World Health Organization [WHO], 1986).

In the mid-1980s, arguments were presented that the health behaviours of individuals were determined by various conditions such as housing, income, social status, employment, and environmental factors. The release of the discussion paper *A Framework for Health Promotion* added social justice and equity as conditions (Epp, 1986). In 1986, Canada held the First International Conference on Health Promotion in Ottawa. This conference was primarily a response to increasing expectations around the world for a new public health movement (Public Health Agency of Canada [PHAC], 2002a). Reutter (2006) explains that the conference "produced a watershed document called the *Ottawa Charter for Health Promotion*, which supported a socio-environmental approach" (p. 5). The socio-environmental approach to health is closely tied to the physical and social environment, such as air and water quality and work hazards, that influence health directly (Reutter, 2006).

reflective **THINKING**   In reflecting upon the socio-environmental approach to health, how would you interpret the meaning of health to a client and family who reside in a northern community?

The Ottawa Charter states several fundamental prerequisites for health (WHO, 1986). Figure 3.1 outlines those prerequisites. An improvement in health requires a secure baseline in these basic prerequisites (WHO, 1986). Being attentive to the prerequisites places responsibility for health on society in general, rather than only on individuals (Reutter, 2006). The Ottawa Charter also outlined five major strategies to promote health (WHO, 1986):

- Build healthy public policy
- Strengthen community action

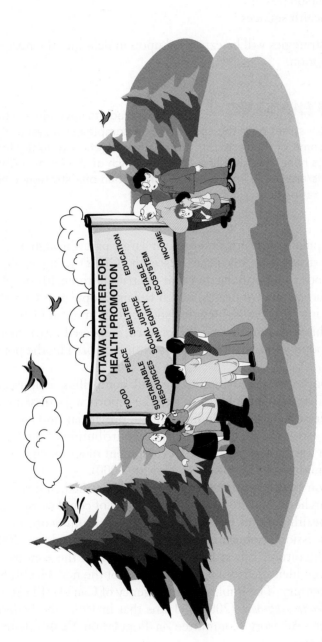

FIGURE 3.1 Fundamental prerequisites for health.

- Create supportive environment
- Develop personal skills
- Reorient health services.

Theses strategies will be expanded upon in detailing the nurse-leader role in health promotion.

> reflective **THINKING**   Many senior adults have either stumbled or fallen on the street near the condominium complex as a result of the poorly lit street. Some of the residents are getting together to lobby for a few street lights near their dwelling. Identify which of the Ottawa Charter strategies is/are being implemented (more than one strategy may apply). State your rationale.

In 1987, population health emerged in large part through the efforts of the Canadian Institute for Advanced Research (CIAR) using epidemiological re-search methods to identify factors that contribute to health (Raphael & Bryant, 2002). The broad view of health, which became popular in Canada in the 1970s and evolved into the 1980s, included social, economic, and political factors that influenced this research. From 1987 onward, respected researchers/members of the CIAR's population health group disseminated broadly the population health perspective.

The reports presented interesting and compelling empirical evidence on nonmedical determinants of health, and the reports were disseminated to a wide range of interested parties, including federal, provincial, and local politicians and other public servants. The most important contribution of the CIAR population health group was thought to be the development of an integrated analysis of the population framework (Legowski & McKay, 2000).

Population health continues to be defined, clarified, and reframed by schol-ars and researchers. Despite a fairly long history of controversy, the concept that population health denotes has continued to gain prominence in Canada amidst extensive discussion (Coburn et al., 2003; Kindig & Stoddart, 2003). In her re-view of the literature, Edwards (1999) claimed that the concept of population health has been identified as a key component of the new Health for All strategy for the 21st century. The Public Health Agency of Canada (PHAC) in *What Is the Population Health Approach* (2002b) claims that in 1997, the Federal, Provincial, and Territorial Advisory Committee on Population Health defined population health as follows:

"Population health refers to the health of a population as measured by health status indicators and as influenced by social, economic, and physical environments; personal health practices; individual capacity and coping skills; human biology; early childhood development; and health services." (p. 2)

Canada has played a leading strategic role in developing the population health concept through its internationally acclaimed work in health promotion (PHAC, 2002b).

The population health perspective has been critiqued on one hand because it is firmly rooted in epidemiological tradition and on the other hand because it lacks values based on such issues as social equity and justice, participation, and community collaboration, as well as emphasis on social change (Raphael & Bryant, 2000; Cohen, 2006). Recently, several Canadian researchers advocated for a critical population health investigation that centres on asking critical questions regarding economic and social causes and on the consequences of health inequalities (Labonte, 2005). The critical population health research seeks to develop an equitable distribution of economic and social conditions that are needed to decrease health inequalities (Labonte, Polanyi, Muhajarine, McIntosh, & Williams, 2005; Cohen, 2006). Labonte, et al. (2005) argue that a critical population health research practice "is a moral praxis built upon explicit social values and analysis" (p. 5). It is an opportunity whereby moral and political necessities for social change become part of our daily life.

> *reflective* **THINKING**   As a nurse leader, how can you make social change a part of your daily work in a health care setting?

Population Health Approach

For several decades, Canada has taken the lead in developing and implementing a population health approach (Lightfoot, Edwards, Fraser-Lee, Kaida, & Predy, 2006). In 1994, the population health approach was endorsed officially by the federal, provincial, and territorial ministers of health in a report entitled *Strategies for Population Health: Investing in the Health of Canadians*. The report summarized the broad determinants of health and outlined a conceptual framework to guide the development of strategies and policies to improve population health (PHAC, 2002c). The population health approach centres on the full scope of individual and collective determinants and on the complex interactions among those factors that determine health and well-being of Canadians (Kushner, 2003).

Population health strategies are based on the assessments of determinants that apply across entire populations or to particular subgroups within the population (PHAC, 2002c). The strategies are designed to improve the health of a population through health promotion interventions and preventive approaches that take into account the determinants of health (MacDonald, 2002; Health Canada, 1998). The goal of a population health approach is to maintain and improve the health status of the population and to decrease inequalities in health status between groups and/or subgroups (PHAC, 2002b).

The Population Health Template: Key Elements and Actions That Define a Population Health Approach was developed by Health Canada Population and Public Health Branch and Strategic Policy Directorate (PHAC, 2002b). The Population Health Template classifies and consolidates the current understanding of population health. The template delineates the processes in a series of steps and procedures intended to implement a population health approach. In brief, the generic processes comprise the following: the analysis of the health issue, priority setting, taking action, and evaluating the results—all of which bring about stronger evidence and knowledge development (PHAC, 2002b).

Figure 3.2 shows the key elements of population health and the generic process steps designed to meet the goals intended to improve the health of the population and decrease health status inequities. The eight key elements are as follows:

1. Assessment of health of populations: the health status and health status inequities of the entire population as well as groups within it, population trends are also examined.
2. Analysis of the determinants of health: addressing the full range of factors and their relationships that determine health.
3. Decision making based on factual evidence: basing decisions on generated knowledge drawn from a variety of data and identifying quality effective interventions.
4. Increase of upstream investments: directing investments to those areas that have the most potential to influence health in a positive manner. However, the choice should always be based on evidence.
5. Application of multiple strategies: using various strategies available in a way that yields the greatest impact on population health outcomes.
6. Collaboration across multiple sectors and levels: coordinating interventions in an integrated way that addresses issues to improve health over the lifespan, engaging health team members to establish shared values, and developing partnerships.
7. Use of mechanisms for public involvement: being politically active to achieve common goals.
8. Accountability for health outcomes: design ways to develop an accountability framework, construct an effective evaluative system, and publicly report the results (PHAC, 2002b; Lightfoot et al., 2006).

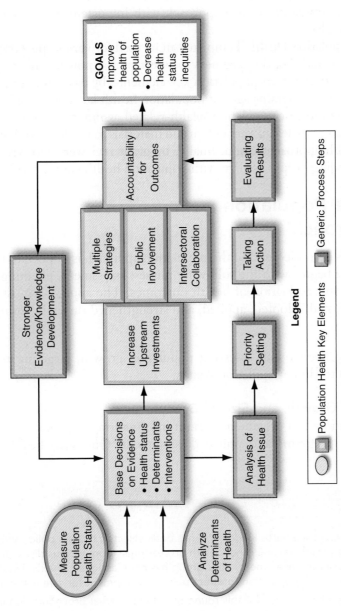

FIGURE 3.2 Key elements of population health. (From "The Population Health Template", reprinted with permission from Public Health Agency of Canada. [2002] Population Health: What Is the Population Health Approach? Ottawa, ON: Author.)

These eight elements are essential for implementing the population health approach. However, key elements 1 and 2 are distinct to the definition of a population health approach. Meanwhile, key elements 3 to 8 consider the implications of a population health approach with important management practices (PHAC, 2002b).

The Population Health Template can be used for various purposes by groups, policymakers, and program planners to ascertain that policies and program development initiatives reflect population key elements; by evaluators to use given criteria to measure programs against population health key elements; by researchers and academics to test population health-related assumptions and hypotheses; by health educators to design curriculum and materials to reinforce and promote population health approaches; and, finally, by grant reviewers and writers to assess whether funding proposals align with population health concepts (PHAC, 2002b).

Enacting the Population Health Approach

The process of implementing the population approach is important in the health care field. It begins with the following phases: assessment, planning and implementation, and evaluation of health outcomes. The approach must be thought through, learned, adopted, applied, and strengthened through "doing."

Assessment

The process begins with assessing population growth, targeting relevant subgroups, and tracking population trends.

Character, Growth, and Size of Groups

The population data provide important information to facilitate the planning of health care programs and policy development. One such health program is

---

Reflections on Leadership Practice

You are a nurse leader who has been selected to be a policy and program planner along with several other health professionals from various disciplines acting for the provincial government. Your group has been assigned to examine the rural community health population to direct policy development for safe water supply.

In preparing yourself for this round of meetings, what procedural input will you be able to offer based on your knowledge of the key elements of the Population Health Template? A summary of the Population Key Elements is found on the PHAC home page at www.phac-aspc.gc.ca/

known as Aboriginal Head Start On-Reserve. It is an early intervention program for First Nations children (ages 0 to 6 years) and their families who live on a reservation. The program is intended to prepare these children for their school years by meeting their emotional, social, health, nutritional, and psychological needs (Government of Canada, 2000).

In Canada, the population grew more rapidly between 2001 and 2006 (+5.4%) than in the previous 5 years (+4.0%). This forward move was due in large part to an increase in international migration. If current fertility, mortality, and international migration trends continue, no population decline is expected over the next 50 years. In 2056, the Canadian population can be expected to number 43 million (Statistics Canada, 2007). When one considers national population growth, the question that arises is: Which group is growing fastest? Figure 3.3 illustrates the population of Canada in the last 50 years and the growth that has occurred.

Regarding the population size of various age groups, the most extensive is the group of individuals known as Baby Boomers, born between 1946 and 1965. This group's ages ranged between 36 and 55 years at the 2001 census and represented nearly one third of the total population (Statistics Canada, 2001). Table 3.1 identifies several birth cohorts that place into perspective population changes by age group that occurred between 1991 and 2001. Projections to 2011 are based on a

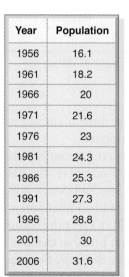

Year	Population
1956	16.1
1961	18.2
1966	20
1971	21.6
1976	23
1981	24.3
1986	25.3
1991	27.3
1996	28.8
2001	30
2006	31.6

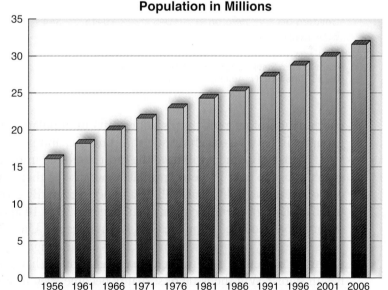

FIGURE 3.3 Population of Canada in the last 50 years. (Adapted from Statistics Canada. [2007]. Portrait of the Canadian Population in 2006, 2006 Census. Catalog No. 97-550-XIE, p. 8. Ottawa, ON: Author.)

TABLE 3.1 SHIFTS IN THE POPULATION SIZE OF VARIOUS AGE GROUPS

Cohort	Year of Birth	Age in 2001	Age in 2011	Average Number of Births Per Year (in thousands)	Size of Cohort
Pre- World War I	Before 1914	88+	98+	201	Relatively small
World War I	1914–1919	82–87	92–97	244	Relatively small
1920s	1920–1929	72–81	82–92	249	Relatively small
Depression Years	1929–1939	62–71	72–81	236	Relatively small
World War II	1940–1945	56–61	66–71	280	Relatively large
Baby Boom	1946–1965	36–55	46–65	426	Very large
Baby Bust	1966–1979	22–35	32–45	362	Relatively small
Children of Baby Boomers	1980–1995	6–21	16–31	382	Relatively large
Children of Baby Bust	1996 on	0–5	10–15	344	Relatively small

Adapted from Statistics Canada. (2001). *2001 Census: Shifts in the population size of various age groups.* Ottawa, ON: Author.

continuation of current trends. The shifts in population size within various age groups will have far-reaching social, economic, and policy impact.

The Baby Boomers will have the most profound impact on the nation's demographics in the next 25 years, primarily because of their large numbers. By 2026, one of every five individuals will be a senior citizen. By 2016, at the latest, Canada will have far more senior citizens than children aged 14 and under, a phenomenon never before recorded (The Health Communication Unit, 2005). Over the coming years, especially as the first Baby Boomers arrive at age 65, is it possible that a new definition of "senior" will replace the current one? What will be the Baby Boomers' health status? Will the issue of sexuality become even more visible for this group? Will more hospitals and personal care homes have to be built, or will the Baby Boomers live in their own communities longer? If they do, what impact will that have for nurse leaders as they collaborate with other health care professionals?

> *reflective* **THINKING**   What do you think will be the impact of an aging population on the collaborative initiatives of nursing leaders with other health professionals in years 2010, 2015, and 2020?

In the population health approach, the assessments of health status and health inequities of the population are critical. In general there are two types of indicators: health status indicators and determinants of health (Braveman, 2003). Each indicator is explained briefly.

Health Status Indicators

The population health approach acknowledges that any analysis of the health of a population must stretch beyond the traditional indicators such as morbidity and mortality. A population health approach establishes indicators related to quality of life, income, satisfaction, mental and social well-being, employment and working conditions, education, and other factors known to influence health (PCAH, 2002d). Health indicators are standardized measures by which health status, health system performance, and characteristics among various jurisdictions in Canada are compared (Canadian Institute for Health Information [CIHI], 2006a).

In 1999, CIHI and Statistics Canada launched a collaborative project on health indicators (CIHI, 2005). The project's goal was to identify indicators that could be used to report on the health of Canadians as well as on the health system and to compile and make this information widely accessible. To improve access to the indicator data, the *Health Indicators e-publication* was created, which is accessible from both the CIHI and Statistics Canada Websites (CIHI, 2005). Updated biannually, this internet publication holds the entirety of regional indicator data developed by the indicator project.

The Canadian Population Health Initiative (CPHI), part of the CIHI group, was created to expand the public's knowledge of population health. CPHI released its Action Plan 2007–2010 (CIHI, 2006b), which focuses on four theme areas (Fig. 3.4).

The focus themes are adopted based on consultation with stakeholders and on criteria used in the past for theme identification. The CPHI works to advance population health by focusing on four complementary functions:

1. Knowledge generation and synthesis: increasing a more comprehensive understanding of the factors affecting health
2. Policy synthesis: contributing to policy development to improve the health and well-being of Canadians

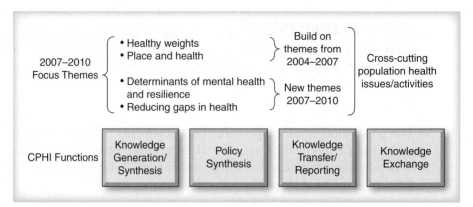

FIGURE 3.4   CPHI key themes for population health for 2007–2010. (From Canadian Institute for Health Information. [2006b]. *The Canadian population health initiative action plan 2007–2010.* Ottawa, ON: Author.)

3. Knowledge transfer and reporting: contributing objective and credible information on population health issues
4. Knowledge exchange: developing collaborative strategies and networks to centre on understanding the determinants of health (CIHI, 2006)

reflective **THINKING**   As a nurse leader, what interventions can you develop to help combat overweight and obesity in your community?

As CPHI moves forward, it will continue to work with leaders in the health sector and beyond to increase understanding of factors affecting the population, with the aim of helping Canadians to stay healthy and live longer. It is crucial that nurse leaders understand the role and functions of CPHI as a key source of valuable data and evidence-based information in the population health field (Bayne & Lewis, 2006).

Socioeconomic, Environmental, and Behavioural Determinants of Health
The assessment of various determinants and their interactive effects are necessary in a population. *Determinants of health* is a collective label applied to the set of multiple complex factors and conditions that continually interact among social and economic factors, the physical environment, and individual behaviour and that influence the health of a population, either as a whole or as a specific subgroup (PHAC, 2003). Table 3.2 outlines the 12 determinants, with explanations provided for each determinant. The relevant social determinants are included as well (PHAC, 2004). Social determinants are the socioeconomic factors that influence the health of individuals, families, communities, and larger jurisdictions as a whole.

TABLE 3.2 | KEY DETERMINANTS OF HEALTH

Key Determinants	Underlying Premises
1. Income and Social Status	Health status improves with each step up the income and social hierarchy. *Key Point:* Income determines living conditions, such as safe housing and the ability to buy sufficient good food.
2. Social Support Networks	Support from families, friends, and communities is associated with better health. *Key Point:* The support of family and friends provides caring relationships. The *result* promotes effective responses to stress, and *it* buffers against health problems
3. Education	Health status improves with the level of education attained. *Key Point:* Education increases opportunities for income and job security and equips people with a sense of control over life circumstances, thereby affecting health.
4. Employment/Working Conditions	Unemployment, underemployment, and stressful work are associated with poorer health. *Key Point:* People tend to be healthier if they have some control over their work circumstances and if the work does not include excessive stress-related demands.
5. Social Environments	The array of values and norms of a society influence in varying ways the health and well-being of individuals and populations. *Key Point:* Social stability, recognition of diversity, safety, good working relationships, and cohesive communities reduce or avoid many potential risks to good health.
6. Physical Environments	Physical factors in the environment, both natural (e.g., air and water quality) and human-built (e.g., housing, community design, roads) are key influences on health. *Key Point:* Environments with adequate housing, clean air, pure water, and safe communities and workplaces promote health and reduce illness.
7. Personal Health Practices and Coping Skills	Certain social environments are key influences that enable and support healthy choices and lifestyles. They include the support of people's knowledge, intentions, behaviours, and coping skills for dealing with life in healthy ways. *Key Point:* There is a growing recognition that personal life choices are greatly influenced by socioeconomic environments in which people live, learn, work, and play.

(table continues on page 68)

TABLE 3.2	KEY DETERMINANTS OF HEALTH (continued)
Key Determinants	**Underlying Premises**
8. Healthy Child Development	The effect of prenatal and early childhood experiences on subsequent health, well-being, coping skills, and competence is very powerful. *Key Point:* Children born in low-income families are more likely than those born to high-income families to have low birth weights, to eat less nutritious food, and to have more difficulty in school.
9. Biology and Genetic Endowment	Basic biology and organic make-up of the human body are fundamental determinants of health. *Key Point:* Genetic endowment influences a wide range of individual responses that affect health status, that is, genetic endowment appears to predispose certain individuals to particular diseases or health problems.
10. Health Services	Certain health services contribute heavily to population health, particularly those designed to maintain and promote health, prevent disease, restore health and function. *Key Point:* The health services continuum of care includes treatment and secondary prevention.
11. Gender	Gender refers to the array of society-determined roles that society ascribes to the two sexes on a differential basis. They include personality traits, attitudes, behaviours, values, and relative power and influence. *Key Point:* "Gendered" norms influence the health system's practices and priorities. For example, women more than men are vulnerable to sexual or physical violence, low income, and lone parenthood, whereas men are more likely than women to die prematurely, largely as a result of heart disease, fatal unintentional injuries, cancer, and suicide.
12. Culture	Some persons or groups face additional health risks related to a particular socioeconomic environment. *Key Point:* Environmental influences are determined largely by dominant cultural values that contribute to the perpetuation of conditions such as marginalization, stigmatization, loss, or devaluation of language and culture.

Adapted from Health Council of Canada (2007). *Health care renewal in Canada: Measuring up?* 2007 Annual Report. Toronto: Author. Used with permission.

In November 2002, a conference was held in Toronto, where more than 400 Canadian social and health policy experts, community representatives, and health researchers came together to address matters dealing with social determinants. The conference was held in response to the increasing evidence that growing social and economic inequalities among Canadians had been and continued to be contributing to higher health costs and other social burdens. As a result of the conference, the Toronto Charter on the Social Determinants of Health was developed. The Charter recommended that the federal and provincial/territorial governments allocate $1.5 billion toward two critical determinants of health for children and families: (1) affordable, safe housing, and (2) a universal system of effective quality educational child care. The Charter is, and will continue to be, a tool for promoting health and social justice (Raphael, Bryant, & Curry-Stevens, 2004).

> reflective **THINKING** In what ways can you as a nurse leader promote affordable housing in your community?

Glouberman and Millar (2003) claim that several Canadian health commissions, such as the Fyke Commission on Medicare, Clair Commission in Quebec, and Romanow Commission on the Future of Health Care in Canada, emphasized the importance of focusing on the determinants of health. The commissions also addressed the incorporation of population health concepts and approaches into the health system so as to improve the health of individuals and communities and to decrease inequities.

> reflective **THINKING** As a nurse leader, which social determinants come to mind that you can address to improve the health of individuals and communities?

In Canada today, the social determinants are of key importance to understanding patterns of health and illness. Raphael (2004) claims:

"Social determinants of health are the economic and social conditions that influence the health of individuals, communities, and jurisdictions as a whole. Social determinants of health determine whether individuals stay healthy or become ill (a narrow definition of health). Social determinants of health also determine the extent to which a person possesses the physical, social, and personal resources to identify and achieve personal aspirations, satisfy needs, and cope with the environment (a broader definition of health). Social determinants of health are about the quantity and quality of a variety of resources that a society makes available to its members." (p. 1)

According to Raphael (2004), many studies indicate that various social determinants of health have far greater influence upon health and the incidence of disease than do the traditional behavioural and biomedical risk factors. For example, McCormack & MacIntosh (2001) explored health experiences of 11 homeless persons in shelters in three New Brunswick cities; they placed particular emphasis on the strategies the people used to attain, maintain, or regain their health. The implications of the study revealed that a fragmented system of help actually hampers access to the services intended to promote health in this population.

Another study by Samuels-Dennis (2006) was conducted to extend the understanding of employment status as a social determinant of psychological distress among single mothers. The results suggest that women's employment status significantly impacts on their psychological well-being. The findings imply that public health nurses are ideally positioned to influence the improvement of public health policies designed to decrease chronic and daily stressors that may exacerbate psychological distress among single mothers. Strong evidence is available to indicate that these factors, which are outside the health care system, strongly affect the quality of health.

The Canadian Nurses Association (CNA, 2005) claims that evidence supports the contention that the socioeconomic circumstances of individuals and groups have a marked influence on health status. This issue is especially important for nurse leaders and all nurses who work on the front lines of the health care system. Everyday, nurses see the impact of the social determinants of health. Nurses can play a most important role in addressing the social determinants of health (CNA, 2005). Box 3.1 outlines specific interventions that nurses can use to advocate for healthy public policies, help reorient the health care system, and work diligently in their individual nursing practices in various settings.

The issue of the social determinants of health is by far the most complex and challenging of all health-related issues (Wilkinson & Marmot, 2003). To that end, nurse leaders and other health care professionals need to make social determinants a priority when addressing matters related to improving the health status of Canadians (CNA, 2005).

Leadership Issue

You are a home care coordinator for a rural community. Today, you are to visit an immigrant family that resides in your area. The family has three school-aged children, one boy and twin girls. The wife's mother, who is ill and frail, lives with the family. The husband works as a mechanic part-time and drives a school bus to supplement his income. He reports feeling stressed and has begun to drink alcohol heavily. The family appears isolated. They have only a few social connections from their church. Their water supply comes from a well. Identify the social determinants that are affecting their health. What strategies will you implement to address these social determinants?

BOX 3.1 SOCIAL DETERMINANTS AND NURSING ACTIVITIES

Nurses can play an important role in addressing social determinants of health by working on their individual practices, helping to reorient the health care system, and advocating for healthy public policies. Possible strategies include the following:

Individual Nursing Practice

- Understand the impact of social determinants on the health of your patients.
- In your assessments of patients, include questions on social determinants—for example, income, housing, food security, and social support.
- Consider social determinants in your treatment and follow-up plans. For example, determine whether patients are financially able to access recommended programs, such as physiotherapy. If not, help the patient to access financial assistance for such programs to make these programs accessible.
- If you work with disadvantaged communities, help people with common health issues to understand the link to social determinants and to organize to take action.
- Know what community and health resources are available to your clients.

Reorienting the Health Care System

- Ensure that health promotion programs go beyond lifestyle and behaviour to take social determinants into account. For example, physical activity programs should be designed so that fees and transportation are not barriers to participation. When access to nutritious food is an issue, refer people to programs such as community gardens and collective kitchens.
- Encourage health departments to take a social determinants approach, including considering the impact of economic inequalities and poverty.
- Advocate for universal access to basic health programs, such as dental care and Pharmacare.

Healthy Public Policies

- Speak from experience. Use stories from your patients to help advocate for policies that address social determinants of health.
- Make decision makers aware of the research on the links between socioeconomic factors and health.
- Look at how structural issues of class, race, and gender affect the way in which populations experience health problems and develop initiatives that address these issues. For example, Aboriginal people are at very high risk for diabetes, yet this is being treated largely as an individual lifestyle issue. Research shows that issues such as poverty, housing, employment, and food security in this population need to be addressed before real progress in dealing with this and other health and social issues can be made.

From Canadian Nurses Association. (2005). *CNA Backgrounder: Social Determinants of Health and Nursing – A Summary of the Issues.* Ottawa, ON: Author.

Planning and Implementation

A population health approach reflects a profound shift in conceptualizing how health is defined and achieved. Population health recognizes that health is a capacity or resource wherein the range of social, economic, and physical environmental factors contribute to health (PHAC, 2002e). Since its inception, population health has acquired new implications for energetic action on measures to improve the health status of a population (Jamieson & Simces, 2001).

Health Promotion Strategies

One way to act on population health is by health promotion. Health promotion is a dynamic process that facilitates, through various services and activities, the engagement of all individuals and groups in various social contexts. Maben & Macleod Clark (1995) argue that "other related concepts of empowerment, equity, collaboration, and participation are the means or methods of achieving health promotion" (p. 1162).

Health promotion strategies focus on reducing differences in current health status and on ensuring fair and equal opportunities and resources to enable people to achieve their fullest health potential. In essence, health promotion goes beyond healthy lifestyles; it achieves well-being (PHAC, 2002f).

Nursing Role: Collaboration

According to Young (2002), health promotion is a highly complex professional practice carried out and practiced by those who value health as being critical. Those professionals include nurses, physicians, nutritionists, and physiotherapists among others. Building alliances with health professionals and other health determining sectors, such as housing, recreation, finance, employment, and social services, is a primary strategy for nurse leaders in improving the health of a population (PHAC, 2002g).

In addition, a population health approach calls for shared responsibility and accountability with health groups and with those who are not normally associated with health. To have meaningful input into the development of health priorities, strategies, and outcomes, the participation of Canadians is crucial at national and international levels. One of the benefits is that those Canadians who are most affected by a health issue can contribute to possible solutions early in the planning process (PHAC, 2002h).

Political Advocacy and Social Support

Nurse leaders are well positioned to act as political advocates for clients and families affected by surmountable health issues. Whitehead (2003) states, "Collectively, nursing is a potentially powerful force that can act for those who are dispossessed of organizational power" (p. 670). He developed an effect model for health promotion that demonstrates activities consistent with sociopolitical approaches to health promotion activities. For example, nurse leaders need to be both politically aware and active to claim the broad role available to them in the health promotion field. By doing so, they can better ensure that their health-related programs are successful. Nurse leaders must also promote collaboration with key health care disciplines and with other agencies to improve the health and well-being of individuals and community (Whitehead, 2003).

Buijs, Ross-Kerr, O'Brien Cousins, & Wilson (2003) conducted a qualitative evaluation of active living in vulnerable elders (Seniors ALIVE), a 10-month health promotion program for low-income senior citizens. One of their findings was that social contact with other program participants and staff contributed to social support, which is one of the determinants of health.

Social support also plays a significant role in developing and maintaining active living. Another relevant finding was that not only strong, but also meaningful, relationships developed between staff and participants. These relationships were enhanced by the readiness and ability of staff to be attentive and listen to the program participants, to encourage autonomy, and to adapt program delivery. It is essential to realize that the Seniors ALIVE program was developed, implemented, and evaluated by an interdisciplinary team of health professionals, with leadership contributions by nurses. Nurses should be encouraged to seek opportunities for interdisciplinary collaboration, because these opportunities provide a rich potential for nurses to be beneficial not only to their profession and their colleagues but also to the larger community (Buijs et al., 2003).

---

reflective **THINKING** Identify a health problem in your community that is of particular interest to you. In what ways can a nurse leader, working within an interdisciplinary team, be politically active to bring about a health-related program as a solution to this issue?

Capacity Building

Labonte and Laverack (2001) claim that for several years, capacity building has been a topic discussed at length in the health promotion literature. It has been argued that capacity building represents a redirection of health promotion activities from population groups to organizations, or to the health system responsible for health promotion, to enhance the ability to initiate, implement, or sustain health promotion programs and, ultimately, to bring about health changes (Hawe, Noort, King, & Jordens, 1997). Furthermore, capacity building promotes problem-solving skills that render people, organizations, and communities more competent to address health and other development issues (Crisp, Swerissen, & Duckett, 2000).

In their article, Joffres et al. (2004) present (1) an operational definition of capacity building for heart-health promotion, (2) three instruments developed to measure organizational capacity for heart-health promotion, and (3) baseline results of capacity for 20 organizations. Joffres et al. (2004) found that the instruments were effective and the data obtained stimulated valuable reflection on the development of a comprehensive framework for heart-health promotion. The writers claim that Alberta and Saskatchewan have adapted the Ontario and Nova Scotia instruments to guide their capacity efforts for heart-health promotion.

The results have implications for policy and practice. For example, nurse leaders who have an interest in promoting heart health should support the development of organizational environments facilitating heart-health promotion. That is, nurse leaders should advocate for organizational policy that supports heart health as an organizational priority, provides sufficient human and financial resources for heart-health activities, and strengthens organizational practices to assess, plan, implement, and evaluate these activities and policy development as well as advocacy (Joffres et al., 2004).

Ebbesen, Heath, Naylor, and Anderson (2004) also wrote an article addressing the collective experiences and insights of four provincial Canadian Heart Health Initiative Projects. They identify issues encountered in measuring capacity, and they provide an insightful discussion on how to address such issues. The importance of understanding and addressing issues in measuring capacity should not be underrated, mainly because these issues may reveal important influences between research and intervention in multiplying health gains significantly.

Raphael (2000) states, "Health promotion is proving to be effective in improving the health of the population" (p. 365). This is mainly because effective health promotion practice is based on principles and values consistent with ethical practice. Box 3.2 outlines the guidelines for making decisions and using evidence in health promotion. These guidelines are most suitable for a nurse leader to use in the field of health promotion mainly because of their effective value-based approach.

---

reflective **THINKING** After reviewing the guidelines for making decisions and using evidence in health promotion, outline a situation in which you as a nurse leader can implement one or more of these guidelines for meaningful input into the development of health priorities, strategies, and outcomes.

Applications for Population Health and Health Promotion

To explain the relationship between population health and health promotion, a three-dimensional population health promotion model was developed by Health

---

BOX 3.2 GUIDELINES FOR MAKING DECISIONS AND USING EVIDENCE IN HEALTH PROMOTION

1. Be as explicit as possible regarding the principles and values that you bring to your health promotion activities.
2. Recognize the tensions and interactions between structural and individual determinants of health and between values and facts.
3. Whenever possible, use multiple sources of evidence.
4. Use truth criteria associated with each form of knowledge.
5. Show awareness of the decisions you make concerning evidence: be a reflexive practitioner.

Reprinted with permission from Raphael, D. (2000). The question of evidence in health promotion. *Health Promotion International, 15*(4), 355–367.

Canada (Hamilton & Bhatti, 1996) called Population Health Promotion: An Integrated Model of Population Health and Health Promotion (PHAC, 2002i). Figure 3.5 outlines the model. To apply this model, it is helpful to visualize it as comprising many interior cubes, each providing a potential blueprint for action with different entry points (PHAC 2002j).

One can begin with the population health determinants that one intends to influence, the health promotion strategies that can be used, and the various levels at which action is to be taken (Cohen, 2006). The model can be used either to focus on health issues of a particular priority group that is at risk for poor health or to address emerging health issues (PHAC, 2002j). Evidence-based decisions are needed to ensure that policies and programs address the correct issues, take effective action, and produce sound outcomes (PHAC, 2002j). (Note: Values and assumptions—the foundation of the model—are especially important and can be examined in depth in the reference cited [PHAC, 2002j].)

Nurse leaders who comprehend the population health promotion model are able to direct health promotion strategies toward individuals, families, communities, and society as a whole (Reutter, 2006). For example, on a community level, nurses can support prenatal programs and programs to prevent or treat sexually transmitted infections. Nurses can use active political tools to address governmental sectors responsible for housing and marginalized groups. Nurses can use these tools to implement healthy public housing and income security policies and advocate for job creation as well (Spenceley, Reutter, & Allen, 2006).

reflective **THINKING** As a nurse leader, what politically active steps could you take to design and implement a harm-reduction program in your community?

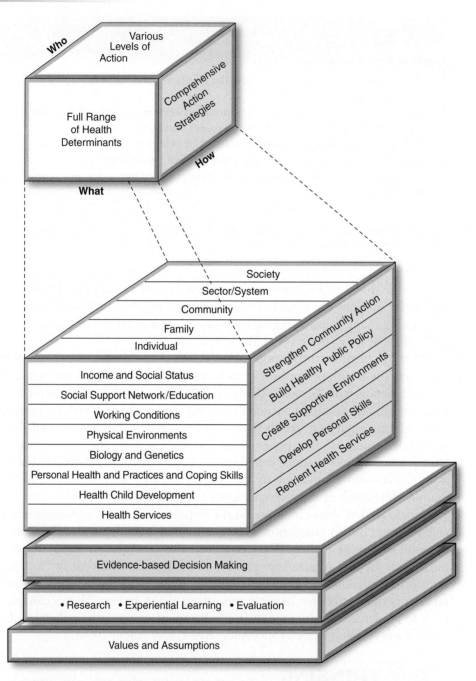

FIGURE 3.5   Population Health Promotion Model. (Adapted from Public Health Agency of Canada. [2002c]. *Population Health Approach—What Determines Health?* Ottawa, ON: Author. Adapted and reproduced with the permission of the Minister of Public Works and Government Services, Canada, 2007.)

The Integrated Pan-Canadian Healthy Living Strategy The Integrated Pan-Canadian Healthy Living Strategy, approved by the Federal, Provincial, and Territorial Ministers of Health, was released in October 2005 (Health Council of Canada, 2007). The strategy, a conceptual framework based on a population health approach, focuses on root causes of poor health outcomes. This approach addresses the working and living environments that affect individuals' health, the conditions that enable and support people in making healthy choices, and the services that promote and maintain health (Intersectorial Healthy Living Network, 2005). The overall goals of the strategy are to:

- Improve overall health outcomes; for example, a population approach to reduce chronic disease offers potentially to significantly improve the health of many people and decrease costs to the system.
- Reduce health disparities (differences in health status that occur among population groups defined by specific characteristics). According to the Intersectorial Healthy Living Network (2005), the most prominent disparities relate to socioeconomic status, Aboriginal identity, gender, disability, culture, and geographic location.

Given the trends in current eating and physical activity patterns, which consequently increase the rates of overweight and obesity, the targets of the Healthy Living Strategy are as follows:

- Healthful eating
- Physical activity
- Healthy body weights (Intersectorial Healthy Living Strategy, 2005)

The Healthy Living Strategy is an integrated approach that involves many sectors working together toward common goals and targets. The strategy describes a way to ensure greater alignment, coordination, and direction for all sectors. In addition, the strategy provides a forum for multiple players to harmonize their efforts and collaborate on ameliorating common risk factors (PHAC, 2005).

Nurse Leader's Role in the Healthy Living Strategy Nurse leaders have countless opportunities to work with other sectors toward the common goals. The success of the Healthy Living Strategy requires that all sectors work together to effect change. For example, the campaign "Drop the Pop" in Nunavut has been a challenge for all sectors (Priest, 2006). Priest states that the campaign encourages students from kindergarten through grade 12 to reduce their consumption of soft drinks. The consumption of soft drinks has had an increasing toll—not only on nutrition and dental health, but also on the cost of health care. As a result of people working together, the campaign is ongoing and reaching out to other areas, such as the Northwest Territories and the Yukon (Priest, 2006).

A group of national nursing leaders was invited to participate in a tour sponsored by the Government of Nunavut's Health and Social Service Department—the first tour of its kind by health professionals. One goal of the tour was for those nursing leaders to explore innovative partnerships that would increase Nunavut's health delivery system. It was found that nursing leaders not only face challenges, but they find ways to overcome those challenges and empower others to do the same (McCarthy, 2006).

> reflective **THINKING**   How can you, as a nurse leader, engage people in an anti-smoking campaign?

Ecological Approach to Health Promotion

Richard et al. (2002) claim that the ecological approach offers an action-and-research framework that emphasizes the complex transactions among individuals, groups, and their environments. Many other authors have contributed to the development and implementation of the concepts underlying the ecological approach in health promotion programs and public health.

Health promotion practiced from an ecological perspective is directed toward developing strategies that target interpersonal, community, organizational, and public policy factors that influence health (Green & Kreuter, 1999). Richard et al. state, "The ecological approach has now gained acceptance and recognition by health promotion researchers and practitioners" (p. 275). Whitehead (2006) adds that a notable shift is occurring in the health promotion literature and specifies that the emphasis is now on the "mainstream" sociopolitical nature of health promotion and on the determinants of health, such as ecological, fiscal, and cultural factors. Maben and Macleod Clark (1995) observe that in addition to information giving, life-skills teaching, and self-empowerment, health promotion means engaging in social and environmental change.

Nurse leaders are called upon to view health promotion as an approach that embraces a set of values including equity, empowerment, participation, and collaboration to improve the health of Canadians (MacDonald, 2002). As leaders, nurses are urged to find ways to equip practitioners with the essential skills and resources for effective practice and ongoing health promotion (Whitehead, 2006).

> reflective **THINKING**   What steps can you as a nurse leader take to incorporate the ecological approach into your nursing practice?

Evaluation

Efforts to improve population health have employed various practical models and tools to evaluate the outcomes of the health of Canadians. Nurse leaders are challenged to evaluate critically the evidence-based strategies applied to individuals, groups, communities, and society at large. Community surveys may be one research method to evaluate how the community views an implemented health promotion program. The important question is what is the health status of that particular population? (Reed, Burdine, & Felix, 2003). For example, nursing staff at community health centres may be interviewed to ascertain the health status of pregnant women from different cultural backgrounds and varying socioeconomic status. Results of the interview may indicate that resources need to be taken into consideration and may have to be redistributed to enhance the well-being of community residents. Canadian attitudes toward health are changing, and the move toward their participation in decision making has become the norm. Nurse leaders must continue to appreciate the role of social factors as a critical determinant in health.

WEBSITES

▓ Social Determinants of Health

www.atkinson.yorku.ca/draphael
Dr. Dennis Raphael is Canada's most influential researcher and advocate for the social determinants of health. There are literally dozens of journal articles and PowerPoint presentations by Raphael in the library on his Website.

▓ Population Health

http://www.phac-aspc.gc.ca/
Located on the Public Health Agency of Canada Website, this link provides an overview on the key determinants of health. It includes links to an annotated bibliography on the social determinants of health and various government agencies.

▓ Canadian Institute for Health Information (CIHI)

http://www.cihi.ca/
CIHI provides high-quality, reliable, and timely health information and is a focal point for collaboration among major health players. It has published many useful resources on the determinants of health, such as "Improving the Health of Canadians," which focuses on income, early childhood development, Aboriginal people's health, and obesity. This report, and others, can be found on their Website.

▓ Public Health Agency of Canada

www.phac-aspc.gc.ca/
PHAC describes key elements of the Population Health Template on the home page.

REFERENCES

Bayne, L., & Lewis, S. (2006). *Retrospect and prospect: Assessment of CPHI's impact in recent years (2004–2007) and possible directions for the future (2007–2010)*. Ottawa, ON: Canadian Population Health Initiative and Canadian Institute for Health Information.

Braveman, P. A. (2003). Monitoring equity in health and healthcare: A conceptual framework. *Journal of Health, Population, and Nutrition, 21*(3), 181–192.

Buijs, R., Ross-Kerr, J., O'Brien Cousins, S., & Wilson, D. (2003). Promoting participation: Evaluation of a health promotion program for low income seniors. *Journal of Community Health Nursing, 20*(2), 93–107.

Canadian Institute for Health Information. (2005). *The health indicators project: The next 5 years*. Ottawa, ON: Author.

Canadian Institute for Health Information. (2006a). *Research & Reports: Health Indicators*. Ottawa, ON: Author. Retrieved May 2007 from http://secure.cihi.ca/

Canadian Institute for Health Information. (2006b). *The Canadian population health initiative action plan 2007–2010*. Ottawa, ON: Author.

Canadian Nurses Association. (2005). CNA Backgrounder. Social Determinants of Health and Nursing: A Summary of the Issues. Ottawa, ON: Author.

Coburn, D., Denny, K., Mykhalovskiy, E., McDonough, P., Robertson, A., & Love, R. (2003). Population health. *American Journal of Public Health, 93*(3), 392–396.

Cohen, B. E. (2006). Population health as a framework for public health practice: A Canadian perspective. *American Journal of Public Health, 96*(9), 1574–1576.

Crisp, B. R., Swerissen, H., & Duckett, S. J. (2000). Four approaches to capacity building in health: Consequences for measurement and accountability. *Health Promotion International, 15,* 99–107.

Ebbesen, L. S., Heath, S., Naylor, P.-J., & Anderson, D. (2004). Issues in measuring health promotion capacity in Canada: A multi-province perspective. *Health Promotion International, 19*(1), 85–94.

Edwards, N. (1999). Population health: Determinants and interventions. *Canadian Journal of Public Health, 90*(1), 10–11.

Epp, J. (1986). Achieving health for all: A framework for health promotion. *Health Promotion International, 1*(4), 419–428.

Glouberman, S., & Millar, J. (2003). Evolution of the determinants of health, health policy, and health information systems in Canada. *American Journal of Public Health, 93*(3), 388–392.

Government of Canada. (2000). *Early childhood development agreement.* Ottawa, ON: Author. Retrieved May 2007 from http://www.socialunion.ca/ecd_e.html

Green, L. W., & Kreuter, M. W. (1999). *Health promotion planning: An educational and environmental approach* (3rd ed.). Mountain View, CA: Mayfield.

Hawe, P., Noort, M., King, L., & Jordens, C. (1997). Multiplying health gains: Health workers talk about capacity-building within health promotion. *Health Policy, 39,* 29–42.

Health Canada. (1998). *Taking action on population health: A position paper for health promotion and programs branch staff.* Ottawa, ON: Author.

Health Council of Canada. (2007). *Health care renewal in Canada: Measuring up?* Toronto, ON: Author.

Intersectoral Healthy Living Network. (2005). *The integrated pan-Canadian healthy living strategy.* Ottawa, ON: Author.

Jamieson, K., & Simces, Z. (2001). *Creative spice: Learning from communities about putting the population health approach into action.* Health Canada, Population and Public Health Branch, BC/Yukon. Vancouver, BC: Social Planning and Research Council of BC.

Joffres, C., Heath, S., Farquharson, J., Barkhouse, K., Hood, R., Latter, C., et al. (2004). Defining and operationalizing capacity for heart health promotion in Nova Scotia, Canada. *Health Promotion International, 19*(1), 39–49.

Kindig, D., & Stoddart, G. (2003). What is population health? *American Journal of Public Health, 93*(3), 380–383.

Kushner, K. E. (2003). Issues in community nursing practice. In J. Ross-Kerr, & M. J. Wood (Eds.), *Canadian nursing: Issues and perspectives* (4th ed., pp. 310–325). Toronto, ON: Elsevier Science Canada.

Labonte, R. (2005). Editorial: Towards a critical population health research. *Critical Public Health, 15*(1), 1–3.

Labonte, R., & Laverack, G. (2001). Capacity building in health promotion, Part 1: for whom? And for what purpose? *Critical Public Health, 11*(2), 111–127.

Labonte, R., Polanyi, M., Muhajarine, N., McIntosh, T., & Williams, A. (2005). Beyond the divides: Towards critical population health research. *Critical Public Health, 15*(1), 5–17.

Lalonde, M. (1974). *A New Perspective on the Health of Canadians.* Ottawa, ON: Information Canada.

Legowski, B., & McKay, L. (2000). *Health beyond health care: Twenty-five years of federal health policy development.* CPRN Discussion Paper. Ottawa, ON: Health Network, Canadian Policy Research Networks, Inc.

Lightfoot, P., Edwards, J., Fraser-Lee, N., Kaida, A., & Predy, G. (2006). A population health approach to planning. In J. M. Hibberd, & D. L. Smith (Eds.), *Nursing leadership and management in Canada* (3rd ed., pp. 43–66). Toronto, ON: Elsevier Mosby.

Maben, J., & Macleod Clark, J. (1995). Health promotion: A concept analysis. *Journal of Advanced Nursing, 22*, 1158–1165.

MacDonald, M. A. (2002). Health promotion: Historical, philosophical, and theoretical perspectives. In L. E. Young, & V. E. Hayes (Eds.), *Transforming health promotion practice: Concepts, issues, and applications* (pp. 22–45). Philadelphia: F. A. Davis.

McCarthy, K. (2006). Understanding the challenges, witnessing primary health care in action. *Canadian Nurse, 102*(4), 9–11.

McCormack, D., & MacIntosh, J. (2001). Research with homeless people uncovers a model of health. *Western Journal of Nursing Research, 23*(7), 679–697.

Priest, A. (2006). Nunavut's drop the pop campaign. *Canadian Nurse, 102*(4), 12–13.

Public Health Agency of Canada. (2002a). *Population health approach – Ottawa charter for health promotion: An international conference on health promotion.* Ottawa, ON: Author. Retrieved May 2007 from http://www.phac-aspc.gc.ca/

Public Health Agency of Canada. (2002b). *Population health: What is the population health approach? Population health template working tool.* Ottawa, ON: Author. Retrieved May 2007 from http://www.phac-aspc.gc.ca/

Public Health Agency of Canada. (2002c). *Population health: Towards a common understanding: Clarifying the core concepts of population health: Executive summary.* Ottawa, ON: Author. Retrieved May 2007 from http://www.phac-aspc.gc.ca/

Public Health Agency of Canada. (2002d). *Population health approach: What determines health? Health status indicators.* Ottawa, ON: Author. Retrieved May 2007 from http://www.phac-aspc.gc.ca/

Public Health Agency of Canada. (2002e). *Population health approach: Population health – What is population health?* Ottawa, ON: Author. Retrieved May 2007 from http://www.phac-aspc.gc.ca/

Public Health Agency of Canada. (2002f). *Population health approach: Implementing the population health approach.* Ottawa, ON: Author. Retrieved May 2007 from http://www.phac-aspc.gc.ca/

Public Health Agency of Canada. (2002g). *Population health approach: Health services and population health.* Ottawa, ON: Author. Retrieved May 2007 from http://www.phac-aspc.gc.ca/

Public Health Agency of Canada. (2002h). *Population health approach: Health is everyone's business.* Ottawa, ON: Author. Retrieved May 2007 from http://www.phac-aspc.gc.ca/

Public Health Agency of Canada. (2002i). *Population health approach: Population health promotion: An integrated model of population health and health promotion.* Ottawa, ON: Author. Retrieved May 2007 from http://www.phac-aspc.gc.ca/

Public Health Agency of Canada. (2002j). *Population health approach: Population health promotion: An integrated model of population health and health promotion: Developing a population health promotion model.* Ottawa, ON: Author. Retrieved May 2007 from http://www.phac-aspc.gc.ca/

Public Health Agency of Canada. (2003). *Population Health: What determines health?* Ottawa, ON: Author. Retrieved May 2007 from http://www.phac-aspc.gc.ca/

Public Health Agency of Canada. (2004). *Population health approach: What determines health? Determinants.* Ottawa, ON: Author. Retrieved May 2007 from http://www.phac-aspc.gc.ca/

Public Health Agency of Canada. (2005). *Health promotion: Healthy living strategy.* Ottawa, ON: Author.

Raphael, D. (2000). The question of evidence in health promotion. *Health Promotion International, 15*(4), 355–367.

Raphael, D. (2004). Introduction to the social determinants of health. In D. Raphael (Ed.), *Social determinants of health: Canadian perspectives* (pp. 1–18). Toronto, ON: Canadian Scholars' Press Inc.

Raphael, D., & Bryant, T. (2000). Putting the population into population health. *Canadian Journal of Public Health, 91*(1), 9–10.

Raphael, D., & Bryant, T. (2002). The limitations of population health as a model for a new public health. *Health Promotion International, 17*(2), 189–199.

Raphael, D., Bryant, T., & Curry-Stevens, A. (2004). Toronto charter outlines future health policy directions for Canada and elsewhere. *Health Promotion International, 19*(2), 269–273.

Reed, J. F., III, Burdine, J. N., & Felix, M. (2003). Aggregate health status: A benchmark index for community health. *Journal of Medical Systems, 27*(2), 177–189.

Reutter, L. (2006). Health and wellness. In P. A. Potter, A. Griffin Perry, J. C. Ross-Kerr, & M. J. Wood (Eds.), *Canadian fundamentals of nursing* (3rd ed., pp. 1–17). Toronto, ON: Elsevier Mosby.

Richard, L., Gauvin, L., Potvin, L., Denis, J.-L., & Kischuk, N. (2002). Making youth tobacco control programs more ecological: Organizational and professional profiles. *American Journal of Health Promotion, 16*(5), 267–279.

Samuels-Dennis, J. (2006). Relationship among employment status, stressful life events, and depression in single mothers. *Canadian Journal of Nursing Research, 38*(1), 58–80.

Spenceley, S., Reutter, L., & Allen, M. N. (2006). The road less traveled: Nursing advocacy at the policy level. *Policy, Politics, & Nursing Practice, 7*(3), 180–194.

Statistics Canada. (2001). *2001 census: Shifts in population size of various age groups.* Ottawa, ON: Author. Retrieved May 2007 from http://www12.statcan.ca/english/census01/products/analytic/companion/age/population.cfm

Statistics Canada. (2007). *Portrait of the Canadian population in 2006, 2006 Census: Population and dwelling counts.* Cat. no. 97-550-XIE. Ottawa, ON: Author.

The Health Communication Unit. (2005). *Audience Analysis: Baby Boomers 2005.* University of Toronto, ON: Author. Retrieved May 2007 from www.thcu.ca/infoandresources/publications/Boomers.Audience.Analysis.v1.2.04.25.05.pdf

Vollman, A. R., Anderson, E. T., & McFarlane, J. (2004). *Canadian community as partner: Theory and practice in nursing.* Philadelphia: Lippincott Williams & Wilkins.

Whitehead, D. (2003). Incorporating socio-political health promotion activities in clinical practice. *Journal of Clinical Nursing, 12,* 668–677.

Whitehead, D. (2006). Health promotion in the practice setting: Findings from a review of clinical issues. *Worldviews on Evidence-Based Nursing, 3*(4), 165–184.

Wilkinson, R., & Marmot, M. (Eds.). (2003). *Social determinants of health: The solid facts* (2nd ed). Copenhagen, Denmark: World Health Organization.

World Health Organization. (1986). *Ottawa charter for health promotion: First international conference on health promotion.* Ottawa, ON: Author. Retrieved May 2007 from http://www.who.int/

Young, L. E. (2002). Transforming health promoting practice: Moving toward holistic care. In L. E. Young, & V. Hayes (Eds.), *Transforming health promotion practice: Concepts, issues, and applications* (pp. 3–21). Philadelphia: F. A. Davis.

DYNAMIC HEALTH CARE ORGANIZATIONS AND THE ROLE OF THE NURSE LEADER

Work empowerment is important to nurses' feelings of respect. Feeling respected on the job is associated with commitment to the job, job satisfaction, and lower stress. Most of these are basic things that don't cost a lot of money. Understanding the nature of respect in organizations can help administrators address this issue in a systematic manner.

—**Heather K. Spence Laschinger, RN, PhD**
University of Western Ontario, London, Ontario.

Adapted with permission from The University of Western Ontario Media Newsroom, The Department of Communications and Public Affairs, Top Stories, September 21, 2004

Dr. Heather Laschinger is Professor and Associate Director of Nursing Research at the University of Western Ontario, School of Nursing, Faculty of Health Sciences in London, Ontario. Since 1992, she has been principal investigator of a research program designed to investigate nursing work environments using Rosabeth Moss Kanter's organizational empowerment theory. Current directions of this research involve extending the workplace empowerment model to nursing practice behaviour and linking it to patient empowerment. In 2003, in recognition of her extraordinary excellence in nursing research, Dr. Laschinger was awarded the Sigma Theta Tau International *Elizabeth McWilliams Miller Award for Excellence in Research* and the Registered Nurses' Association of Ontario *Leadership Award in Nursing Research*. Currently, Dr. Laschinger is co-principal investigator on a Canadian study entitled *A Profile of the Structure and Impact of Nursing Management in Canadian Hospitals* that will profile nursing leadership/management structures in teaching and nonteaching hospitals across the country.

(Selected from Dr. Laschinger's home page: http://publish.uwo.ca/~hkl/. Used with permission.)

Overview

It is essential today that a nurse leader comprehends the dynamics of a health care organization. The vision and mission statements and set of values, together with a list of goals, provide the framework for the health care organization. This framework can be used for choosing, creating and developing, and evaluating services. Other essential areas of interest are the funding and delivery systems of health care services that are in place to assist clients and their families make appropriate choices of care.

Additional challenges for nurse leaders include understanding the forces that impact and transform health care delivery and facilitating staff nurse empowerment to improve their health and well-being and job satisfaction. Responding to the need for nurses to be accountable professionals is critical for promoting staff nurse leadership skills.

Objectives

By critically reflecting upon and processing knowledge throughout this chapter, you will be able to respond effectively to the following objectives:

1. Critique the definition of organization.
2. Design a health care organization that contributes to the quality of life of all individuals and their families.
3. Compare and contrast the public and private sources of health care funding.
4. Examine how influential forces impact the health care systems.
5. Create a scenario illustrating how the nurse leader copes on the unit, or in general practice, with recent technological changes.
6. Describe strategies the nurse leader can implement to retain nursing staff in a health care organization.
7. Apply your knowledge of empowerment to the nursing staff around you in your clinical area of nursing practice.
8. State how, in a community health care centre, you as a nurse leader can facilitate the empowerment of nurses.
9. Replicate a research study conducted by Laschinger, Almost, Purdy, & Kim (2004) in your work setting.
10. After reviewing the consolidated list of actions from the Canadian Nursing Leadership Study (CNLS) that could be attempted by nurse leaders, decide what strategies you would begin to implement in your work setting.
11. Critique the categories of leadership-empowering behaviours.
12. Describe a unit that has implemented shared governance as an organizational framework on its care unit.

The Modern Health Care Organization

The nurse leader needs to gain a thorough understanding of the essential components of the organization in various settings. Doing so will promote staff workplace satisfaction and effective health care delivery for clients and their families. To begin the learning process on organizations, the nurse leader needs a working definition of an organization and its organizational dimensions, such as vision and mission statements, values, and goals.

Definition and Dimensions of An Organization

In reviewing several definitions of organizations, a few common denominators seem to be critical. These denominators include the following:

- A social system
- Two or more interacting participants
- Coordination of group efforts
- A defined environment
- Common goals (Yoder-Wise, 2007; Kreitner, Kinicki, & Cole, 2007; Johns & Saks, 2008).

In an organization, such as a health care delivery system, which is continually shifting, changing, and evolving, employees must:

- Be motivated to enter and remain to be socialized in the organization.
- Carry out their practice effectively, in terms of quality and service.
- Be willing to learn and expand their knowledge and skills.
- Be flexible, innovative, and adaptable to change (Johns & Saks, 2008).

It is critical that all nurses demonstrate these behaviours within a hospital, in a home care agency, in community health care resources, or in other health care organizations. The challenge for nurse leaders is to be visible and attentive to relationship issues. The nurse leader must value diversity, respect boundaries, and encourage open communication among team members. It is important that the nurse leader builds a healthy workplace environment in the organization by supporting team activities as they productively focus on carrying out the mission statement and achieving the goals of the health care organization.

reflective **THINKING**   What does the concept of an organization mean to you? What other behaviours, activities, and intentions can a nurse leader demonstrate in an organization to encourage team collaboration?

Vision, Mission Statement, and Values

Hibberd, Doody, and Hennessey (2006) state that the *vision statement*, which is usually brief, not only reflects the values of the organization But also provides a common direction for providing health services. An organization's vision statement reflects its vision of the future (Kelly-Heidenthal, 2004). For example, the Canadian Nurses Association (CNA) vision statement is the following: "Registered Nurses: leaders and partners working to advance health for all" (CNA, 2007).

All organizations, including health care organizations or departments within an organization or community-based health centres, have a purpose and stated direction. Typically, these are expressed in the *mission statement*, which should be clear and brief. The statement communicates who the organization is, who it serves, what it values, and what activities it performs (Dressler & Starke, 2004). All team members working in a department should participate in developing the mission statement to ensure that the statement is meaningful and achievable. The completed statement should be written down and made visible to all staff to empower them to work together as they strive to meet the organization's mission (Kelly-Heidenthal, 2004).

To assist both the staff and the organization in interpreting the vision and in achieving the mission, the board of directors may affirm a *set of values*. Such values facilitate organizational decision making and other relevant activities (Hibberd, Doody, & Hennessey, 2006). Box 4.1 outlines the Vision, Mission Statement, and Values of the Hospital for Sick Children, an Ontario health care, teaching, and research hospital affiliated with the University of Toronto.

Goals

Goals should be developed by the health care organization to reflect the mission statement. A *goal* is a specific aim, or target, that the organization wishes to attain. Kreitner, Kinicki, & Cole (2007) state that "goal accomplishment is the most widely used effectiveness criterion for organizations" (p. 255). Frequently, organizational results are compared with stated goals and objectives. That is, the mission statement and goals serve as benchmarks against which an organization's performance is evaluated (Ellis & Hartley, 2004). It becomes imperative that the nurse leader know these ideals in the organization and reflect them in the management and delivery of quality health care services (Hibberd, Doody, & Hennessey, 2006).

---

reflective **THINKING**   Gather a few classmates together and write a vision and mission statement of a paediatric unit in an urban hospital. State a few goals for the unit. As an option, try the same task for your class.

BOX 4.1   HOSPITAL FOR SICK CHILDREN: VISION, MISSION, AND VALUES

Vision
Healthier children. A better world.

Mission
As innovators in child health, we will lead and partner to improve the health of children through the integration of care, education, and research.

Values
- Providing the best in complex and specialized health care for children
- Creating ground-breaking scientific and clinical advancements
- Sharing our knowledge and expertise worldwide
- Championing the development of an accessible, comprehensive, and sustainable child health care system

Innovation
. . .in creating, evaluating, and disseminating new knowledge; in developing and implementing creative approaches for family-centred care, research, and education; and in responding to the unique and changing needs of children and of the health care system.

Excellence
. . . in compassionate family-centred care and service that embraces diversity; in management and decision making; in promoting teamwork and encouraging leadership; and in a safe and healthy environment.

Collaboration
. . . in all our relationships; with families and children throughout the care process; building knowledge and capabilities across the health care system; and supporting transitions of care and service.

Integrity
. . . in our commitment to accountability and transparency; in respect for all; in effective communication; and in our ethical practices.

From The Hospital for Sick Children. (2006). *Website: Vision, Mission & Values.* Retrieved from http://www.sickkids.ca/ Used with permission.

Health Care Funding and Delivery: Role of Public and Private Sectors

When health care organizations are examined regarding funding and delivery of health services, important distinctions should be made regarding what is "public" and "private" in the health care context. Several levels exist within both the public and private sectors, as noted in Table 4.1. The public sector refers to governments and government agencies, where government may be national, provincial/territorial, or municipal. Presently, most hospitals in Canada continue to be public and not-for-profit health care organizations (Smith, Klopper, Paras, & Au, 2006).

Meanwhile, the private sector is broad and includes the corporate for-profit sector, small business and entrepreneurial entities, and charitable or voluntary not-for-profit organizations, as well as individuals and families (Madore & Tiedemann, 2005). The private for-profit organizations aim to make profits for owners and shareholders. Some surgical procedures (e.g., cataract surgery), cortisone injections, laboratory services, and some community and home care services are other examples of for-profit organizations. An example of a voluntary not-for-profit organization is the Victorian Order of Nurses (Smith, Klopper, Paras, & Au, 2006).

The public and private sectors are involved in both the funding and delivery of health care. Table 4.2 illustrates various combinations of public and private sector involvement in health care. For example, as shown in Box 4.1, public health is a responsibility of the public sector: the government funds and provides

TABLE 4.1	CATEGORIES OF PUBLIC AND PRIVATE SECTORS
Category	**Level**
Public	• National • Provincial/territorial • Regional • Local
Private	• Corporate for-profit • Small business/entrepreneurial • Charity (non-profit) with paid employees or volunteers • Family/individual

From Deber, R. B., et al. (1998). The public-private mix in health care. In *Striking a balance: Health care systems in Canada and elsewhere* (p. 433). Papers commissioned by the National Forum on Health, Vol. 4, Éditions MultiMondes, Saint-Foy, Quebec.

TABLE 4.2	PUBLIC- AND PRIVATE-SECTOR INVOLVEMENT IN HEALTH CARE		
Financing	**Delivery**		
	Public	**Private Not-for-Profit**	**Private for-Profit**
Public	• Public health • Provincial psychiatric institutions • Home care in some provinces	• Most hospitals • Addiction treatment	• Primary health care physicians • Ancillary services in hospitals (laundry services, meal preparation, and maintenance) • Laboratories and diagnostic services in most provinces • Some hospitals
Private	• Enhanced nonmedical (e.g., private room) and medical (e.g., fibreglass cast) goods and services in a publicly owned hospital	• Some home care and nursing homes in some provinces	• Cosmetic surgery • Long-term care • Extended health care benefits such as prescription drugs, dental care, and eye care in some provinces • Some magnetic resonance imaging and computed tomography scan clinics • Some surgery clinics

From Deber, R. B. (1999). *Delivering Health Care Services: Public, Not-For-Profit, or Private?* Discussion Paper No. 17. Ottawa, ON: Commission on the Future of Health Care in Canada. Used with permission of Public Works and Government Services Canada.

public health services, such as the National Immunization Strategy, which provides standardized coverage across the country, including four new vaccines (Health Council of Canada, 2007).

In contrast, as shown in Table 4.2, cosmetic surgery is an area left entirely to the private sector. In this case, the individual and/or the individual's private insurance company pays for the full cost of the surgery performed by a private for-profit provider. Other examples include free-standing private hospitals that provide surgical procedures for which the client must pay the entire cost associated with the surgery. Examples include the Cambie Surgery Centre in Vancouver and the Maple Surgical Centre in Winnipeg. The reason that clients, or their private insurance company, must pay the whole cost is that the procedures are performed by physicians who have opted out of the publicly funded system, which every

Reflections on Leadership Practice

You are a nurse manager in a neurological paediatric unit. A preschool child has been on your unit with a primary head injury caused by a motor vehicle accident. The child has regained consciousness but has difficulty concentrating and needs assistance in starting and finishing tasks. The family would like to take the child home immediately. Using your knowledge about public and private funding, what steps can you take to successfully orchestrate additional home care for this child?

province's health care insurance legislation permits (Madore & Tiedemann, 2005). As health care funding and delivery become more complex, nurse leaders must continue providing staff with a healthy work environment that is also effective and safe for clients and their families (see *Reflections on Leadership Practice*).

Influential Forces on Health Care Systems

Many factors become forces that influence the evolution of the health care delivery system. Among these factors are demographic, social, and technological forces.

Demographic Forces

As the Canadian population grows and ages, clients in hospitals and the community require more complex and specialized care. Immigration, regional access to care, and the incomes of the population are a few demographic factors that are influencing health care (Yoder-Wise, 2007). New roles for nurses as leaders are evolving in managing the care of clients and their families. For example, with the aging of the population, the demand for specialized gerontological nursing is increasing (Kaasalainen et al., 2006). The CNA Certification Program, which continues to grow in the number of nursing specialities, has the greatest number of certified nurses in gerontology (CNA, 2006a), reflecting the importance of caring for the elderly and their families.

Social Forces

A prime issue affecting the health care delivery system significantly now and in the future is that the Aboriginal population is expected to grow about four times the rate of the non-Aboriginal population (Villeneuve & MacDonald, 2006). Although the Aboriginal governments are forming their own health, education, and social services, enormous health disparities still exist between Aboriginal and non-Aboriginal people. Many disparities are attributable to preventable disease (Reading, Ritchie, Victor, & Wilson, 2005). Diabetes, for example, is a chronic disease that is three times more prevalent in the Aboriginal population (Health Council of Canada, 2007; Health Canada, 2007). Many other chronic conditions and illnesses that require continuing care have begun to appear in the 45 to 64 years age group in the general population (Roscelli, 2005). The need exists to implement preventative community-based programs to target this vulnerable group (Reading, Ritchie, Victor & Wilson, 2005).

Currently in Aboriginal communities, the lack of health care service providers, such as nurses, poses problems. The average length of community stay for nurses is 2 years. This deficiency in available nurses will contribute to serious resource problems at the Aboriginal community level, where health care services are, in most instances, provided by nurses (Health Council of Canada, 2005).

To promote health care services and help relieve the shortage of health care professionals among Aboriginal communities, nurse leaders can be advocates in provincial associations and educational and community settings for nursing in Aboriginal communities. Recruitment measures may be undertaken to guide young people from the Aboriginal communities into the profession of nursing. Nurse leaders need to be aware that an important element regarding health care services is that the First Nations and Inuit Health Branch (FNIHB) of Health Canada provides public health services and health promotion and disease prevention activities to Aboriginal communities. However, services are not provided to those First Nations and Inuit communities that have opted for transfer of health services. By way of transfer, communities can assume control over community-based programs that were formally managed by FNIHB (Health Council of Canada, 2005). The factors that determine the health of an Aboriginal community are multifaceted and complex, which consequently places nurses in a strong position to assume leadership roles. Although it is important to adapt services that are culturally appropriate, it is also important to pursue effective traditional or alternative health care methods (Srivastava, 2007).

Other social forces affecting the delivery of health care must not be underestimated. The health needs of culturally diverse populations, as well as the Aboriginal population, including home care, primary health care, and mental health care, are important issues. The role of the nurse leader is in taking steps to ensure that quality health care is delivered in an integrated and coordinated manner.

reflective **THINKING** You are a community health nurse recently employed in a First Nations Community Health Centre, whose health services are controlled by the community. You have been asked to plan activities and strategies to achieve health outcomes for the community. In what ways can you use your leadership skills and knowledge to plan a comprehensive health program based on primary health care principles?

Technological Forces

Health care services will continue to be affected by technology. Villeneuve and MacDonald (2006) state that "Emerging quantum technology (e.g., nanotechnology [the study and science of building something from miniscule materials such as atoms or molecules]) will transform illness care by increasing the proportion of outpatient procedures and making many surgeries less invasive, or avoidable altogether" (p. 77). As Canada continuously seeks to improve the effectiveness of the health care system, nurse leaders, in addition to improving their own competence in using information and communications technology, need to encourage their team members to do so as well. Information and communications technology initiatives, such as telehealth, databases, electronic health records, e-mail, and Internet resources, affect the process of decision making, which results in better health outcomes (CNA, 2006b). The Canadian Healthcare Association states that the accelerated implementation of the pan-Canadian electronic health record will improve access to care and high-quality services and increase the efficiency of the health care system (Canadian Healthcare Association, 2006).

The Human Genome Project has great potential to transform health, as well as illness care, because essentially, all diseases and conditions have a genetic, or genomic, component. The future of health care for all individuals includes identifying specific diseases, targeting diagnostic tests, and selecting modes of treatment specific to underlying causes (rather than only to symptoms) and monitoring the treatment and care given (Grady & Collins, 2003). Bottorff et al. (2005) state that an urgent need exists for all Canadian nurse leaders, in all settings, to be informed and involved in the incorporation of this new knowledge in the health care delivery system.

Canada, like every country in the developed world, is struggling for solutions to the forces that create challenges to the health care delivery system. Nurse leaders are ideally positioned to be at the forefront, applying their knowledge and skills to ensure safe care for clients and their families.

> reflective **THINKING** Identify other dynamic forces that you think influence the health care delivery system. Give reasons for your choices. What are the effects of these forces on the role of the nurse leader in the health care delivery system?

Human Health Resources

Canadians want timely access to effective, high-quality, client-centred, and safe health care delivery and services. To meet these expectations, jurisdictions across Canada must not only plan but also effectively manage their health care delivery systems. This includes planning for the human health resources required to provide effective care within the system (Federal/Provincial/Territorial Advisory Committee on Health Delivery and Human Resources, Health Canada, 2004).

Regarding human health resources, nurses comprise the majority of health care professionals who give care in the health care delivery system. However, the ongoing massive restructuring of the Canadian health care delivery system has impacted negatively in many ways on the personal and professional life of nurses (Blythe, Baumann, & Giovannetti, 2001). Cummings and Estabrooks (2003) conducted a study "to assess the evidence on the effects of hospital restructuring that included layoffs, on nurses who remained employed, using a systematic review of the research literature to contribute to policy formation" (p. 8). The findings indicated that significant decreases occurred in personal efficacy, job satisfaction, ability to provide quality care, and physical and emotional health. Increases occurred in turnover and disruption to health care team relationships. Negative impacts on nurses are also outlined in Box 4.2. The toll of such impacts on the nursing workforce has created a resource crisis (O'Brien-Pallas et al., 2004). Restructuring actually disempowers nurses by reducing their autonomy in the workplace (Blythe, Baumann, & Giovannetti, 2001).

A project, called "Building the Future: An Integrated Strategy for Nursing Human Resources in Canada," was developed to provide the first comprehensive account of the state of nursing human resources in Canada. The goal of the project was to create an informed, long-term strategy to ensure an adequate supply

---

BOX 4.2 NEGATIVE IMPACTS ON NURSING RESULTING FROM RESTRUCTURING OF THE HEALTH CARE SYSTEM

- The labour market in nursing has fluctuated over the years from periods of oversupply to serious shortages.
- Today, quality of patient care across Canada is seriously threatened as a nursing shortage challenges all health care settings.
- Other negative impacts affecting nurses are as follows:
    1. Increases in workload
    2. Non-nursing duties
    3. Overtime
    4. Use of unregulated health care providers
    5. Patient acuity, coupled with casualization of the nursing workforce
    6. Massive layoffs
    7. Wage and compensation freeze
    8. Decline in the number of senior nursing positions along with the aging of the nursing workforce

Reprinted with permission from O'Brien-Pallas, L., Murphy, G. T., White, S., Hayes, L., Baumann, A., Higgin, A., et al. (2004). *Building the future: An integrated strategy for nursing human resources in Canada-Research synthesis report.* Ottawa, ON: The Nursing Sector Study Corporation.

of knowledgeable and skilled nurses to meet the evolving health care needs of all Canadians. To oversee such a complex project, the Nursing Sector Study Corporation was created in 2001. The 5-year study, comprising two phases, examined all three regulated groups of the nursing workforce (licensed practical nurses, registered nurses, and registered psychiatric nurses) (O'Brien-Pallas et al., 2004). Phase I dealt with research about the labour market for nurses in Canada. Phase II was the development of a pan-Canadian human resource strategy in consultation with government and non-government stakeholders. Phase II built upon the findings and recommendations presented at the completion of Phase I (O'Brien-Pallas et al., 2004).

In the fall of 2005, Phase II of the project got underway to build a pan-Canadian nursing human resource (HR) strategy. The document *Toward a Pan-Canadian Planning Framework for Human Health Resources* (2005), published jointly by the CNA and Canadian Medical Association, set out the discussion for 10 core principles and associated strategic directions that might clearly underpin such an approach in Canada under the themes of client-centred care, planning, and career cycle (CNA/Canadian Medical Association, 2005). A report summarizing the consultation formed the basis of the final step of Phase II.

In the spring of 2006, nursing stakeholders from across the country met to review the strategies that were identified by previous consultations. Six main strategies (Box 4.3) were identified as priorities for implementation (Med-Emerg Inc., 2006).

The report urged that HR planning should not be conducted in isolation. The report emphasized the examination of other health HR (HHR) initiatives that had been underway in Canada. Such initiatives were the work of the Advisory Committee on Health Delivery and Human Resources and Task Force Two (a study of physician HR). Theses two studies had many features in common with the Nursing Sector Study. The reports of all three studies recommended that needs-based HHR planning be established as a national standard. Furthermore, both nurses and physicians recommended that an infrastructure for HHR planning be established with the analytical capacity, infrastructure support, and a governance model to coordinate a pan-Canadian needs-based approach to HHR planning (Med-Emerg Inc., 2006). The need to implement this pan-Canadian approach at the community and jurisdictional level is consistent in all reports. Another evident and common theme is the emphasis on the importance of collaborative practice through interdisciplinary teams. Finally, a heavy emphasis is placed on one further matter. That is the need to develop comprehensive approaches to the recruitment and retention of health professionals to ensure access to quality health care in Canada (Med-Emerg Inc., 2006).

The nursing sector has provided an increased understanding of nursing HR issues, and, more importantly, consensus has been reached on the key strategies for implementation. Although implementation plans still need to be developed,

BOX 4.3	TOP PRIORITIES FOR IMPLEMENTATION SELECTED BY NURSING STAKEHOLDERS FROM ACROSS CANADA

Nurses identified six strategies as priorities for implementation:

1. There is a need to move away from the language of "scope of practice" and focus on developing management policy to facilitate nurses to practice [sic] to their level of competency in various clinical settings.

2. There is a need to broaden the nursing HR [human resources] planning framework to be inclusive of other health professions; i.e., develop an integrated health professional health human resource strategy.

3. Given that forecasting models predict a large number of nurses leaving the nursing professions in the coming years (through normal attrition, retirement, etc.), there is a need to devote adequate funding to increase the supply of nurses by increasing the capacity of nursing education programs in Canada.

4. Compile "Best Practices" that outline effective workplace strategies that create effective working environments and maximize nurse and systems outcomes.

5. Create a coordinated pan-Canadian strategy to inform health system managers and policy-makers regarding the relationship between workload and quality patient care and nurse health.

6. Address issues related to workplace health and safety and working environments to ameliorate the effects of overwork and burnout.

From Med-Emerg Inc. (2006). *Building the future: An integrated strategy for nursing human resources in Canada- Phase II final report* (p. iii). Ottawa, ON: The Nursing Sector Study Corporation. Used with permission.

linkages have been established to ensure that nursing HR is tied into the greater Canadian HHR picture. Most importantly, this momentum needs to be continued to ensure that the important work of the Nursing Sector Study benefits clients and their families as well as the Canadian health care system (Med-Emerg Inc., 2006). Nursing leaders must continue to encourage relevant action to implement the strategies put forth. Doing so will be instrumental to retain nursing as a viable health care profession in Canada and to secure the health and well-being of Canada (O'Brien-Pallas et al., 2004).

reflective **THINKING**   What changes can a nurse leader implement in a personal care home to help retain nursing staff?

Human health resources, management, and social structures in health care organizations are key variables influencing the delivery of care by health professionals, especially nurses, across the health care continuum (O'Brien-Pallas et al., 2004). In fact, access to organizational social structures influences the work outcome of nurses in a satisfactory manner (Almost & Laschinger, 2002). In nursing, *empowerment* is a process whereby nurses feel confident they can successfully implement a course of action given their access to the following social structures in an organization: opportunities, resources, information, and support. To attain all of the available professional and personal benefits in their nursing practice, nurse leaders must use their degree of power to allow all nurses access to various social structures in the health care delivery system. Empowerment enables nurses to take control over, and make decisions in, their workplace so that they can practice more effectively and attain job satisfaction, as well as improve client outcomes (Dooher & Byrt, 2005).

Empowerment

Empowerment is an abstract concept that has been defined in a variety of ways by different disciplines. Empowerment is about the conscious striving for increased participation by individuals and groups for effective decisions and choices affecting their lives (Menon, 2002).

In analyzing the concept of empowerment, Rodwell (1996) states that empowerment is a helping process, a partnership valuing self and others, mutual decision making, and freedom to make choices and accept responsibility (Figure 4.1).

The Empowerment Paradigm shows empowerment as a continuum. Empowered nurses are more likely to achieve their goals, acknowledge personal expectations, and recognize the value that their goals will have on their life. Such an understanding of empowerment falls in direct contrast to nurses who experience helplessness and feel apathetic (Dooher & Byrt, 2005).

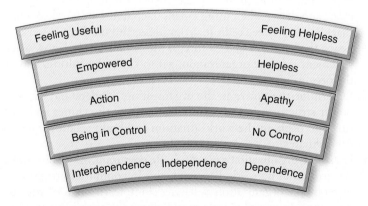

FIGURE 4.1 The empowerment paradigm. (From Dooher, J., & Byrt, R. [2005]. A critical examination of the concept of empowerment. In J.R. Cutcliffe & H. P. McKenna [Eds.], *The essential concepts of nursing: Building blocks for practice* [pp. 109–122]. Toronto, ON: Elsevier Churchill Livingstone.)

> *reflective* **THINKING** Describe instances of your own professional empowerment. What are some ways, events, or situations that can cause you to experience empowerment in your clinical or educational setting?

Personal Empowerment Strategies

It is important to note that each individual nurse must comprehend the concept of empowerment and then experience the development of personal power strategies that lay the foundation of empowerment. Laschinger and Sabiston (2000) and Marquis and Huston (2006) have provided strategies whereby individual nurses can experience the effective use of a personal power base. Box 4.4 outlines several such strategies and provides brief explanations.

BOX 4.4 PERSONAL POWER STRATEGIES

1. Present a powerful profile to others. Be assertive, articulate, well-groomed, and rested. Display a positive attitude and be flexible and be willing to negotiate.
2. Enhance professional knowledge and skills. Attend professional conferences, bring resources in from the outside, read professional nursing literature and research studies to enhance evidence-based practice, share information to build trust and co-operation, and ask for information.
3. Use facilitative communication skills. Effective listening and verbal skills are important. Follow professional format for writing letters; keep messages simple, clear, and direct when using email, telephones, or wireless email devices (e.g., BlackBerries); take credit for your ideas; and maintain a sense of humour.
4. Learn the language and culture of the organization. Know what the mission statement is in the organization, get to know the culture, and be socialized into the organization.
5. Determine the power in the organization. Understand the formal and informal power structures in the organization; know the names and faces of administration and peers in the work situation; and build relationships with superiors and subordinates.
6. Learn the organization's priorities. Be cognizant of organizational goals and vision.
7. Be visible and network. Become active in committees or groups that are recognized by the organization as having clout; learn to "toot your own horn"; accept compliments as well as give compliments to others who are deserving of their accomplishments.
8. Empower others. Support others. Value the profession.

reflective **THINKING**   As a nurse, what strategies other than those mentioned in Box 4.4 can you use as part of a personal power base?

Kanter's Theory of Structural Empowerment

The definition of empowerment provided above is aligned with Kanter's (1977, 1993) Theory of Structural Empowerment in Organizations. Kanter believes that access to information regarding organizational goals and policies, support (guidance and feedback) from superiors or peers, access to resources needed to accomplish work, and opportunities to learn and develop professionally by participating on committees and task forces are essential to the growth of employee empowerment (Laschinger, Finegan, & Shamian, 2001; Almost & Laschinger, 2002). Kanter posits that the impact of organizational social structures on the behaviours of employees is more prominent than either the impact of the employee's personality characteristics or socialization processes (Kanter, 1977, 1993).

Power, the central concept of Kanter's theory, affects organizational behaviours and attitudes. Kanter (1993) claims that access to these organizational structures is influenced by the degree of formal, as well as informal, power that the individual has in the organization. Formal power results from having a job characteristic that promotes visibility, encourages decision making, offers recognition, and contributes to key organizational goals. On the other hand, informal power refers to the stable connections and alliances that the individual has with sponsors, peers, and subordinates. It is they who provide approval and support so that the individuals can reach their goals in collaborative work environments that promote success and increase work effectiveness (Siu, Laschinger, & Vingilis, 2005).

Kanter's Theory Expanded in Nursing

Considerable support for Kanter's theory exists in the nursing literature. The Workplace Empowerment Research Program, led by Dr. Heather K. Spence Laschinger at the University of Western Ontario, has contributed considerable support for, and knowledge about, Kanter's organizational theory as a model for creating healthy work environments in nursing practice settings (Laschinger, 1996). Recently, Kanter's (1993) theory was expanded to include psychological empowerment as both an outcome of structural empowerment and as an intervening variable between empowerment and the effective work behaviours of employees (Kluska, Laschinger, & Kerr, 2004; Kramer, Siebert, & Liden, 1999). Psychological empowerment is defined as the psychological state that the individual must experience for empowerment interventions to be successful (Spreitzer, 1995). In fact, Spreitzer (1995) describes four components of psychological empowerment:

1. Meaning, which entails harmony between the employee's values and job requirements
2. Competence, which refers to being secure in one's job performance abilities
3. Self-determination, which refers to feelings of control related to one's work
4. Impact, which is a sense of being able to exert influence upon important outcomes within the organization

Laschinger, Finegan, Shamian, & Wilk (2001) tested an expanded model of Kanter's structural empowerment, which specified the relationships among structural and psychological empowerment, job strain, and work satisfaction. The results of this study provide support for an expanded model of organizational empowerment, supporting a broader understanding of the empowerment process. Psychological empowerment has been linked empirically to certain work behaviour outcomes and to client outcomes through cautious manipulations of the hospital environment (Manojlovich & Laschinger, 2002). The work environment is an important and significant milieu for staff work effectiveness. Administrators and managers need to be able to focus on the work environment with the direct intention to empower their employees by providing resources, opportunity, information, and support. Manojlovich & Laschinger (2002) state: "Nurses who view their work environments as empowering are more likely to provide high quality care" (p. 594). Figure 4.2 summarizes the tenets of work empowerment.

Several empirical studies cite the importance of structural empowerment in the workplace. One study of nurse managers indicated that high levels of structural empowerment were related to lower levels of emotional exhaustion and higher levels of energy (Laschinger, Almost, Purdy, & Kim, 2004). The researchers conclude that an empowering workplace can be an effective way of reducing organizational stress for nurses. The findings of a recent study of new graduate nurses indicated that structural empowerment has a direct effect on the quality of work life. That is, when new graduate nurses experience access to empowerment structures, they feel more engaged in their work and more committed to the organization (Cho, Laschinger, & Wong, 2006).

Figure 4.3, a crossword puzzle, provides an overview of the empowerment concept for nurses. The puzzle was developed by a group of fourth-year students completing a Leadership for Nursing Practice course in the baccalaureate program for nursing. The students used the puzzle as a teaching tool for their fellow students during a presentation on empowerment for nurses. The solution is provided at the end of the chapter (see Figure 4.4).

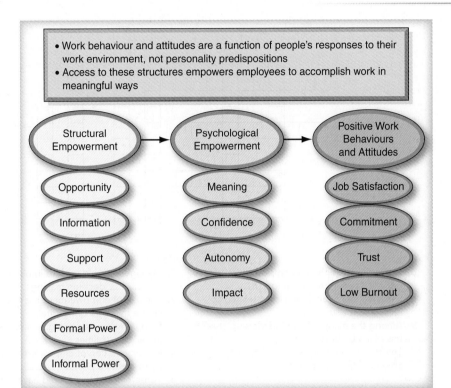

FIGURE 4.2 Summary of tenets of work empowerment theory. (From Laschinger, H. K. S. [2004]. *Tenets of Work Empowerment. Canadian Nursing Leadership Study.* London, ON: University of Western Ontario. Used with permission.)

reflective **THINKING** You are a nurse leader at a community resource health centre. In what ways can you empower your staff in your work setting?

A study was conducted using a model derived from Kanter's Theory of Structural Empowerment (1993) in a unique nursing population, examining the relationship between the First Nations and Inuit Health Branch (FNIHB) nurses' perceptions of workplace empowerment and their commitment to the organization (Scott, 2006). The findings indicated that nurses had moderate empowerment scores, indicating the need to improve the structures of power in nurse work settings. Nurses in this group perceived themselves as having greatest access to opportunity but lesser access to information. In addition, access to

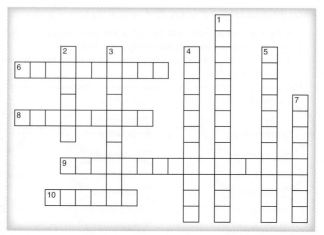

Across:
6. Strategies to implement empowerment focus on LEB: Leader Empowering _____.
8. Empowerment can solve issues related to recruitment and _____.
9. Among the many different leadership styles this could be best used.
10. This theorist developed The Theory of Structural Empowerment.

Down:
1. Managers should seek to implement the use of _____ decision making.
2. The use of empowerment has the ability to create this type of hospital.
3. Being empowered can give a nurse _____ in her own abilities.
4. Implementation of empowerment has the ability to create a positive _____.
5. Those empowered should have the _____ for growth, mobility, and the chance to increase knowledge and skills.
7. Empowerment is a process of _____ others.

FIGURE 4.3 Empowerment in nursing. (From Fletcher, L., Mathieson, H., DeRuyck, K., & Ross, L. [2007] Empowerment Crossword Puzzle. Winnipeg, Manitoba: Students BN Program, Faculty of Nursing, University of Manitoba.)

support and resources were concerns to these nurses. The nurses perceived greater informal power but lower than average levels of formal power. A related finding of this study was that male respondents perceived greater access to informal power than did female respondents. Results regarding commitment indicated that the FNIHB nurses were more likely to maintain organizational membership due to a belief that they *need* to (continuance commitment) rather than *want* to (affective commitment) or *ought* to (normative commitment). Scott (2006) claims that further research of the perception of power in FNIHB nursing managers and leaders would contribute to a further understanding of nursing power in this unique work environment.

Evidence from empirical studies indicates that organizational structure impacts the quality of the work of nurse leaders in work environments. Good organizational structures contribute to a more professional practice, especially in the presence of strong nursing leadership. However, developing one's own personal power strategies is particularly important for the nurse leader's sense of empowerment.

Canadian Nursing Leadership Study

Over the last decade, dramatic changes have occurred in nursing leadership roles. These changes have been noted in several aspects of the nurse leader's responsibilities. They include a wider scope of responsibility and control, a significant reduction in the number of managerial positions, and reduced visibility and availability of mentoring.

Only a few studies have examined how nursing leadership roles differ across Canada or how nurse leadership roles affect professional services. Laschinger and Wong (2007) conducted a study entitled "A Profile of the Structure and Impact of Nursing Management in Canadian Hospitals." The purpose of this study was to profile nursing leadership structures in Canadian hospitals in relation to organizational and structural characteristics of nursing management roles.

The findings indicated that the mean age of nurse leaders at all levels ranges between 47 and 50 years. They are positive about their work and have the ability to be effective and are very experienced with enormous responsibility for client care in the health care delivery system. In addition, they found that nurse leaders have large spans of control at all levels of management and that the role responsibilities of senior nursing leaders are seen as the authority (having power) in clinical programs.

At an invitational symposium, the research team shared the findings of the study with nursing leaders from across Canada. This generated discussion resulting in the identification of key issues and directives. The participants were challenged to act on the proposed actions within their own spheres of influence and responsibilities. The consolidated list of actions that could be attempted by most symposium participants in their own workplace is shown in Box 4.5.

Leadership Issue

You are one of the individual managers who has been invited to the symposium to consider the research results of the study conducted by Laschinger and Wong (2007). You have contributed in the discussion and are aware of the consolidated list of actions that could be tackled in your own workplace. To improve the leadership skills of staff nurses on your geriatric unit, which of those individual actions would you tackle first? Explain the steps you would take to accomplish this action. Write down your rationale in each case.

> ## BOX 4.5   INDIVIDUAL WORKPLACE ACTIONS FOR LEADERS
>
> 1. Profile front line leaders in your organization through available media channels: bulletin boards, newsletters, Websites, e-mail, etc.
> 2. Promote the development of an organization-wide plan for succession planning.
> 3. Deliberately build age diversity into your leadership and management team.
> 4. Create capacity in your organization for protected staff development time (including building in opportunities for participation in decision making).
> 5. Create mutual-gain processes that involve young nurses and managers so that they might address topics of shared interest.
> 6. Create opportunities and education for staff nurses to build leadership skills through "stretch" opportunities, i.e., an experience that challenges staff nurses and provides growth and learning opportunities that are beyond the scope of their usual work expectations.

From Laschinger, H. K. S., & Wong, C. (2007). *Canadian Nursing Leadership Study Invitational Symposium: Final report.* February 4th, 2007 (p. 2), by H. K. S. Laschinger and C. Wong, Co-Principal Investigators. Ottawa, ON: Nursing Leadership Study. Retrieved from http://publish.uwo.ca/~hkl/national_leadership_study/index.htm

Leadership Empowering Behaviours

It is well known that the empowering behaviours of nurse leaders can be of paramount importance in the way staff nurses react to their work environment. Greco, Laschinger, and Wong (2006), in their study "Leader Empowering Behaviours, Staff Nurse Empowerment and Work Engagement/Burnout," state that other investigators have identified particularly significant categories of leadership-empowering behaviours in the work setting (Greco, Laschinger, & Wong, 2006). These categories are as follows:

■ *Enhancing meaningfulness of work*: providing staff nurses with a sense of meaning and purpose of their work increases nurses' self-worth
■ *Fostering participation in decision making*: seeking nurses' participation in the decision-making process
■ *Facilitating goal attainment and providing autonomy and freedom from bureaucratic constraints*: allowing for the best way to use nurses' qualities and resources for best possible work performance outcomes, promoting nurses' work autonomy despite the possible existence of bureaucratic rules and restriction

Other researchers have found that the active endeavour toward empowering leadership behaviours is necessary to job satisfaction, productivity, turnover intentions, and organizational commitment (Gillis, Jackson, & Beiswanger, 2004; Kleinman, 2004).

Empowerment has become a highly desirable and valued reciprocal process in health care. It enables nurse leaders to interact professionally with colleagues to share opportunities, information, and resources. Finally, empowerment enhances the autonomy and self-worth of nurses so they can recognize and exercise more freely their valuable expertise to make effective decisions in their nursing practice.

Shared Governance

Professional nurses have long identified shared governance as a key indicator in nursing practice (Porter-O'Grady, 2001). Shared governance can be viewed as a philosophy of management, a model of professional practice and accountability that focuses on staff involvement in decision making—especially in decisions that affect professional practice in health care organizations (Finkelman, 2006). Organizational theories from the HR era have been credited with setting the initial foundation for shared governance (Anthony, 2004). Many definitions of shared governance exist; one is considered here.

O'May and Buchan (1999) address the core definition of *shared governance* as "a decentralized approach which gives nurses greater authority and control over their practice and work environment; engenders a sense of responsibility and accountability; and allows active participation in the decision-making process, particularly in administrative areas from which they were excluded previously" (p. 281). Shared governance relies on the nurse's autonomy, authority, and control to lead effectively in the implementation of nursing practice (Upenieks, 2000).

Shared governance involves having the courage and capacity to challenge the existing structures and their impediments with determination and persistence to create a healthy organization that values collateral interactions and relationships and allows and encourages participation in decision making and resolving conflicts. Finkelman (2006) states, "It is important to recognize that to move toward a shared governance model the organization must take a comprehensive change approach and not an incremental approach" (p. 150). That is, all parts of the organization and all staff are expected to change. At times it is a difficult but necessary process if shared governance is the goal. However, a change in nursing culture will support the viability of a governance model (Dunbar et al., 2007). Contemporary nursing leadership is necessary for the transformation of hierarchical structures and processes into those structures that are inclusive and empowering (Herrin, 2004). One critical factor in shared governance is that management and staff work together to reinforce new patterns of interaction, shared decision making, and accountability (Porter-O'Grady, 2001).

reflective **THINKING**   In your own words, what is one critical outcome of shared governance in health care organizations?

Kanter (1977, 1993), in her theory on structural power, proposed assumptions suggesting that formal and informal power permit access to work empowerment structures (opportunity, resources, support, and information) that enable employees to accomplish their work (Anthony, 2004). One study based on Kanter's (1977, 1993) Model of Structural Empowerment found that shared governance, which relies on individual autonomy, authority, and control, has the potential to enhance work effectiveness (Buckles-Prince, 1997). Recently, other studies (Erickson, Hamilton, Jones, & Ditomassi, 2003; Laschinger, Almost, & Tuer-Hodes, 2003) found that a relationship exists between structural empowerment and characteristics of shared governance (autonomy and control over practice environments), resulting in the nurses' sense of empowerment, which, in turn, positively affects job satisfaction. Shared governance provides organizational support for direct-care nurses and allows them to become committed to quality nursing practice within their organizations (Green & Jordon, 2004). However, visionary and creative nursing leadership is needed to sustain the changes in the organization. Shared governance has attracted the attention of organizations and nurses because it is perceived as an avenue for maintaining job satisfaction, quality care, and fiscal viability.

> reflective **THINKING**   In the work setting, how can you as a nurse leader enable the clinical nurses' opportunities to pursue their nursing practice and at the same time gain greater job satisfaction?

Empowerment and Accountability in Education and Practice Settings

The need exists to socialize student nurses about accepting professional accountability. Leader nurses acting as positive role models can mentor students in various health care settings. By doing so, the leader nurse exposes the student nurse early on to the accountable, empowered nurse role model and the structures in which these nurses participate (Herrin, 2004).

Nurse Leaders as Agents of Change

Herrin (2004) states that senior nurse leaders must set the stage for change and guide the practicing nurse into a framework of the acceptance of accountability before empowerment and involvement in governance can occur. Nurse leaders must have the skills to guide changes in the work environment, provide tools for nurses to do their nursing practice well, and assist them to feel successful (Porter-O'Grady & Mallock, 2002). Rietdyk (2005) claims that, for nursing staff, a nursing professional practice council (NPPC) improves the quality of workplace environment. The NPPC concept was developed and implemented in the Ontario Public Health Unit to create an environment where nurses are valued, supported, and empowered. Although further research is required to document the relationship between the NPPC and outcomes for nurses, clients, and the health care organization, it appears that the benefits experienced in the first few months of NPPC outweigh the costs involved. Organizations must be encouraged to ensure that environments are provided in which nurses can practice in a safe, competent, and ethical way (CNA, 2005). The CNA and the Canadian Federation of Nurses Union in their joint position statement *Practice Environments: Maximizing Client, Nurse and System Outcomes* (2006) believe that practice environments are essential in all domains of nursing (clinical practice, education, research, administration, and policy) (CNA/Canadian Federation of Nurses Union, 2006). These environments have a direct impact on work production, job satisfaction, recruitment and retention, quality of care, and client outcomes (College of Registered Nurses of British Columbia, 2005).

A special aspect of shared governance is that it provides an organizational framework and an opportunity for staff nurses to become committed more effectively to their nursing practice (Upenieks, 2000). Major keys in making the transition from traditional to shared governance has been nurse leaders' flexibility, their efforts to listen critically, and their willingness to trust and support the transition process (Dunbar et al., 2007). The ability of organizations and nurses to improve the workplace partnership is vital to health care (Green & Jordan, 2004).

108

Section 1   Restructuring the Canadian Health Care System: Role of the Nurse Leader

WEBSITES

▓ The Health Action Lobby

http://www.physiotherapy.ca/HEAL/english/index.htm

The Health Action Lobby (HEAL) is a coalition of national health and consumer associations and organizations dedicated to protecting and strengthening Canada's health care system. It represents more than half a million providers and consumers of health care. HEAL was formed in 1991 out of concern over the erosion of the federal government's role in supporting a national health care system.

▓ The Canadian Healthcare Association

http://www.cha.ca/

The Canadian Healthcare Association (CHA) is the federation of provincial and territorial hospital and health organizations across Canada. Through its members, CHA represents a broad continuum of services provided by regional health authorities, hospitals, facilities, and agencies that are governed by board members and trustees who act in the public interest. CHA is a leader in developing, and advocating for, health policy solutions that meet the needs of Canadians and is committed to a publicly funded health system that provides access to a continuum of comparable health services throughout Canada. CHA was founded in 1931 and this year is celebrating its 75th Anniversary. To mark this special occasion, CHA is publishing a history of the organization, which will reflect the history and evolution of health care in Canada.

▓ The Hospital for Sick Children (SickKids)

http://www.sickkids.ca/

SickKids, affiliated with the University of Toronto, is Canada's most research-intensive hospital and the largest centre dedicated to improving children's health in the country. As innovators in child health, SickKids improves the health of children by integrating care, research, and teaching. With a staff that includes professionals from all disciplines of health care and research, SickKids provides the best in complex and specialized care by creating scientific and clinical advancements, sharing knowledge and expertise and championing the development of an accessible, comprehensive, and sustainable child health system. Check out the virtual tour.

REFERENCES

Almost, J., & Laschinger, H. K. S. (2002). Workplace empowerment, collaborative work relationships, and job strain in nurse practitioners. *Journal of the American Academy of Nurse Practitioners, 14*(9), 408–420.

Anthony, M. K. (2004). Shared governance models: The theory, practice, and evidence. *Online Journal of Issues in Nursing, 9*(1), Manuscript 4. Retrieved July 2007 from http://www.nursingworld.org/ojin/

Blythe, J., Baumann, A., & Giovannetti, P. (2001). Nurses' experiences of restructuring in three Ontario hospitals. *Journal of Nursing Scholarship, 33*(1), 61–68.

Bottorff, J. L., McCullum, M., Balneaves, L. G., Esplen, M. J., Carroll, J. C., Kelly, M., et al. (2005). Canadian nursing in the genomic era: A call for leadership. *Nursing Research, 18*(2), 56–72.

Buckles-Prince, S. (1997). Shared governance: Sharing power and opportunity. *Journal of Nursing Administration, 27*(3), 28–35.

Canadian Health Care Association. (2006). *A strong publicly-funded health system: Keeping Canadians healthy and securing our place in a competitive world. A brief submitted to the House of Commons Standing Committee on Finance.* Ottawa, ON: Author.

Canadian Nurses Association. (2006a). Certification statistics for 2005. *Certification Bulletin, Number 3*(April). Ottawa, ON: Author.

Canadian Nurses Association. (2006b). *E-nursing strategy for Canada.* Ottawa, ON: Author. Retrieved July 2007 from http://www.cna-aiic.ca/

Canadian Nurses Association. (2005). *Fact Sheet: The nursing perspective on patient safety.* Ottawa, ON: Author.

Canadian Nurses Association. (2007). *About CNA: Vision and mission.* Ottawa: Author.

Canadian Nurses Association/Canadian Federation of Nurses Unions. (2006). *Joint position statement: Practice environments: Maximizing client, nurse and system outcomes.* Ottawa, ON: Canadian Nurses Association.

Canadian Nurses Association/Canadian Medical Association. (2005). *Toward a pan-Canadian planning framework for health human resources: A green paper.* Ottawa, ON: Canadian Nurses Association.

Cho, J., Laschinger, H. K. S., & Wong, C. (2006). Workplace empowerment, work engagement and organizational commitment of new graduate nurses. *Nursing Leadership, 19*(3), 43–60.

College of Registered Nurses of British Columbia (2005). *Guidelines for a quality practice environment for nurses in British Columbia.* Vancouver, BC: Author.

Cummings, G., & Estabrooks, C. A. (2003). The effects of hospital restructuring that included layoffs on individual nurses who remained employed: A systematic review of impact. *International Journal of Sociology and Social Policy, 23*(8/9), 8–53.

Deber, R. B., et al. (1998). The public-private mix in health care. In *Striking a balance: Health care systems in Canada and elsewhere*, Papers commissioned by the National Forum on Health, Vol. 4, Éditions MultiMondes, Saint-Foy, Quebec.

Deber, R. B. (1999). *Delivering Health Care Services: Public, Not-For-Profit, or Private?* Discussion Paper No. 17. Ottawa, ON: Commission on the Future of Health Care in Canada.

Dooher, J., & Byrt, R. (2005). A critical examination of the concept of empowerment. In J. R. Cutcliffe, & H. P. McKenna (Eds.), *The essential concepts of nursing: Building blocks for practice* (pp. 109–122). Toronto, ON: Elsevier Churchill Livingstone.

Dressler, G., & Starke, F. A. (2004). *Management principles and practices for tomorrow's leaders* (2nd Canadian ed.). Toronto, ON: Pearson Prentice Hall.

Dunbar, B., Park, B., Berger-Wesley, M., Cameron, T., Lorenz, B., Mayes, D., et al. (2007). Shared governance: Making the transition in practice and perception. *Journal of Nursing Administration, 17*(4), 177–183.

Ellis, J. R., & Hartley, C. L. (2004). *Nursing in today's world: Trends, issues & management* (8th ed.). Philadelphia: Lippincott Williams & Wilkins.

Erickson, J. I., Hamilton, G. A., Jones, D. E., & Ditomassi, M. (2003). The value of collaborative governance/staff empowerment. *Journal of Nursing Administration, 33*(2), 96–104.

Finkelman, A. W. (2006). *Leadership and management in nursing.* Upper Saddle River, NJ: Pearson Prentice Hall.

Gillis, A., Jackson, W., & Beiswanger, D. (2004). University nurse graduates: Perspectives on factors of retention and mobility. *Canadian Journal of Nurse Leadership, 17*(1), 97–110.

Grady, P. A., & Collins, F. S. (2003). Genetics and nursing science: Realizing the potential. *Nursing Research, 52*(2), 69.

Greco, P., Laschinger, H. K. S., & Wong, C. (2006). Leader empowerment behaviours, staff nurse empowerment and work engagement/burnout. *Canadian Journal of Nursing Leadership, 19*(4), 41–56.

Green, A., & Jordan, C. (2004). Common denominators: Shared governance and work place advocacy—strategies for nurses to gain control over their practice. *Online Journal of Issues in Nursing, 9*(1), Manuscript 6. Retrieved June 2007 from http://www.nursingworld.org/ojin/

Health Canada. (2004). Advisory Committee on Health Delivery and Human Resources. Retrieved November 2007 from http://www.hc-sc.gc.ca/

Health Canada. (2007). First Nations and Inuit health. Retrieved July 2007 from http://www.hcsc.gc.ca/

Health Council of Canada. (2005). *The health status of Canada's First Nations, Métis and Inuit peoples.* Toronto, ON: Author.

Health Council of Canada. (2007). *Health care renewal in Canada: Measuring up?* Ottawa, ON: Author.

Herrin, D. M. (2004). Shared governance: A nurse executive response. *Online Journal of Issues in Nursing, 9*(1), Manuscript 1b. Retrieved June 2007 from http://www.nursingworld.org/ojin/

Hibberd, J. M., Doody, L. M., & Hennessey, M. (2006). Business planning and budget preparation. In J. M. Hibberd & D. L. Smith (Eds.), *Nursing leadership and management in Canada* (3rd ed., pp. 691–695). Toronto, ON: Elsevier Canada.

Johns, G., & Saks, A. M. (2008). *Organizational behaviour: Understanding and managing life at work* (7th ed.). Toronto, ON: Pearson Prentice Hall.

Kaasalainen, S., Baxter, P., Martin, L. S., Prentice, D., Rivers, S., Ploeg, J., et al. (2006). Are new RN graduates prepared for gerontological nursing practice? Current perceptions and future directions. *Perspectives, 30*(1), 4–9.

Kanter, R. M. (1977). *Men and women of the corporation.* New York: Basic Books.

Kanter, R. M. (1993). *Men and women of the corporation* (2nd ed.). New York: Basic Books.

Kelly-Heidenthal, P. (2004). *Essentials of nursing leadership & management.* New York: Thomson Delmar Learning.

Kleinman, C. S. (2004). Leadership: A key strategy in staff nurse retention. *Journal of Continuing Education, 35*(3), 128–132.

Kluska, K. M., Laschinger, H. K. S., & Kerr, M. S. (2004). Staff nurse empowerment and effort-reward imbalance. *Nursing Leadership, 17*(1), 112–128.

Kramer, M. L., Siebert, S. E., & Liden, R. C. (1999). Psychological empowerment as a multidimensional construct: A test of construct validity. *Educational Psychological Measurement, 59*, 127–142.

Kreitner, R., Kinicki, A., & Cole, N. (2007). *Fundamentals of organizational behaviour: Key concepts, skills, and best practices* (2nd ed.). Toronto, ON: McGraw-Hill Ryerson.

Laschinger, H. K. S. (1996). A theoretical approach to studying work empowerment in nursing: A review of studies testing Kanter's theory of structural power in organizations. *Nursing Administration Quarterly, 20*(2), 25–41.

Laschinger, H. K. S., Almost, J., & Tuer-Hodes, D. (2003). Workplace empowerment and magnet hospital characteristics: Making the link. *Journal of Nursing Administration, 33*(7/8), 410–422.

Laschinger, H. K. S., Almost, J., Purdy, N., & Kim, J. (2004). Predictors of nurse managers' health in Canadian restructured healthcare settings. *Nursing Leadership, 17*(4), 88–105.

Laschinger, H. K. S., Finegan, J., & Shamian, J. (2001). Promoting nurses' health: Effect of empowerment on job strain and work satisfaction. *Nursing Economics, 19*(2), 42–52.

Laschinger, H. K. S., Finegan, J., Shamian, J., & Wilk, P. (2001). Impact of structural and psychological empowerment on job strain in nursing work setting: Expanding Kanter's model. *Journal of Nursing Administration, 31*(5), 260–272.

Laschinger, H. K. S., & Sabiston, J. (2000). Staff nurse empowerment and workplace behaviours. *Canadian Nurse, 96*(2), 18–22.

Laschinger, H. K. S., & Wong, C. (2007). *Canadian nursing leadership study invitational symposium: Final report.* February 4th, 2007, by H. K. S. Laschinger and C. Wong, Co-Principal Investigators. Ottawa, ON: Nursing Leadership Study. Retrieved November 2007 from http://publish.uwo.ca/;hkl/national_leadership_study/index.htm

Madore, O., & Tiedemann, M. (2005). *Private health care funding and delivery under the Canada Health Act.* Ottawa, ON: Library of Parliament.

Manojlovich, M., & Laschinger, H. K. S. (2002). The relationship of empowerment and selected personality characteristics to nursing job satisfaction. *Journal of Nursing Administration, 32*(11), 586–595.

Marquis, B. L., & Huston, C. J. (2006). *Leadership roles and management functions in nursing: Theory and application* (5th ed.). Philadelphia: Lippincott Williams & Wilkins.

Med-Emerg Inc. (2006). *Building the future: An integrated strategy for nursing human resources in Canada – Phase II final report.* Ottawa, ON: The Nursing Sector Study Corporation.

Menon, S. (2002). Toward a model of psychological health empowerment: Implications for health care in multicultural communities. *Nursing Education Today, 22*, 28–39.

O'Brien-Pallas, L., Murphy, G. T., White, S., Hayes, L., Baumann, A., Higgin, A. et al. (2004). *Building the future: An integrated strategy for nursing human resources in Canada- Research synthesis report.* Ottawa, ON: The Nursing Sector Study Corporation.

O'May, F., & Buchan, J. (1999). Shared governance: A literature review. *International Journal of Nursing Studies, 36*, 281–300.

Porter-O'Grady, T. (2001). Is shared governance still relevant? *Journal of Nursing Administration, 31*(10), 468–473.

Porter-O'Grady, T., & Mallock, K. (2002). *Quantum leadership: A textbook of new leadership.* Gaithersburg, MD: Aspen.

Reading, J., Ritchie, A. J., Victor, J. C., & Wilson, E. (2005). Implementing empowering health promotion programmes for Aboriginal youth in two distinct communities in British Columbia. *Promotion & Education, 12*(2), 62–65.

Rietdyk, A. (2005). Nursing professional practice councils: The quest for nursing excellence. *Nursing Leadership, 18*(4), 47–53.

Rodwell, C. M. (1996). An analysis of the concept of empowerment. *Journal of Advanced Nursing, 23*, 305–313.

Roscelli, M. (2005). Political advocacy and research both needed to address federal-provincial gaps in service: Manitoba First Nations personal care homes. *Canadian Journal of Public Health, 96*, S55–S59.

Scott, T. (2006). *The relationship of workplace empowerment and organizational commitment among First nations and Inuit health branch nurses.* Unpublished master's thesis, University of Manitoba, Winnipeg, Manitoba, Canada.

Siu, H. M., Laschinger, H. K. S., & Vingilis, E. (2005). The effect of problem-based learning on nursing students' perceptions of empowerment. *Journal of Nursing Education, 44*(10), 459–469.

Smith, D. L., Klopper, H. E., Paras, A., & Au, A. (2006). Structure in health agencies. In J. Hibberd & D. L. Smith (Eds.), *Nursing leadership and management in Canada* (3rd ed., pp. 163–179). Toronto, ON: Elsevier Canada.

Spreitzer, G. (1995). Psychological empowerment in the workplace: Dimensions, measurement, and validation. *Academy of Management Journal, 38*(5), 1442—1462.

Srivastava, R. (2007). Culture: Perspectives, myths, and misconceptions. In R. H. Srivastava (Ed.), *The health professional's guide to clinical cultural competence.* Toronto, ON: Elsevier Canada.

Upenieks, V. (2000). The relationship of nursing practice models and job satisfaction outcomes. *Journal of Nursing Administration, 30*(6), 330–335.

Villeneuve, M., & MacDonald, J. (2006). *Toward 2020: Visions for nursing.* Ottawa, ON: Canadian Nurses Association.

Yoder-Wise, P. S. (2007). *Leading and managing in nursing* (4th ed.). St. Louis, MO: Mosby Elsevier.

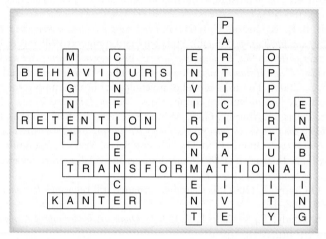

FIGURE 4.4   Solution to Empowerment in Nursing crossword puzzle.

CHAPTER 5

UNDERSTANDING ORGANIZATIONS AND THE PROCESS OF CHANGE: A CHALLENGE FOR NURSE LEADERS

hange can't be managed. Change can be ignored, resisted, responded to, capitalized upon, and created. But it can't be managed and made to march to some orderly step-by-step process. However, whether change is a threat or an opportunity depends on how prepared we are. Whether we become change victims or victors depends on our readiness for change.

—Jim Clemmer,
The Clemmer Group, Canada.

Adapted with permission from Jim Clemmer, August 22, 2007.

Jim Clemmer is a best-selling author and internationally acclaimed keynote speaker, workshop/retreat leader, and management team developer on leadership, change, customer focus, culture, teams, and personal growth. During the last 25 years, he has delivered more than 2,000 customized keynote presentations, workshops, and retreats. Jim is listed in half a dozen Canadian, American, and international *Who's Who* publications.

Overview

Comprehending and appreciating the historical evolution of organizational theories, from the traditional to the contemporary approaches, greatly facilitates the understanding of organizational structure and performance. The study of organizational culture, in a constantly changing restructured environment, is a challenge. It is important, actually, for the nurse leader to attend to cultural attributes to ensure that organizational goals can be achieved. Organizations, which are dynamic in nature, react profoundly in times of change and stress, for example, during the restructuring process. As organizations work to restore equilibrium, the tone may be set by a strong, steadfast, and visionary nurse leader who can act decisively in times of turbulence and challenge. It is imperative that nurse leaders develop insight and openness to organizational dimensions as restructured workplace environments move forward to promote quality health care delivery. At the same time, nurse leaders need to work toward increasing job security and boosting the morale of the nursing staff and interdisciplinary health care team.

Objectives

By critically reflecting upon and processing knowledge throughout this chapter, you will be able to respond effectively to the following objectives:

1. Compare and contrast principles, benefits, and limitations of organizational theories.
2. Analyze the principles that nurse leaders can use in organizations and that are inherent in organizational theories.
3. Design a unit in an organization based on one of the organizational theories.
4. Interpret the meaning of complexity science.
5. Examine the importance of the principles of complexity science as applied to a complex adaptive system, such as the health care organization.
6. Critique the change model and its six distinct functions.
7. Implement the change model for an issue you wish to change in a clinical practice unit within the organization.
8. Describe the impact of restructuring on staff nurses in health care organizations.
9. Differentiate the benefits and limitations of tall and flat organizations.
10. Construct a nursing practice model in a unit within a health care organization.
11. Develop a research proposal to examine the benefits of nursing practice models.
12. Determine the importance of organizational culture in the practice environment.
13. Devise a plan to promote cultural diversity in an organization.
14. Conduct a debate about generational differences in the organization.

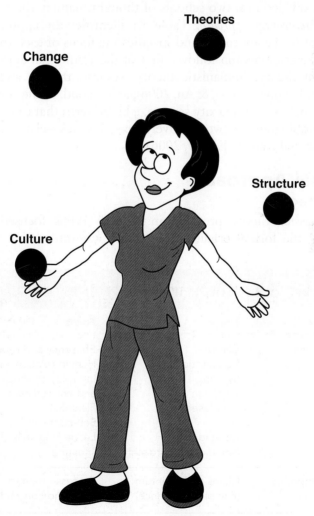

Dynamic Elements of the Organization

Nursing leadership is critical in complex organizations. Nurse leaders can orchestrate effective organizational changes by taking risks and by challenging the establishment to maintain professional standards of excellence in client and family care (Broughton, 2001). The combined abilities to partner and to build relationships and networks are related skills that a nurse leader must possess (Canadian Nurses Association, 2002). However, first and foremost, nurse leaders must comprehend the theoretical dimensions and elements of an organization that make the organization fluid and efficient. Figure 5.1 pinpoints the most important elements of an organization.

FIGURE 5.1 Dynamic organizational elements.

> *reflective* **THINKING**   What nurse leadership skills are required to promote the development of professional nursing standards in the practice environment of a health care organization?

Theoretical Perspectives

Organizations are a part of everyday life. Their intent is to carry out an established mission to meet organizational goals. Sullivan and Decker (2005) state that understanding the health care organization begins with comprehending organizational theory—a crucial element for nurse leaders. The relevant theories can be divided into two schools of thought, namely the *traditional approach* and the *contemporary approach*. Table 5.1 identifies the approach, lists the theories relevant to the approach, and specifies the focus of each theory.

A brief discussion follows, first of the traditional approach, which includes classical theory, humanistic theory, systems theory, and contingency theory (Smith, Klopper, Paras, & Au, 2006); and second, of the contemporary approach, which includes complexity science, a broad term that can be thought as being of the combination of two relatively new theories—chaos and quantum theories (Barker, Sullivan, & Emery, 2006).

Traditional Approach
Classical Theory

The classical theory, prevalent in the early 1900s, focused mainly on the structure of the formal organization, which was intended to boost efficiency and

TABLE 5.1   THEORETICAL PERSPECTIVES OF ORGANIZATIONS

Approach	Theory	Focus
Traditional	Classic	Efficiency and productivity
	Humanistic	Human-relations oriented
	Systems	Interplay of structure, technology, worker,
	• Open	and environment
	• Closed	Flexible
		Self-contained
	Contingency (situational approach)	Leadership style depends on the situation
Contemporary	Chaos and quantum (complexity science)	Process-oriented Fluid and constant renewal

productivity (Sullivan & Decker, 2005). Those who contributed to this theory included Fredrick Taylor, the founder of scientific management; Frank and Lillian Gilbreath, who focused on the specialization of labour through their famous time–motion study principles; and Henri Fayol, who stated that managers in organizations perform five basic functions: planning, organizing, commanding, coordinating, and controlling (Dessler & Starke, 2004). Classical theory is, in turn, built around four elements:

1. *Division and specialization of labour:* Specific parts of the work to be completed are assigned to different individuals. Meanwhile, the manager endeavours to keep the workers' production accurate and efficient to improve the organization's product (Johns & Saks, 2008). In the health care organization, an example may be that nurses, physicians, occupational therapists, dieticians, and social workers, experts in their fields, all provide portions of health care to the client and family. The nurse unit manager oversees the safety of the care provided by these professionals.
2. *Unity of command:* Here authority refers to the right of power that is the power of one person to give orders. Responsibility is the obligation to fulfill the objectives or perform certain functions. Workers are responsible to report to one supervisor ranked immediately above the employee. This situation is known as the unity of direction (Grohar-Murray & DiCroce, 2003). For example, health care aides usually follow the direction of and report to the staff nurse. On the other hand, student nurses, although they are part of the health care team and interact accordingly, are responsible ultimately to report to their clinical supervisor.
3. *Organizational structure:* This refers to the way a group is formed, its line of communication, and its means for channelling authority and making decisions (Marquis & Huston, 2006). The design of the organization is to foster organizational success and survival. Max Weber created what he believed to be the most ideal "pure form" of organizational structure. Weber's system (1969) was an intentionally rational form of organization, which he called *bureaucracy*. Weber described bureaucracy as having certain special characteristics, including well-defined hierarchy of authority, clear division of labour, system of rules and regulations covering the rights and duties of individuals, and impersonality of interpersonal relationships (Dessler & Starke, 2004). Weber (1969) envisioned bureaucracy as a theoretical model that would standardize behaviour in an organization and provide workers with a sense of purpose and security. Some degree of bureaucracy is characteristic of the formal operation in almost every organization, such as hospitals, because it promotes smooth operations within a large and complex group of individuals (Tappen, Weis, & Whitehead, 2004).

4. *Span of control:* This concept relates to the number of employees a manager can effectively and efficiently supervise. The larger the span, the less potential there is for coordination by direct supervision. That is, as the span increases, the attention that a supervisor can devote to each subordinate decreases (Johns & Saks, 2008). When addressing this concept, many variables must be considered, such as the managerial experience of the manager or the skill level of the employees (Grohar-Murray & DiCroce, 2003).

Classical theory offers a structured approach to organizations. However, the principles have been criticized as being more intellectual inventions than the results of empirical research (Grohar-Murray & DiCroce, 2003).

> reflective **THINKING**   What are your thoughts regarding classical theory? In the organizational setting where your nursing practice takes place, are you finding a few, or many, elements of bureaucracy? Explain.

Humanistic Theory

Wide criticisms of classical theory led to the development of the humanistic theory, an approach identified with the human relations movement in the 1930s (Sullivan & Decker, 2005). The Hawthorne studies at the Western Electric Company in Chicago began with the concern of the effects of lighting (illumination), fatigue, and rest pauses on the productivity of the workers. In the first study, the effect of illumination on productivity was studied. The findings indicated that no relationship existed between the two variables. However, the researchers observed that although there was no effect on the workers' physical condition, there were psychological and social effects on productivity and work adjustment (Johns & Saks, 2008). That is, the researchers concluded that the social setting created by the research itself—the special attention given to the workers—enhanced productivity (Sullivan & Decker, 2005). The ability of the group to influence workers has come to be known as the *Hawthorne Effect* (Grohar-Murray & DiCroce, 2003).

Other theorists who contributed to the human relations movement include Douglas McGregor, Fredrick Herzberg, and Chris Argyris. Douglas McGregor's *Theory X* and *Theory Y* together provide an interesting example of the contrast between scientific management and the human relations movement. In brief, Theory X stated that most people do not want to work hard, and it is the manager's responsibility to make certain that they produce efficiently. Meanwhile, Theory Y states that managers believe that the work itself can be motivating and that the individuals will work hard when their managers provide a supportive

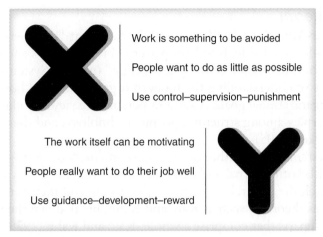

Work is something to be avoided

People want to do as little as possible

Use control–supervision–punishment

The work itself can be motivating

People really want to do their job well

Use guidance–development–reward

FIGURE 5.2 Theory X versus Theory Y. (Reprinted with permission from Tappen, R. M., Weiss, S. A., & Whitehead, D. K. [2004]. Essentials of nursing leadership and management [3rd ed., p. 13]. Philadelphia: F.A. Davis.)

climate (Tappen, Weis, & Whitehead, 2004). See Figure 5.2 for several points relevant to Theory X and Theory Y.

More recently, leaders such as Jim Clemmer from Canada and Stephen Covey from the United States have provided insights into personal and organizational success. Leaders such as these, with different and revolutionary insights, share a common optimistic view of the worker in the workplace. They advocate open communication, more employee participation in decision making, and less rigid, more decentralized control. They believe that the individual has the potential to be self-directed and is highly capable of enhancing productivity. A blend of structured principles, however, and a favourable climate need to exist to allow individuals to perform and achieve goals (Grohar-Murray & DiCroce, 2003).

Using the human relations perspective, the nurse leader believes that the attitudes, opinions, and hopes, as well as fears, of the staff nurses are important as they care for their clients and families. Considerable effort is expended by all who are involved to resolve conflicts and promote professional and personal growth among staff so that they can work in an atmosphere where caring becomes the prime motivator of nursing practice (Tappen, Weis, & Whitehead, 2004).

reflective **THINKING**   View Jim Clemmer's Website at www.clemmer.net/. Create a small group discussion session in your seminar. Determine how Clemmer's approach to leadership and personal growth might actually influence you in the practice of nursing.

Systems Theory

Grohar-Murray and DiCroce (2003) state that "the social nature of organizations allows individuals to have patterned relationships and to play a specific part in the overall mission of the organization" (p. 130). Systems theory is an insightful way of understanding the modern organization and how workers accomplish the organizational goals. A systems perspective views productivity as the function of interplay among structure, people, technology, and the environment (Sullivan & Decker, 2005).

Systems can be either *closed*—self-contained, or *open*—interacting and adapting with both internal and external forces. Systems theory provides a framework by which the interrelated parts of the system and their functions can be studied. Systems theorists, such as Katz and Kahn, break down the modern organization into subparts that comprise a whole. Katz and Kahn (1978) focus on the interrelation of the dynamic concepts in a framework of *inputs*—resources such as individuals, material, and money are imported from the environment; *throughputs*—the processes that produce a product from the inputs, such as work process; and *outputs*—the product of inputs and throughputs. The products of the work process, *outputs*, are then exported to the environment (Yoder-Wise, 2007; Sullivan & Decker, 2005). An organization, then, is a recurrent dynamic cycle of input, throughput, and outputs. See Table 5.2 for the key framework concepts for systems theory.

One of the tools of systems theory is systems thinking. Systems thinking requires that organizations be viewed from a broad-brush perspective. That is, the focus on the interrelatedness of the subsystems is an essential aspect of systems thinking (Dessler & Starke, 2004). Individual departments, such as human resources, or processes, such as quality assurance, can be considered as organizational subsystems. Because the overall behaviour of a system is more than the

TABLE 5.2	SYSTEMS THEORY: KEY CONCEPTS OF FRAMEWORK (KATZ & KAHN, 1978)
Input	Resources from environment, i.e., people, money, material
Throughput	Process that produces product from input, i.e., work process
Output	Product of inputs and throughputs, i.e., product of the work process

Adapted from Yoder-Wise, P. S. (2007). *Leading and managing in nursing* (4th ed.). St. Louis, MO: Mosby Elsevier; Sullivan, E. J., & Decker, P. J. (2005). *Effective leadership and management in nursing* (6th ed.). Upper Saddle River, NJ: Pearson Prentice Hall.

sum of its parts, nurse leaders need to see the broader scheme of things. Smith, Klopper, Paras, and Au state that this is sometimes described as "seeing the big picture," "strategic thinking," or "thinking outside the box" (p. 171). The nurse leader can apply systems theory to modern health care organizations through planning and evaluation activities, such as client and family satisfaction surveys.

---

reflective **THINKING** Design a brief example of a client and family satisfaction survey that would assist you, as a nurse leader, to determine the perceived quality of care received in the hospital.

Contingency Theory

Contingency theory (also called the situational approach) was developed in the 1960s. It recognizes that an appropriate leadership style depends on the demands of the situation. These dependencies are called *contingencies*. That is, theorists observed that certain leadership styles worked well in one situation, but often failed to work when applied in another situation (Dessler & Starke, 2004). Therefore, the central premise of contingency theory is based on the idea that the leadership style to be used depends mostly on the situation at hand (McShane, 2006).

The first comprehensive *contingency model* for leadership was developed by Fred Fiedler. This model proposes that effective group performance depends on the proper match between the leader's style and the degree to which the situation gives control to the leader. Another leadership model was developed by Hersey and Blanchard, and was called the *situational leadership theory*, whereby the effective leader adapts his or her leadership style according to how willing and able a follower is to perform tasks. Both the contingency theory and the situational leadership theory have received little empirical support. Fiedler's contingency model has been found to be quite difficult to apply in the work situation (Langton & Robbins, 2007).

One contingency theory that has withstood scientific critique better than others is the path–goal leadership theory (McShane, 2006). The theory was initially developed in the late 1960s by Martin Evans from the University of Toronto. The essence of the theory is that the leader's job is to assist followers in attaining their goals and to provide the necessary direction and/or support to ensure that followers' personal goals are compatible with the overall goals of the group or the organization (Langton & Robbins, 2007). This leadership theory will be discussed in chapter 6, "Nursing Leadership for Today."

Contingency theory has many theoretical and practical applications. For example, Kanter's (1993) Theory of Organizational Empowerment explains that

Reflections on Leadership Practice

*R*eview Kantor's Theory of Structural Empowerment. Then, take time to reflect on your experience in the clinical setting.

Which contingencies in the clinical setting affect your work performance in a positive way? Do you need to develop other organizational contingencies? If so, what are they? What particular strategies do you as a nurse leader need to develop?

work behaviours are not due to personal characteristics. Rather, high-quality work behaviours are shaped by organizational contingencies, such as mobilizing support, resources, and information, which Kanter called structural empowerment. Dr. Heather Spence Laschinger at the University of Western Ontario School of Nursing has used Kanter's concepts extensively in management research and practice (Laschinger, Finegan, & Shamian, 2001). This contingency theory provides a framework for nurse leaders to use as they contemplate such issues as nursing practice models (Lankshear, Laschinger, & Kerr, 2007).

Contemporary Approach: Complexity Science

According to Barker (2006), "Complexity science is a broad term that can be thought of as a combination of new theories and concepts about how the world works, including chaos, complexity, and quantum theories" (p. 57). Complexity science is thought to be the new science of the 21st century. It has surfaced as a way to deal with people in real-life, complex organizations and situations and has the potential to revolutionize leadership practices. Complexity science examines the unpredictable, nonlinear, disorderly, and uncontrollable ways that human organizations actually behave that are not predictable by traditional evidence (Martin & Sturmberg, 2005). That is, complexity may be understood in contrast to a linear, simple, and equilibrium-based system (Zimmerman, Lindberg, & Plsek, 1998). At the core of complexity science are complex adaptive systems that denote a set of interdependent agents that are not totally predictable. One such complex adaptive system is the health care organization (Plsek, 2003).

A framework that is useful for comprehending complexity science and its relationship to health care leadership is *Edgeware's Nine Emerging and Connected Organizational and Leadership Principles From The Study of Complex Adaptive*

Systems (Zimmerman, Lindberg, & Plsek, 1998; Burns, 2001). A brief description of the nine principles follows:

1. *Lens of complexity*: Viewing the organization through the lens of complexity means alternating mechanistic activities with leadership behaviours that create environments to produce highly unpredictable outcomes.
2. *Good enough vision*: Providing a general sense of direction to the organization rather than detailed planning, because interactions among members are highly unpredictable.
3. *Clockware and swarmware*: Using rational planned and standardized ways of management while exploring new possibilities through trial and error in the organization.
4. *Tune to the edge*: Fostering the correct degree of information flow, diversity, connectivity and difference instead of controlling information and forcing agreement among members in the organization.
5. *Paradox and tension*: Exposing tension and encouraging the organization to find new and innovative ways to move forward. Leaders, who believe that stereotypical questions are better than wicked questions, can prevent the organization from reaching its full potential. Take time to challenge sacred cows.
6. *Multiple actions*: Focusing on multiple actions within an organization; reflecting on responses that worked and on those that did not work; shifting time and energy to actions that worked best.
7. *Shadow system*: Understanding that organizations have two networks. First, the formal system, which is managed by mechanistic styles of management and focuses on stability; second, the informal system, or the shadow system, which is a network of informal relationships generating creativity and innovation.
8. *Chunking*: Allowing complex systems to emerge out of various simple links among systems that work well and are capable of operating independently; that is, when the simple link operates independently, it chunks—links with other simple systems to create complexity.
9. *Balance cooperation and competition*: Allowing members to engage in cooperative behaviours. However, when they respond supportively to another member's action, it enables them to compete productively with that member in the organization (Burns, 2001).

Table 5.3 illustrates the principles, meaning, and application for nurse leaders.

Burns (2001) conducted a survey of 103 administrative staff in a health care system. The findings revealed that health care leaders intuitively support principles of complexity science. Further, leaders who use complexity principles offer ways to focus less on control and more on fostering relatedness and creating

TABLE 5.3	PRINCIPLES FOR NURSE LEADERS: MANAGING COMPLEX ADAPTIVE SYSTEMS	
Principle	**Meaning**	**Application to Clinical Community Setting**
Lens of complexity	View the organization as complex and acknowledge that change is unpredictable.	Allow issues on the unit to emerge.
Good enough vision	Provide minimal number of specifications and a general sense of direction, rather than extensive detail.	Allow for individualization and innovative approaches.
Clockware and swarmware	Balance data and intuition.	Circulate about the unit. Give support. Suggest a new direction for a problem.
Tune to the edge	Foster the right degree of information flow, resources, and relatedness.	Observe. Promote relatedness within the interdisciplinary team.
Paradox and tension	Expose differences that occur between the organizational goals and reality.	Ask "wicked" questions that have no obvious answers. Challenge "sacred cows."
Multiple actions	Take action in small successive steps. Experiment. Adapt. Change. Reflect. Attend to what works.	Notice small, successive successes. Energize people. Calm doubters.
Shadow system	Be aware of the informal and formal networks that exist among members.	Encourage the visibility of relatedness in informal networks. Explore and validate diverse views.
Chunking	Allow complex systems to form from links that work well.	Reinforce successful links in the community, e.g., Reh-Fit programs.
Balance cooperation and competition	Activate the simple strategy meaning "tit" for "tat." Know when to cooperate and when to compete.	Activate and promote cooperation and productive competition among staff.

Adapted from Zimmerman, B., Lindberg, C., & Plsek, P. (1998). *Edgeware: Insights from complexity science for health care leaders.* Irving, TX: Veterans Health Affairs; Matlow, A. G., Wright, J. G., Zimmerman, B., Thomson, K., & Valente, M. (2006). How can the principles of complexity science be applied to improve the coordination of care for complex pediatric patients? *Quality & Safety in Health Care, 15,* 85–88; Burns, J. P. (2001). Complexity science and leadership in healthcare. *Journal of Nursing Administration, 31*(10), 474–482.

conditions in which complex adaptive systems can evolve to produce creative results. Burns (2001) suggests "that more research is needed to clarify the skills and competencies leaders need to apply effectively complexity principles in the chaotic health care environment" (p. 482). Findings of Aherne and Pereira (2005) indicate that the Canadian health policy context is complex and requires innovative solutions to achieve desired changes. As time progresses, the concepts of complexity science will continue to emerge, with a capacity to generate new solutions within organizations. Nurse leaders are core players in understanding the key principles of complex adaptive systems (Penprase & Norris, 2005). Nurse leaders must create environments where trust, risk-taking, and flexibility thrive and countless possible new ideas are allowed to emerge.

reflective **THINKING** Generate ideas about an innovative project you wish to create to bring about a new practice in your clinical unit. What risk behaviours might you need to consider to implement this project? Discuss a sacred cow that you need to challenge.

Change

Change is a natural process of society, organizations, groups, and individuals (Yoder-Wise, 2007). Change today is constant, pervasive, and variable in rate and intensity. The term *permanent white-water* has been used to describe the environment of chaotic change prevalent in most organizations (Vaill, 1989). The volume of change affecting the health care organization is immense, as well, and places pressure on the way these organizations are managed.

Types of Change

According to Skelton-Green (2006), change may take three forms: spontaneous, developmental, or planned. Briefly, *spontaneous change* can occur either from internal or external forces. The outbreak of severe acute respiratory syndrome (SARS) in Toronto Hospital is such an example of unplanned spontaneous change that affected every department in the organization (Loutfy, Wallington, Rutledge, Mederski, et al., 2004). *Developmental change* takes place as the organization grows and becomes more complex. *Planned change* occurs when a plan is created and implemented to achieve better outcomes. One such change in clinical units is the implementation of nursing practice models, where nurses can be more involved in making decisions for implementing quality care.

Change Model

Barker (2006) illustrates a model that can be used as a framework for change. This model can be modified depending on the nature of change and the complexity of change. Change agents selectively use change management functions to assist in the creation and management of change to reach specific or innovative functions (Yoder-Wise, 2007).

Figure 5.3 illustrates five distinct functions that are cyclical rather than linear. Briefly, the function of creating dissatisfaction is described first. Other functions will be addressed in clockwise order.

1. *Create dissatisfaction:* The first and foremost task of the nurse leader is to create the urgency and rationale for change. Change does not happen unless staff members are dissatisfied with the status quo. Find out why they are dissatisfied. Although the term dissatisfaction has a negative connotation, staff members do not change until they become dissatisfied with the status quo. The leader could help create the dissatisfaction, create a vision that the area will improve, and implement actions to initiate the change.

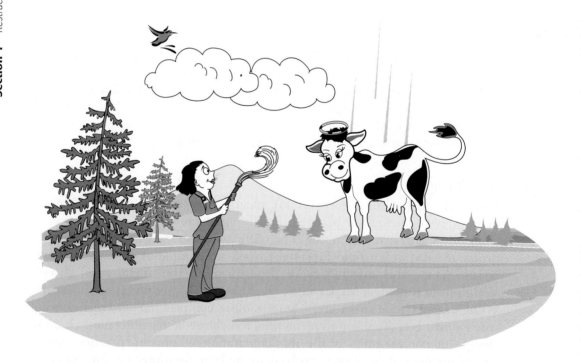

FIGURE 5.3   Change model. (Reprinted with permission from Barker, A. M., Sullivan, D. T., & Emery, M. J. [2006]. *Leadership competencies for clinical managers: The renaissance of transformational leadership.* Toronto, ON: Jones and Bartlett Publishers.)

2. *Form a change team:* It is critical that connections are made among the team members so that the final outcome is greater than any one individual can make. Organizational culture and staff readiness influence responses to change. However, responses may range from full readiness to participate to open rejection.

3. *Create vision and expectations:* The vision will provide a general direction, simplifying more detailed decisions as forward steps are taken and aligning actions of the team. Be aware of common patterns in individual behavioural responses that can either facilitate or hinder change.

4. *Take action:* Use complexity science to determine plans for change. That is, formalize a few strategies, such as assigning responsibilities, and then allow other strategies to emerge during the process. Take small and multiple steps at the same time. Use trial and error.

5. *Evaluate outcomes:* Measure outcomes achieved either with surveys or focus groups. Talk to clients and their families for their observations. Their data are rich with patterns and themes (Barker, 2006).

L e a d e r s h i p   I s s u e

In your clinical practice setting, apply the change model to implement a change that you would like to have happen. List and evaluate both the positive and negative aspects of this change.

Nurse leaders who wish to promote and facilitate the change process in an organization need to be knowledgeable about change process, to possess a set of flexible tools and strategies they can implement, and to model a positive attitude toward change (Skelton-Green, 2006).

Restructuring

The impact of restructuring on staff nurses in health care organizations has been devastating. Many nurses report feelings of disempowerment and dissatisfaction with their degree of input into changes and concerns regarding the provision of optimal levels of client care (Ritter-Teitel, 2002). Because of developing nursing shortages, nurses may have greater leverage within organizations. That is, the shortage may enable them to advocate empowering strategies that give them input into decisions (Blythe, Baumann, & Giovannetti, 2001). However, it is of utmost importance that nurse leaders implement initiatives that can foster change to structures and processes that enhance the practice of nursing.

Organizational Structures in Transition

Organizational structure is an important tool that nurse leaders can implement to increase organizational efficiency in attaining the mission, goals, and lines of communication in the environment.

Traditional to Innovative

Using a classic perspective, Mintzberg and his colleagues at McGill University described five types of organizational designs (Mintzberg, 1989). One design, the *professional bureaucracy*, is of particular interest in the health field. This organizational design allows professionals to work relatively independently of their team members but closely with the clients and families they serve.

Another highly flexible organizational design is *adhocracy*. Adhocracy represents a fluid structure wherein management, staff, and experts work together in teams. Sullivan and Decker (2005) state that, in this design, "power, coordination, and control are constantly shifting" (p. 13). This organizational configuration lends itself especially to the management of projects and innovations (Smith, Klopper, Paras, & Au, 2006). Both professional bureaucracy and adhocracy can be witnessed in hospital settings. Although nurses (registered nurses) are central to providing hospital services and have a broad educational preparation, the structures governing their practice environments do not typically provide for professional autonomy (Smith, Klopper, Paras, & Au, 2006).

Lankshear, Laschinger and Kerr (2007) state that because of significant organizational restructuring, the implementation of program management and the elimination of profession-specific departments have occurred. Health care organizations across Canada have been prompted to implement professional practice structures. Matthews and Lankshear (2007) describe several elements of the professional practice structures, one being the role of the professional practice leader (PPL). The PPL role is to address concerns from professionals regarding the lack of professional identity, development, and input into organizational decision making that could affect practice.

A prime indicator in the widespread implementation of this role was the emergence of the Professional Practice Network of Ontario (PPNO). The PPNO provides an interprofessional forum for communication and collaboration among leaders in professional practice. However, PPNO members express frustration stemming from a lack of clarity regarding the professional role, challenges in demonstrating outcomes associated with the role, and varying degrees of organizational support (e.g., lack of formal authority and time allocation) for the role. Lankshear, Laschinger, and Kerr (2007) conducted a review of the PPL role. On the basis of their findings, they recommend the use of Kanter's theory, which can act as a decision-support framework for implementing the PPL role, especially when designing new PPL roles or reviewing existing ones.

On the other hand, Dunbar, Park, Berger-Wesley, Cameron, et al., (2007) believe that a change in nursing culture will support either the variability of shared governance or the nursing practice model. That is, nursing management flexibility—the willingness to trust and support the transition—is key in making the transition from a traditional to a shared governance model. Herrin (2004) emphasizes that "contemporary nursing leadership is essential for the transformation of traditional hierarchical structures and processes into those that are inclusive and empowering" (p. 1).

The main premise is that nursing practice models (shared governance) provide an organizational framework that enables staff nurses to become more committed to their practice. The importance of shared governance cannot be underestimated, because these models actually allow nurses to participate with an active role in decision making, with maximal participation and with accountability for the outcomes of those decisions (Upenieks, 2000).

> *reflective* **THINKING**   What vision do you hold for nursing in the future? What strategies can you, as a nurse leader, develop to support your vision?

Tall (Centralized) to Flat (Decentralized) Structure

Complex organizations usually have numerous departments that are highly specialized and differentiated. Authority is *centralized*, resulting in a *tall structure* with many work groups. Less complex organizations have *flat structures*, whereby authority is *decentralized*, with several managers supervising large work groups (McShane, 2006). This type of structure has controls that are less rigid, and in this structure, more freedom is available to the employees. This situation results in administrative staff with wide spans of control and nurse leaders with increased authority (Grohar-Murray & DiCroce, 2003). The terms *centralized* and *decentralized* refer to the degree to which an organization has spread its line of authority, power, and communication (Kelly-Heidenthal, 2004). See Figure 5.4 to view the relationship between the span of control and tall and flat organizations.

Nurse leaders need to be aware of the structure prevalent in their organization. The work environment that is comfortable and nonthreatening as well

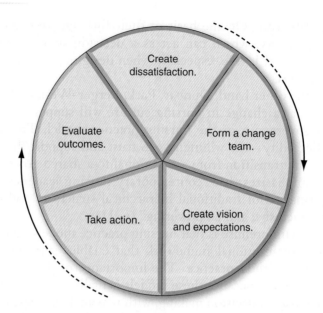

FIGURE 5.4   Span of control and tall/flat structures. (Reprinted with permission from McShane, S. L.
[2006]. *Canadian organizational behaviour* (6th ed.).
Toronto, ON: McGraw-Hill Ryerson.)

as participatory and engaging can enhance one's professional commitment to
the organization.

Organizational Culture

Organizational culture is a system of symbols, connectedness, and interactions
unique to each organization (Marquis & Huston, 2006). That is, it represents the
shared beliefs, values, expectations, norms, and assumptions that are manifest
in attitudes and behaviour and that bind people to the organization (Crow &
Hartman, 2002). Organization culture is fluid and dynamic and is considered to
drive the employee's attitudes and organizational effectiveness and performance
(Waters, 2004). It is shaped and formed by the combination and integration of
all who work in the organization.

Functions

The organization's culture fulfills four functions, as outlined in Box 5.1. The
role of culture in influencing employee behaviour appears to be increasingly important in today's workplace. Culture can also influence the ethical behaviour
of employees and emphasize the importance of a team culture where everyone
feels involved (Langton & Robbins, 2007).

BOX 5.1 FUNCTIONS OF ORGANIZATIONAL CULTURE

1. Develops a sense of organizational identity—sets tone and informs employees of who they are within the organization.
2. Facilitates collective commitment—facilitates shared meaning that all employees are venturing forth in the same direction.
3. Enhances social stability—provides a "social glue" that helps hold the organization together by providing vision, mission, and values.
4. Shapes attitudes and influences behaviours of employees—assists them to make sense of the organization and how it intends to accomplish its long-term goal.

Adapted from Langton, N., & Robbins, S. P. (2007). *Fundamentals of Organizational Behaviour* (3rd Canadian ed., pp. 332–334). Toronto, ON: Pearson Prentice Hall; and Kreitner, R., Kinicki, A., & Cole, N. (2007). *Fundamentals of organizational behaviour: Key concepts, skills, and best practices.* (2nd Canadian ed., pp. 273–275). Toronto, ON: McGraw-Hill Ryerson.

Socialization Processes

Organizational socialization is an important process by which employees learn values, norms, and required behaviours in the organization. Kreitner, Kinicki, and Cole (2007) describe a three-phase model of organizational socialization that may be characterized by a sequence of three identifiable steps. In addition, the model specifies behavioural and affective outcomes that can be used to evaluate how well the individual has been socialized. The length of time required to complete the three-phase sequence depends on individual differences and the complexity of the situation. The phases follow:

1. *Anticipatory socialization*: The organizational process of socialization begins before the individual joins the organization. Anticipatory socialization comes from a variety of sources, such as advertisements, human resource Websites, and even word of mouth. All of this information—formal or informal—assists the individual to anticipate realities about the organization and the new job.
2. *Encounter*: This phase begins when the employment contract has been signed. It may be an anxiety-ridden experience as the newcomer enters the unfamiliar environment. Many organizations use orientation programs to socialize employees during this phase. As the new recruit discovers what the organization is really like, values, skills, and attitudes begin to shift. The recruit becomes increasingly more familiar with task and group dynamics.
3. *Change and acquisition*: The mastery of important skills and the resolution of role conflicts signal the beginning of this final phase of the socialization process. The employee adjusts to values and norms of the work group. Those who do not journey to this phase usually leave either voluntarily or involuntarily, or they become isolated from social networks (Kreitner, Kinicki, & Cole, 2007).

Behavioural and affective outcomes occur as the employee performs role assignments and remains with the organization and is generally satisfied and motivated to work. The degree of cooperation and high job involvement are also important outcomes that can be evaluated. These phases occur when either a new graduate or a seasoned nurse enters a new health care environment. Nurse leaders can play a key role by helping staff to integrate within the organizational culture. They can model proactive behaviours and be attentive to the socialization process of all of their staff.

Mentoring

Mentoring can also be used to facilitate the socialization process for nurses. According to Donner and Wheeler (2007), mentoring is an effective leadership development strategy that has been used in the nursing profession for a many years. Mentors encourage and support protégés as they develop and grow in their careers. They focus on role-modeling and guiding, rather than on supervising and instructing. The Canadian Nurses Association has developed a *Guide to Preceptorship and Mentoring* (2004). This guide is important to assist nurses and other health professionals to develop and revise programs that use preceptors and mentors to enhance the quality of the nurse's work environment and nursing practice. Kane-Urrabazo (2006) conducted a study to address the importance of the manager's role in the development and maintenance of organizational culture. The findings indicated that one of the critical components was mentorship. Managers who provide mentors to new employees help to alleviate some of the anxiety of new employees that goes along with being in the new environment.

reflective **THINKING**   What is your experience with the mentoring process? In what ways can you as a nurse leader encourage the staff on your unit to participate in mentoring?

Cultural Diversity

In organizations, cultural diversity includes ethnicity, culture, gender, lifestyle, and career stages of employees (Tappen, Weiss, & Whitehead, 2004). The term *cultural diversity* is used to describe a vast range of cultural differences among individuals or groups working in an organization. Workforce diversity presents a challenge in the workplace. To understand, value, and use diversity, nurse leaders need to approach each staff member as an individual. Even though differences exist among people, a common element that prevails is that staff members want to be treated with respect and fairness (Yoder-Wise, 2007).

Failure to address cultural diversity leads to negative effects in performance and in staff interactions. Nurse leaders hold the key to implementing strategies that address cultural diversity and enrich staff experiences. One way is to build on the valuable culture associated with each staff member. For example, considerable enrichment can be experienced by having several staff members present a client-centred conference or share their views on client care (based on their values) (Yoder-Wise, 2007). The key element is that cultural diversity be recognized and valued in the organization.

> *reflective* **THINKING** What other strategies can be used to value cultural diversity on a clinical unit or in a community setting?

Generational Diversity

An organization's culture is a composite of the previous and current generation's attitudes and values (Leuenberger & Kluver, 2005–2006). The impact of understanding all generations on organizational culture is often underestimated. Table 5.4 presents general characteristics of the various generations.

TABLE 5.4	GENERATIONAL CHARACTERISTICS	
Generation	**Years of Birth**	**General Characteristics**
Traditionalists	1900–1945	• Loyalty to and faith in institutions • Belief in a top-down approach • Stress on the reward of retirement for years • Value hard work
Baby Boomers	1946–1964	• Economically optimistic • Driven by competition and by material rewards • Hard working, driven, and dedicated • Focused on the "big picture"
Generation X	1965–1980	• Skeptical about the safety and the predictability of the world • Independent • Resourceful and clever • Media savvy
Generation Y (frequently called Millennials)	1981–2002	• Realistic and assertive • Self-controlled • Collaborative • Driven by meaning in their work • Experts in the use of technology

From Leuenberger, D. Z., & Kluver, J. D. (2005–2006). Changing Culture: Generational collision and creativity. *The Public Manager, 34*(4), 16–21.

Generations X and Y are key to understanding the types of employees the nursing staff will have *in* and will also attract *to* the profession. Although these individuals are comfortable with change, they are at times vocal, resist organizational loyalty, and do not stay in the same job if their demands are not met. Understanding generational characteristics provides nurse leaders some further insight into how these nurses will adapt to the practice settings. Nurse leaders need to appreciate and recognize generational perspectives that can both decrease tension and enhance personal and professional growth in various health care settings (Johnson & Romanello, 2005).

Working with nurses from different generations offers opportunities to explore new and innovative ways of thinking about nursing care (Weston, 2006). In fact, learning diverse points of views, leveraging strengths, and valuing differences in colleagues from different generations can enable nurse leaders to form creative, adaptable, and cohesive work groups. Employees from generations X and Y may provide the impetus needed to encourage other nurses to develop their personal power. Incorporating the perspective of colleagues from younger generations forces an examination of past assumptions and enhances nurses' control over their practice.

Nurse Leaders

Nurses are the largest group of health care professionals and are accountable for providing "quality care." Nurse leaders can empower others by sharing knowledge, valuing the profession, and supporting employees within health care teams. The leaders must take an active role in creating organizational cultures that endure sustainability in the present and future.

WEBSITES

■ Voluntary Sector Knowledge Network (VSKN)

http://www.vskn.ca/

VSKN is a Web-based service intended as a resource that assists managers of nonprofit organizations. It is intended to be of specific interest to smaller organizations, such as those that are volunteer-led and those in rural and remote areas. It was created in 2001 with funds from the New Partnerships in Learning Technology program of Human Resources Development Canada and the InVOLve Program of the government of British Columbia.

■ Jim Clemmer

http://www.clemmer.net/

For more than 25 years Jim Clemmer's practical leadership approaches have been inspiring action and achieving results. His keynote presentations and workshops/retreats, five best-selling books, columns, and newsletters have helped people worldwide. Jim is a popular columnist and a regular guest on radio and television programs. Jim lives in Kitchener, Ontario. Visit Jim's daily blog of leadership tips and ideas.

■ I.H. Asper School of Business

http://www.umanitoba.ca/asper/

The primary purpose of the I.H. Asper School of Business is to provide management education in Manitoba by creating and disseminating leading-edge knowledge and developing skills relevant to current and future managers in organizations operating in a global environment. The School strives to achieve recognition by producing high-quality undergraduate, graduate, and executive programs while fulfilling its commitment to university, community, and professional service.

REFERENCES

Aherne, M., & Pereira, J. (2005). A generative response to palliative service capacity in Canada. *International Journal of Health Care Quality, 18*(1, Leadership in Health Services), iii–xxi.

Barker, A. M. (2006). Complexity science and change: A path to the future. In A. M. Barker, D. Taylor Sullivan, & M. J. Emery (Eds.), *Leadership competencies for clinical managers* (pp. 57–75). Boston: Jones & Bartlett Publishers.

Blythe, J., Baumann, A., & Giovannetti, P. (2001). Nurses' experiences of restructuring in three Ontario hospitals. *Journal of Nursing Scholarship, 33*(1), 61–68.

Broughton, H. (2001). *Nursing leadership: Unleashing the power.* Ottawa, ON: Canadian Nursing Association.

Burns, J. P. (2001). Complexity science and leadership in healthcare. *Journal of Nursing Administration, 31*(10), 474–482.

Canadian Nurses Association. (2002). *Position Statement: Nursing leadership.* Ottawa, ON: Author.

Canadian Nurses Association. (2004). *Achieving excellence in professional practice: A guide to preceptorship and mentoring.* Ottawa, ON: Author.

Crow, S. M., & Hartman, S. J. (2002). Organizational culture: Its impact on employee relations and discipline in health care organizations. *Health Care Manager, 21*(2), 22–28.

Dessler, G. & Starke, F. A. (2004). *Management: Principles and practices for tomorrow's leaders* (2nd Canadian ed.). Toronto: Pearson Prentice Hall.

Donner, G. J., & Wheeler, M. M. (2007). Mentoring as a leadership development strategy. *Canadian Nurse, 103*(2), 24–25.

Dunbar, B., Park, B., Berger-Wesley, M., Cameron, T., Lorenz, B. T., Mayes, D., & Ashby, R. (2007). Shared governance: Making the transition in practice and perception. *Journal of Nursing Administration, 37*(4), 177–183.

Grohar-Murray, M. E., & DiCroce, H. R. (2003). *Leadership and management in nursing.* Upper Saddle River, NJ: Prentice Hall.

Herrin, D. (2004). Shared governance: A nurse executive response. *Online Journal of Issues in Nursing.* Retrieved May 24, 2007 from http://www.nursingworld.org/ojin/

Johns, G., & Saks, A. M. (2008). *Organizational behaviour: Understanding and managing a life at work* (7th ed.). Toronto, ON: Pearson Prentice Hall.

Johnson, S. A., & Romanello, M. L. (2005). Generational diversity: Teaching and learning approaches. *Nurse Educator, 30*(5), 212–216.

Kane-Urrabazo, C. (2006). Management's role in shaping organizational culture. *Journal of Nursing Management, 14,* 188–194.

Kanter, R. M. (1993). *Men and women of the corporation* (2nd ed.). New York: Basic Books.

Katz, D., & Kahn, H. (1978). *The social psychology of organizations.* New York: Wiley.

Kelly-Heidenthal, P. (2004). *Essentials of nursing leadership & management.* Clifton Park, NY: Thomson Delmar Learning.

Kreitner, R., Kinicki, A., & Cole, N. (2007). *Fundamentals of organizational behaviour: Key concepts, skills, and best practices* (2nd Canadian ed., pp. 273–275). Toronto, ON: McGraw-Hill Ryerson.

Langton, N., & Robbins, S. P. (2007). *Fundamentals of organizational behaviour* (3rd Canadian ed.). Toronto, ON: Pearson Prentice Hall.

Lankshear, S., Laschinger, H. & Kerr, M. (2007). Exploring a theoretical foundation for the professional practice leader role. *Nursing Leadership, 20*(1), 62–71.

Laschinger, H. K. S., Finegan, J., & Shamian, J. (2001). The impact of workplace empowerment, organizational trust on staff nurses' work satisfaction and organizational commitment. *Health Care Management Review, 26*(3), AB/INFORM Global pg.7, 7–23.

Leuenberger, D. Z., & Kluver, J. D. (2005–2006). Changing culture: Generational collision and creativity. *The Public Manager, 34*(4), 16–21.

Loutfy, M. R., Wallington, T., Rutledge, T., Mederski, B., Rose, K., Kwolek, S. et al. (2004). Hospital preparedness and SARS. *Emerging Infectious Diseases 10*(5), 771–776. Retrieved from http://www.cdc.gov/eid

Marquis, B. L., & Huston, C. J. (2006). *Leadership roles and management functions in nursing: Theory and application* (5th ed.). Philadelphia: Lippincott Williams & Wilkins.

Martin, C. M., & Sturmberg, J. P. (2005). General practice—chaos, complexity and innovation. *The eMedical Journal of Australia 183*(2), 106–109.

Matthews, S., & Lankshear, S. (2003). Describing the essential elements of a professional practice structure. *Canadian Journal of Nursing Leadership, 61*(2), 63–71.

McShane, S. L. (2006). *Canadian organizational behaviour* (6th ed.). Toronto, ON: McGraw-Hill Ryerson.

Mintzberg, H. (1989). *Mintzberg on management: Inside our strange world of organizations.* New York: Free Press.

Penprase, B., & Norris, D. (2005). What nurse leaders should know about complex adaptive systems theory. *Nursing Leadership Forum, 9*(3), 127–132.

Plsek, P., & Paul E. Plsek & Associates, Inc. (2003, January). *Complexity and the adoption of innovation in health care.* A paper presented at Accelerating Quality Improvement in Health Care Strategies to Speed the Diffusion of Evidence-Based Innovations, Washington, DC.

Ritter-Teitel, J. (2002). The impact of restructuring on professional nursing practice. *Journal of Nursing Administration, 32*(1), 31–41.

Skelton-Green, J. (2006). Leading and managing change. In J. M. Hibberd, & D. L. Smith (Eds.), *Nursing leadership and management in Canada* (3rd ed., pp. 549–556). Toronto, ON: Elsevier Canada.

Smith, D. L., Klopper, H. E., Paras, A., & Au, A. (2006). Structure in Health Agencies. In J. M. Hibberd, & D. L. Smith (Eds.), *Nursing leadership and management in Canada* (3rd ed., pp. 163–198. Toronto, ON: Elsevier Mosby.

Sullivan, E. J., & Decker, P. J. (2005). *Effective leadership & management in nursing* (6th ed.). Upper Saddle River, NJ: Pearson Prentice Hall.

Tappen, R. M., Weiss, S. A., & Whitehead, D. K. (2004). *Essentials of nursing leadership and management.* Philadelphia: F. A. Davis.

Upenieks, V. (2000). The relationship of nursing practice models and job satisfaction outcomes. *Journal of Nursing Administration, 30*(6), 330–335.

Vaill, P. B. (1989). *Managing as a performing art: New ideas for a world of chaotic change.* San Francisco: Jossey-Bass.

Waters, V. L. (2004). Cultivate corporate culture and diversity. *Nursing Management, 35*(1), 36–37, 50.

Weber, M. (1969). Bureaucratic organization. In A. Etzioni (Ed.), *Readings on modern organizations.* Englewood Cliffs, NJ: Prentice-Hall.

Weston, M. J. (2006, June 29). Integrating generational perspectives in nursing. *Online Journal of Issues in Nursing 11*(2). Retrieved from http://www.nursingworld.org/ojin/

Yoder-Wise, P. S., (2007). *Leading and managing in nursing* (4th ed.). St. Louis, MO: Mosby Elsevier.

Zimmerman, B., Lindberg, C., & Plsek, P. (1998). *Edgeware: Lessons from complexity science for health care leaders.* Irving, TX: Veterans Health Affairs, Inc.

REFOCUSING ON THE LEADERSHIP ROLE

6

NURSING LEADERSHIP FOR TODAY

o out from this place with new partners and serve your communities. Go where there is disunity and despair, and speak the language of reconciliation and hope. Go out and create space for reflection and innovation, and change the world.

—Kaaren Neufeld, RN, MN,
Speaking on the Evolving Role of Nursing Leadership.

Canadian Nursing Leadership Conference, February 14, 2005.
With permission of Canadian Nurses Association,
Toward 2020: Visions for Nursing (2006).

Kaaren Neufeld is chief quality officer for the Winnipeg Regional Health Authority, responsible for quality improvement and accreditation, client relations, the patient experience, and quality analysis and audits. She has served as executive director and chief nursing officer for the St. Boniface General Hospital. Neufeld is Assistant Professor, Faculty of Nursing, at the University of Manitoba, and she is on the board of directors of the St. Boniface Hospital and Research Foundation and the Canadian Patient Safety Institute. Neufeld has experience at the governance level of several national initiatives, including an executive position of the Academy of Canadian Executive Nurses and as a member of the national advisory committee on SARS. Neufeld graduated with a Bachelor of Nursing degree in 1978 and a Master of Nursing degree in 1986. Neufeld's 2-year term of presidency of Canadian Nurses Association began in June 2008.

Overview

Leadership resides in every nurse. Today, complex changes are occurring in the health care delivery system. Because of those changes, it is imperative that nurses at all levels read the spirit of the time. In this new century, knowledge about and the skills related to such matters as globalization, gender-related issues, and cultural diversity are central challenge issues that nurse leaders need to embrace. However, nurse leaders must also embark on a spiritual journey of self-discovery so that they encourage others to help shape an environment that promotes excellence and satisfaction. Current challenges require the nurse leader to develop emotional intelligence, first, to create a climate that encourages staff to become life-long learners, and second, to further health outcomes in the organization. Leadership competencies are essential for nurse leaders today. Nurse leaders are being challenged to develop special qualities and attitudes that will enable them to become effective change agents. Transformational leaders strive for excellence, and they shape their environment so that followers can be motivated to share the future of nursing practice.

Objectives

By critically reflecting upon and processing knowledge throughout this chapter, you will be able to respond effectively to the following objectives:

1. Evaluate the necessity of self-development as an important aspect of leadership development.
2. Find a specific example of a leader who portrays emotional intelligence.
3. Describe how you would apply Goleman's theory of emotional intelligence in your daily work with other members of a health team on a nursing unit.
4. Compare and contrast dissonant leaders with resonant leaders.
5. Write your thoughts and feelings about relational capacity.
6. Identify times or instances when you respond reflexively toward a client and his or her family.
7. Design a clinical unit that includes nurse leaders and other health team members. Illustrate ways in which Kouzes and Posner's leadership practices can be exemplified.
8. Use the Leading Change Framework to pursue a change initiative on a clinical unit.
9. Examine eight attributes of transformational leadership used by nurse leaders.
10. Discuss the importance of leadership competencies in health care organizations.

Primal Dimensions of a Nurse Leader

In the restructuring process of health care today, nursing leadership is increasingly important during times of rapid change. Villeneuve (2006) states that "nurse leaders must focus on health and the health system rather than on nurses and nursing" (p. 84). That is, a shift must occur from traditional paths of nursing to a broader perspective that involves client- and system-focused approaches in the health care arena.

Nurses will be expected to be advocates for clients, families, and communities, as well as for various social issues, such as homelessness. Professional nurses find themselves in an excellent position to provide leadership within their work setting, their professional associations, their communities, and in society at large (Grossman & Valiga, 2005).

Nurses will need also to be more representative of the Canadian population—both from a gender and ethnic perspective (Villeneuve, 2006). To attain the needed diversity, nurses must continue on the path of being transformed from unequal to equal partners by having an active rather than a passive voice and by seeking out opportunities to be visible instead of being invisible nursing leaders in the health care system (Broughton, 2001; Buresh & Gordon, 2006).

> *reflective* **THINKING** What are a few social issues that an effective nurse leader can advocate for clients and families?

Self-Development

It has been proposed that at the very heart of today's nurse leadership lies the process of self-discovery (Amendolair, 2003). This process of increasing one's self-awareness needs to be initiated and developed, both at individual and collective levels. Several scholars have identified self-awareness as the key to empowerment and leadership (McBeth, 2003; Sherwood, 2003; Porter-O'Grady & Malloch, 2007). Fletcher (2006) claims that every nurse leader needs to find a path that is appropriate for this journey. In walking this path of self-discovery, personal work, which is actually one's spiritual work, must be accomplished. In other words, the effective nurse leader must develop self-awareness during the journey to find the true self. Figure 6.1 reflects one's quest during such a spiritual journey.

Spiritual Principles

In her book entitled *Finding Our Way: Leadership for an Uncertain Time*, Margaret Wheatley (2005) states that several spiritual principles describe the essential work for leaders in this era. These principles are as follows:

- *Life is uncertain:* the world is ever-changing and it is easier to move on than to cling desperately to old practices.

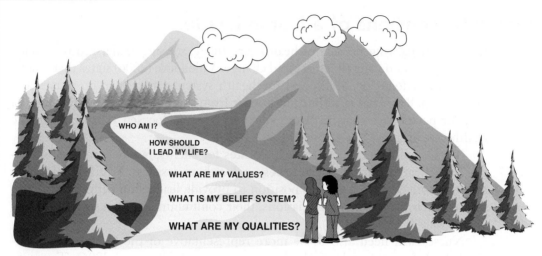

WHO AM I?

HOW SHOULD
I LEAD MY LIFE?

WHAT ARE MY VALUES?

WHAT IS MY BELIEF SYSTEM?

WHAT ARE MY QUALITIES?

FIGURE 6.1   Spiritual path to self-awareness.

- *Life is cyclical:* life uses cycles to create newness; leaders can help individuals stay with the chaos and look for new insights.
- *Meaning is what motivates people:* it is critical for the leader to arrange time for individuals to remember why they are doing this work and whom they are serving. It is important, especially in the health profession, to pause now and then to remember the initial idealism and desire to serve.
- *Service brings joy:* the joy and meaning of service is found in every spiritual tradition.
- *Courage comes from the heart:* when leaders are deeply affected, when their hearts respond to a person or an issue, courage pours from the open heart.
- *We are interconnected with all life:* every spiritual tradition speaks about oneness. Leaders need to act on this truth at such times when they are willing to notice how a decision might affect others and when they think systemically about how they might be affecting future generations.
- *We can rely on human goodness:* this is the value of Berkana Institute, the Leadership Foundation that Wheatley cofounded in 1992. Even though the prevalence of human badness exists, this perspective on human goodness motivates leaders to rely to great heights on human goodness.

The spiritual principles listed above teach leaders to find a peace of mind and an acceptance, which is a prime prerequisite for wellness.

reflective **THINKING**   Describe how Wheatley's spiritual principles resonate for you as a nurse leader?

Spiritual Journey

McBeth (2003) states "leading is giving of one's spirit that propels a reciprocal process as others give of themselves" (p. 38). This cycle of interaction demonstrates the extent of commitment and care that are essential to spiritual growth and development. The human spirit is one's inner essence, the power that motivates one to find real human happiness (Vanier, 2001). For example, to attain true happiness, the leader must choose what is just and take into account the interests of others. The workplace in the organization can be transformed only as the leader is able to change his or her own life and is able to nurture and inspire others to begin their own journey (Bolman & Deal, 2001). Box 6.1 outlines the nurse leader's actions to nurture the human spirit.

Effective leaders have a deep sense of comfort with themselves, and they manifest an engaging attitude about life that is generative and harmonizing. The attributes of self-discipline, resolve, insight, and a sense of direction are important keys to prepare for empowering others to embrace life that contributes to wellness. Consequently, leaders, by the smallest of their actions, can exert a significant and meaningful impact on others at every level of the organization (Porter-O'Grady & Malloch, 2007).

Through self-awareness, the concepts of caring and inner security contribute to being open to knowing each other through listening, understanding, and acceptance. The nurse leader and the members of the health care team demonstrate concepts of caring by being present to one another and by appreciating and respecting one another's uniqueness and diversity. Professional health team members, who know they will be treated with trust, can empower others to give of themselves more creatively and openly while building a common spirit in the organization (Sherwood, 2003). The nurse leader's spiritual journey of self-discovery and fidelity to her or his own values and certitudes can contribute to the healing process within the maze of fragmentation in the health care delivery system.

> *reflective* **THINKING**   What is your response to the statement that personal development is a spiritual work in progress and requires a lifetime commitment?

Emotional Intelligence

Scholarly literature describes emotional intelligence as being critical to the success of leaders. Nurse leaders require a combination of skills when working with clients, their families, physicians, departmental managers, and other leaders and members of their own health care team (Reeves, 2005). Emotional intelligence ranks as one of the most prime concepts encompassing interpersonal skills, effective leadership, partnership building, networking, and critical thinking skills

BOX 6.1   NURTURING THE HUMAN SPIRIT

Self-Care Options
- Reflect/meditate daily
- Prioritize rather than wait for things to happen
- Think positively and limit negative thoughts
- Practice gratitude
- Schedule time to just be
- Find the humour in situations and laugh
- Eat healthy food and exercise
- Maintain nurturing friendships and outside interests

Leadership Strategies
- End meetings positively
- Limit negative talk
- Post periodic achievement lists
- Practice gratitude
- Have interactive conversations with colleagues
- Reflect with others on stories/events
- Celebrate success
- Encourage self-renewal

Sustaining Change
- Be specific about what to change and how
- Practice daily for 3 weeks to instill new behaviours
- Get a coach/mentor or partner for support
- Analyze previous times of high achievement
- Recognize daily work contributions
- Document progress
- Reflect on changes
- Share, or challenge, new goals with others

Adapted from Sherwood, G. (2003). Leadership for a healthy work environment: Caring for the human spirit. *Nurse Leader, 1*(5), 36–40.

(Snow, 2000). *Emotional intelligence* is the ability to monitor and discriminate among emotions and to use the data to guide thought and action. It is substantial, and it is described as the primal aspect of leadership (Herbert & Edgar, 2004).

Mayer and Salovey's Theory of Emotional Intelligence

In 1997, Mayer and Salovey developed a theory of emotional intelligence that has been framed within a model of intelligence. The use of this frame is significant in that emotional intelligence is defined as the ability to perceive and appraise emotions, to access and generate emotions to facilitate thought, to comprehend emotions and emotional knowledge, and to regulate emotions to promote emotional and intellectual growth (Mayer & Salovey, 1997). These abilities are organized hierarchically, with the most basic psychological process being the ability to perceive and express emotions; the most complex ability is the management and regulation of emotions in oneself and others (Herbert & Edgar, 2004). In fact, the development of these abilities is tied directly to professional and personal growth (Moss, 2005).

reflective **THINKING**   Reflect on a situation in the clinical area where you encountered personal frustration and you reacted. Considering your knowledge of emotional intelligence, how will you be inspired to respond to similar situations in the future?

Research by Mayer and Salovey, Goleman, and others has identified that thinking skills, measured as intelligence quotient, and emotional skills, measured as emotional intelligence (EI), are critical for leaders to engage in the skills needed to meet the challenges posed by chaos and growth in the health care organization (Emmerling & Goleman, 2003).

Goleman's Model of Emotional Intelligence

Goleman's theory is specific to the domain of work performance and how an individual's potential for mastering the skills found in each of the following four domains translates into success in an organization. These four major domains of EI are *self-awareness, social awareness, self-management*, and *relationship management* (Goleman, Boyatzis, & McKee, 2002). Goleman's Model of Emotional Intelligence, outlined in Box 6.2, briefly describes the competencies included in the four major components.

Goleman postulates that each of these domains becomes that foundation of learned abilities, or competencies, that depend on the underlying strength in the relevant EI domain. All emotional competencies can be learned and developed. The core competencies—emotional self-awareness, accurate self-assessment, self-confidence, emotional self-control, and empathy—are the most critical because they are fundamental (Taft, 2006). For example, the EI domain of self-awareness provides the underlying basis for the learned competency of "accurate self-assessment" of strengths and limitations pertaining to the role of leadership. Meanwhile, the EI domain of social awareness provides the underlying basis for the competency of empathy. The competency level of this framework is based on a content analysis of capabilities that have been identified through internal research on work performance in several hundred companies and organizations globally (Emmerling & Goleman, 2003).

BOX 6.2 GOLEMAN'S MODEL OF EMOTIONAL INTELLIGENCE

Self-Awareness
- *Emotional self-awareness:* Able to read one's emotions and to recognize their impact; using "gut-sense" to guide decisions
- *Accurate self-assessment:* Knowing one's strengths and limits
- *Self-confidence:* Having a sound sense of one's self worth and capabilities

Self-Management
- *Emotional self-control:* Keeping disruptive emotions and impulses under control
- *Transparency:* Displaying honesty, integrity, and trustworthiness
- *Adaptability:* Demonstrating flexibility in adapting to changing situations or in overcoming obstacles
- *Achievement:* Having the drive to improve performance to meet inner standards of excellence
- *Initiative:* Being ready to act and to seize opportunities
- *Optimism:* Seeing the "up side" in events

Social Awareness
- *Empathy:* Sensing others' emotions, understanding their perspectives, and taking active interest in their concerns
- *Organizational awareness:* Reading the currents, decision networks, and politics at the organizational level
- *Service:* Recognizing and meeting follower, client, or customer needs

Relationship Management
- *Inspirational leadership:* Guiding and motivating with a compelling vision
- *Influence:* Using a range of tactics for persuasion
- *Developing others:* Bolstering others' abilities through feedback and guidance
- *Change catalyst:* Initiating, managing, and leading in a new direction
- *Conflict management:* Resolving disagreements
- *Building bonds:* Cultivating and maintaining a web of relationships
- *Teamwork and collaboration:* Fostering cooperation and team building

Adapted from Herbert, R., & Edgar, L. (2004). Emotional intelligence: A primal dimension of nursing leadership? *Nursing Leadership, 17*(4), 56–63; Boyatzis, R., & McKee, A. (2005). *Resonant leadership: Renewing yourself and connecting with others through mindfulness, hope, and compassion.* Boston: Harvard Business School Press.

Resonance

Goleman, Boyatzis, and McKee (2002) formulated two types of leaders: *dissonant leaders,* who are not in touch with their feelings or the feelings of others, and *resonant leaders,* who are in touch with their own and others' feelings.

149

Chapter 6 Nursing Leadership for Today

Dissonant Versus Resonant Leaders

Dissonant leaders create an environment that allows people to feel more depressed and off balance, leading to burnout and marginal work performance. Either they are abusive and humiliate team members, or they are charming and manipulative only for their own ambitions. In nursing, this interferes in a negative way with the nurses' ability to sense the client's feelings. It increases the risk for medication errors and results in overall poor quality health care.

On the other hand, resonant leaders are those leaders for whom people are eager to work. They inspire organizations and communities to reach for their dreams (Boyatzis & McKee, 2005). Resonant leaders demonstrate EI by being in touch with their emotions as well as those of the workers. Developing resonant leadership requires finding the ideal and the real self and being able to differentiate between the two. After the differences are discovered, efforts to build the strengths and reduce the gaps are essential within the realm of self-directed learning and discovery. That is, newly learned abilities emerge through experimentation and practice. With the support of others, new understanding evolves into changed behaviours, and the gap between the ideal and real self narrows (Amendolair, 2003). In nursing, the practice area thrives as the team members feel respected and their enthusiasm is ignited. Nursing care soars and the clients and families cherish the environment where spirits are uplifted and the most stressful events are lightened.

> *reflective* **THINKING** Review Goleman's Model of Emotional Intelligence. Take time to discern what learned abilities in the four domains you are demonstrating in your clinical setting toward becoming a resonant leader.

Research Supports Emotionally Intelligent Nursing Leadership

Cummings and her colleagues (2005) conducted a study in Alberta to develop a theoretical model of the impact of hospital restructuring on nurses and determine the extent to which emotionally intelligent nursing leadership mitigated these impacts. Their findings indicated that nurses working for resonant leaders reported significantly less emotional exhaustion and psychosomatic symptoms, better emotional health, greater work group collaboration and teamwork with physicians, more satisfaction with supervision and their work, and fewer unmet client care needs than did nurses working with dissonant leaders. Resonant leaders know how to deal with complexities and challenges in the organization by having EI as a determining factor in leadership (Boyatzis & McKee, 2005).

Researchers and developers of EI training programs have agreed that it is possible to learn how to increase EI in participants (Goleman, Boyatzis, & McKee, 2002). Evans and Allen (2002) state that incorporation of EI training into the

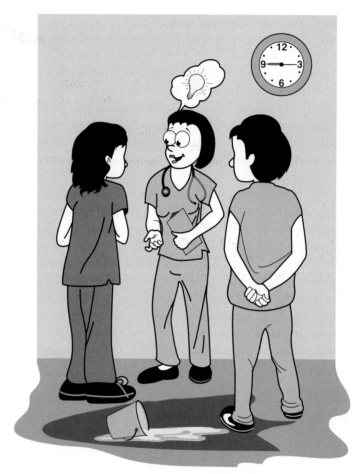

FIGURE 6.2 Emotionally intelligent leader.

nursing curriculum has been identified as essential for nursing education. Figure 6.2 portrays the enlightened and emotionally intelligent nurse.

It is important for nurse leaders to study EI because it can provide a framework for understanding ways that a nurse leader's behaviours can contribute to positive and quality practice environments. EI is critical to professional success and personal well being in nursing. Box 6.3 outlines the steps for improving emotional competencies. See also *Reflections on Leadership Practice*.

Relational Capacity

Relatedness is a prime competency for nurse leaders. Effective interactive skills allow leaders to guide, direct, motivate, and inspire those around them (Barrett, 2006). Such skills are essential to foster and develop the understanding and respect necessary to encourage others to follow a leader. Ferguson-Paré, Mitchell,

BOX 6.3 STEPS TO IMPROVE EMOTIONAL COMPETENCIES

Step 1
- Practice self-reflection by asking, "What am I feeling now?"
- Soon, the identification of feelings that are triggered by certain individuals and events will occur.
- The knowledge of how to respond will come to you.
- Build on and engage your strengths.
- Develop clear, manageable goals; have them reflect your personal vision for self-development.

Step 2
- Increase your self-awareness:
  1. of the dynamics that exist among specific individuals in varying contexts.
  2. of your own feelings and responses to them.
- Understand that self-development will take time and sustained focus. It doesn't happen overnight!

Step 3
- Develop empathy for others and a sense of organizational awareness about the culture and climate of the organization.
- Seek feedback from others as possible.
- Read; think on your own behaviour and developmental goals.
- Keep a written record of thoughts, feedback, insights, difficulties, and successes.

Step 4
- Increase your skill at managing different or challenging relationships, such as interactions in multidisciplinary teams and conflicts that can arise.
- Give yourself credit for evidence of developmental improvements; reinforce your growth.
- Seek ways to further sharpen your developmental progress.
- Assess your continued commitment to behaviour change.
- Assess your continued commitment.

Adapted from Stichler, J. (2006). Emotional intelligence: A critical leadership quality for the nurse executive. *The Nurse Executive, 10*(5), 422–425; Taft, S. H. (2006). Emotionally intelligent leadership in nursing and health care organizations. In L. Roussel, R. C. Swansburg, & R. J. Swansburg (Eds.), *Management and leadership for nurse administrators* (4th ed., pp. 28–44). Mississauga, ON: Jones and Bartlett Publishers Canada.

Perkin, and Stevenson (2002) state that nurse leaders, at all levels, are presented with opportunities to explore meanings embedded in nursing practice and nurse-client relationships. They should take the time for self-reflection and to recognize the values and goals within each situational context. To enhance nurse-client relationships, harmony must be present in terms of a pleasant environment, feelings of satisfaction, positive self-concepts, and effective nursing interventions (Easley, 2007).

Reflections on Leadership Practice

You are a nurse unit manager on a geriatric unit. You overhear a nurse speaking in harsh tones to Mrs. Jones, who has a degree of cognitive impairment. You also know that the nurse's husband died a few weeks ago. When the nurse leaves the room, you ask her to come in for a talk. What would initially be the most appropriate approach in interacting with this nurse? How would you then deal with her behaviour toward the client?

Human Conversations

The most important aspect for nurse leaders to know and experience is that the core principles of trust, respect, and integrity begin with human conversations (McBeth, 2003). In her book *Turning to One Another: Simple Conversations to Restore Hope in the Future*, Margaret Wheatley (2002) states that: "Human conversation is the most ancient and easiest way to cultivate the conditions for change—personal change, community and organizational change, planetary change. If we can sit together and talk about what's important to us, we begin to come alive. We share what we see, what we feel, and we listen to what others see and feel." (p. 3)

In caring and being fully present to this listening process, a common bond of trust is developed and a capacity to experience the deep connectedness of one another unfolds. Creativity spills, giving birth to new visions for health care services. The key ingredient for these conversations includes courage, simplicity, listening, and diversity (Wheatley, 2002).

Social Intelligence

In conversations with members of the health care team or clients and others, the socially intelligent nurse leader begins by being fully present to the other. Once the leader is engaged and then senses how people feel, shifting people to a positive state becomes more of a reality (Goleman, 2006). Further, Goleman (2006) states that no magic recipe exists for what to do or what method to use in every situation. No five-steps-to-social-intelligence-at-work exists. Every person has a built-in bias toward cooperation, empathy, and altruism—provided that they develop the social intelligence to nurture these capacities in themselves and others (Goleman, 2006).

reflective **THINKING** What do you sense are the personal qualities that you bring into a relationship? What can you do to develop your social intelligence?

Effective Relationships

Several research studies have emphasized the connection between effective nurse–client relationships and the level of client care through effectively engaging with the client and implementing interactive skills. For example, an evaluation of communication-enhancement interventions on staff and client in a complex continuing-care facility was conducted by McGilton, Irwin-Robinson, Bascart, and Spanjevic (2006). The researchers' results indicate that the nursing staff feel better about the work and about their clients as they enhance their communication skills. Meanwhile, Morse et al. (2006) present a model describing the responses of nurses to clients who are suffering. They claim that the nurse's level of engagement with the client is affected by whether or not the caregiver is focused on himself or herself or on the sufferer and whether or not the caregiver is responding reflexively or with a learned response. Four types of interactive patterns are identified:

1. Sufferer-focused, first-level responses are triggered by the emotional insight of the caregiver being engaged in the sufferer's experience.
2. Patient-focused, second-level responses are characterized by decreasing of emotional responses, initiating second-level responses, such as the learned professional responses of reassurance and/or distraction.
3. Self-focused, first-level responses relate to protecting the caregiver from being embodied with the suffering experience with the client.
4. Self-focused, second-level responses feature the blocking of engagement, leaving the caregiver without feelings for the client.

The authors argue that the essence of the nurse–client relationship is engagement, that is, the identification of the nurse with the client, because the first-level responses are evoked reflexively and without premeditation. These responses are always appropriate and without premeditation. The responses are on target; they relieve distress and produce comfort (Morse et al., 2006).

This model is important for the nurse leader to know because linking nurse–client engagement with nursing actions in an explanatory model is new and significant. This model not only provides the theoretical basis for teaching and interacting, but also acts as an explanatory model for understanding nurses' responses to suffering in the clinical area.

Nurse leaders must take risks and be willing to foster collaborative conversations. They must challenge the established order to move forward (Bednash, 2003). Doing so means being clear regarding one's values, as well as one's commitment to a common good in relatedness with others.

---

reflective **THINKING** Take time to reflect on how you engage clients and enter a conversation with them. Describe your responses.

Dynamic Process of Leadership for Nurses

Many nurses, whether they are students, recent graduates, or seasoned working nurses, ponder the question "What is leadership?" Primarily, *leadership* is a process used to persuade and to influence the thoughts, feelings, and behaviours of others regarding certain outcomes (Kouzes & Posner, 2007). A nurse leader is important in developing connections among followers to promote a high level of performance and to achieve purposeful goals. Leaders display EI and are skilled in engaging others in relationships, mentoring, and empowerment. They play a significant role in creating positive work environments that can have a prime impact on how nurses respond to their working condition (Greco, Laschinger, & Wong, 2006).

Leadership Competencies

Shirey (2007) states that "Benner's novice-to-expert research has significant application in the nursing leadership context" (p. 167). Patricia Benner's skill acquisition model has most frequently been applied to nurses in clinical, and not administrative, practice (Benner, 1984). The model is built on the assumption that learners, in acquiring and developing a skill, pass through five levels of proficiency. These proficiencies are as follows:

1. *Novice stage:* a beginning nurse leader who has no background in a particular competency.
2. *Advanced beginner:* a nurse leader who may deal with a variety of nursing leadership situations yet may need the frequent guidance of a mentor.
3. *Competent:* a nurse leader who has been in the same or similar situation for a period of time. The skill acquisition in a role is more important than the time in the role.
4. *Proficient:* a nurse leader who focuses on a holistic understanding of the situation and approaches decision making from this perspective.
5. *Expert:* a nurse leader who has an extensive background and repertoire of experiences. The expert is able to zero in on problems. This leader has an intuitive grasp from a deep understanding of the total situation and a sense of knowing what is best.

According to Shirey (2007), these levels of proficiency have a particularly strong relevance to nursing leadership practice.

Leadership Practices

According to Kouzes and Posner (2007), five fundamental leadership practices contribute to exemplary leadership. Box 6.4 briefly describes these practices that provide the hope needed to seize opportunities that can lead to extraordinary accomplishments in an organization (Tourangeau, 2004).

BOX 6.4 FIVE PRACTICES OF EXEMPLARY LEADERSHIP

Challenge the Process
- The leader must venture out and be willing to take risks in uncharted waters.
- Search for opportunities to innovate, grow, and improve.
- Learn from successes as well as from failures.

Inspire a Shared Vision
- Be willing to dream and share visions and believe in those dreams.
- Envision exciting and ennobling possibilities—have a desire to make something happen.

Enable Others to Act
- Realize that leadership is a team effort. Leaders must be able to influence others.
- Foster collaboration and build trust. Work to make people feel strong, capable, and committed.

Model the Way
- Serve as role models through personal example and be dedicated to action.
- Exemplify the leadership role in a confident manner.
- Find one's own voice and clearly give voice to one's values.

Encourage the Heart
- Care and support others. Encouragement can take many forms, from simple gestures to lavish celebrations. Genuine acts of caring uplift the spirit and draw people forward to celebrate values and victories.
- Understand that a community spirit can carry others through extraordinarily difficult times.

Adapted with permission from Kouzes, J. M., & Posner, B. Z. (2007). *The leadership challenge* (4th ed., pp. 14–18). San Francisco: John Wiley & Sons.

The leader's enthusiasm must radiate from a strong belief in the purpose and a willingness to express his or her conviction of that purpose. The most effective leaders are involved with others in deep, caring ways (Pangman, 2004). Followers want leaders to demonstrate interest and understanding; they want leaders to value everyone's contribution. Prospective leaders need to be aware of their own strengths, qualities, and limitations, and they need to use their abilities to assist their followers to achieve the desired goals (Pangman, 2004).

To measure both self-reported and observer-reported leadership practices, Kouzes and Posner (1995) developed the Leadership Practice Inventory (LPI) tool. The LPI is a reliable and well-validated instrument comprising 30 statements—six statements for measuring each of the five leadership practices (Kouzes & Posner,

1995). Both a self and an observer form of the LPI have been developed. All who participate in seminars, coordinated by facilitators, first complete the LPI-self form and then invite approximately five or six people who are familiar with their general behaviour to complete the LPI-observer form. The LPI-observer form is voluntary and generally unsigned (anonymous). The tools are then returned to the seminar facilitators for scoring and evaluation (Kouzes & Posner, 1995).

Leadership Issue

The behaviours that characterize the five practices of leadership promoted by Kouzes and Posner (2007) are sometimes difficult or subtle to observe in leaders. Think of one nursing leader who has demonstrated, or is demonstrating, at least two of the leadership practices. Describe briefly what the leader did to demonstrate the leadership practice.

Dorothy Wylie Nursing Leadership Institute

The rationale for developing the Dorothy Wylie Nursing Leadership Institute (DWNLI) became apparent because of the critical need for leadership development in Canada. Visionary and transformational leadership skills were deemed necessary at different levels of health care organizations (Simpson, Skelton-Green, Scott, & O'Brien-Pallas, 2002). The Institute was named after Dorothy M. Wylie, who is a long-standing leader in the Canadian nursing community. She is well known by nurses for her activities as teacher, mentor, coach, volunteer, risk-taker, and friend. DWNLI was designed to assist nurse leaders to develop attitudes, knowledge, and a set of core leadership competencies as well as to strengthen leadership abilities of current leaders and identify emergent leaders (Tourangeau, 2004).

Tourangeau and her co-investigators (2004) conducted a study to increase their understanding of the effectiveness of leadership development interventions for nurses. The objective of the study was to determine empirically immediate through long-term effects on participants of the DWNLI.

One of the data instruments used was the LPI developed by Kouzes and Posner (1995). The results indicated that DWNLI was effective in strengthening leadership behaviours performed by established, as well as aspiring, nurse leaders. In addition, particularly in the short-term evaluation, changes in leadership behaviours by Institute participants were more visible to observers than to participants themselves. That is, peer observers of study participants reported significant improvements in leadership practices from the pretest to the posttest time periods in all five leadership practices. No significant differences were noted, however, in how study participants rated their own performance in leadership behaviours from pretest to posttest time periods. The rationale of these results may result from processes of how one views oneself when changing one's self-concept. It may take less time for others to change the manner in which they

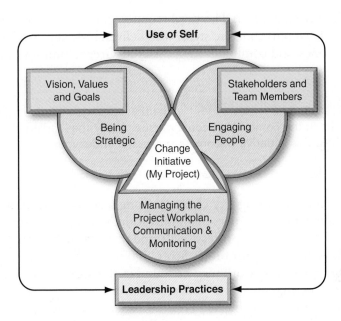

FIGURE 6.3 Leading change framework. (Reprinted with permission of Longwoods Publishing from Skelton-Green, J., Simpson, B., & Scott, J. [2007]. An integrated approach to change leadership. *Nursing Leadership, 20*[3], Online Exclusive.)

view another's behaviour. Tourangeau et al. (2004) state that it is also possible that others may detect smaller shifts or changes in behaviours of those they observe as compared with self-observation.

One of the key features of the DWNLI is that the participants bring a change initiative that they wish to pursue in their organization. The facilitators assist them in developing that project to the point where it has a strong likelihood of success. Skelton-Green, Simpson, and Scott (2007), who were instrumental in developing the Institute with O'Brien-Pallas, developed an integrated conceptual framework and methodology for leading change initiatives so that participants could use this tool in future change projects. Figure 6.3 outlines the leading change framework. As the dynamic framework indicates, there are three possibly overlapping requirements, as follows:

1. *Being strategic:* The first requirement for successful change is choosing the project and the timing of it and developing vision and values to guide the change as well as the desired outcomes.
2. *Engaging people:* The second requirement involves identifying, analyzing, and enlisting the support of stakeholders and enlisting the strengths and skills that different team members bring.

3. *Managing the project:* The third requirement is to ensure that the vision is translated into concrete steps, with deliverables, key activities, accountabilities, timelines, and communication (Skelton-Green, Simpson & Scott, 2007).

reflective **THINKING**   Identify a change initiative that you, as a nurse leader in the community, could pursue. Apply the leading change framework to help this initiative become a successful endeavour.

In implementing any change, strong leadership skills are required, as well as insights into one's personal motivation. One of the essential core competencies of health care professionals today is leading change in organizations (Skelton-Green, Simpson, & Scott, 2007). Further activities to assist leaders in applying the framework may be found in the articles cited in the reference section of this chapter.

The recently established Health Leaders Institute was designed for all health professionals, not just nurses. It follows some of the design features that have proved effective at the DWNLI. For more information, access the Website at http://www.healthleaders.ca.

Nursing Leadership Competency Development Project

A group of senior nurse leaders from the Winnipeg Regional Health Authority (WRHA) were involved in developing a nursing leadership competency program. This project was based on the notion that research is scarce regarding specific knowledge and skills required to maximize leadership performance. In addition, the expectations of the leader are not clear at any point along the continuum from novice to expert, as noted in a model developed by Benner (1985).

This project explores the potential use of a framework developed by the DWNLI. The framework first defines competencies necessary for high performance, and second, examines four interrelated components—*profession of nursing, business of health care, use of self,* and *competencies of leadership.* This framework also includes a novice-to-expert skill level continuum illustrating the behaviours of the leader. Outlined throughout the framework are key leadership behaviours that have been analyzed through focus groups, interviews, and roundtable discussions.

This Nursing Leadership Development Framework will benefit those nurses within the WRHA currently holding leadership positions, as well as those nurses who are aspiring to become nurse leaders of the future (WRHA,

Nursing Leadership Council, April 2006). This initiative is a Web-based program and is available online at http://www.hsc.mb.ca/.

---

reflective **THINKING** What are your thoughts about the Nursing Leadership Competency Development Project?

Nursing leadership is increasingly challenging in health care organizations. Leadership competencies are warranted to target not only better client and family outcomes but to empower, as well as inspire, nurses in their nursing practice.

Leadership Theories: Past and Present

The concept of leadership has changed over time. Initially, the premise was that a trait marked a leader—but evidence is scarce to justify the concept that leaders are born. The study of leadership shifted to behavioural styles as a source of leadership effectiveness. Although the term *style* was helpful, it was not a sufficient guide for leaders. It failed to provide the thorough understanding needed of the leadership phenomenon (Pangman, 2004). Many researchers called for a more comprehensive approach to leadership—a theory to focus on competencies, skills, and knowledge. Again, however, the picture of leadership was incomplete because it failed to describe fully what leaders really do. It became important to emphasize the results of leadership effectiveness (Pangman, 2004). Leadership "expression" calls for a set of skills that are different from those that have been successful in the past (Porter-O'Grady, 2003).

Transformational Leadership

Transformation leadership focuses on creating a vision in line with the organization's mission (Finkelman, 2006). It is a new leadership paradigm that encompasses the emotional and intuitive nature of people by placing emphasis on interpersonal relationships. On the other hand, a transactional leader prefers risk avoidance, focuses on efficiency, and uses the exchange-reward paradigm (Nahavandi, 2003).

According to Ward (2002), there are eight attributes of transformational leadership, as follows:

1. *Self-knowledge:* being aware of personal values, strengths and weaknesses
2. *Authenticity:* being genuine and indicating consistent behaviour with one's belief system
3. *Expertise:* having the skills, knowledge, and technical ability required for the chosen endeavour
4. *Vision:* having the abilities to form a clear vision and to articulate expectations for the future

5. *Flexibility:* being able to find comfort with chaos and complexity
6. *Shared leadership:* equalizing power among the health team members. An environment of shared leadership supports personal and professional development among group members
7. *Charisma:* having personal charm and a positive attitude that energizes people
8. *Inspiration:* being able to inspire and motivate people and to instill confidence in them

reflective **THINKING**   Evaluate your leadership effectiveness on the unit and in the classroom. Identify a few of the attributes of transformational leadership you have and a few that you need to improve.

Johns (2004) states that over time these characteristics become internalized and, in the process, are increasingly practiced by the nurse leader. Nurse leaders can be taught transformational leadership through education and professional development in key leadership competencies within the organization (McGuire & Kennerly, 2005; Murphy, 2005).

In working within Aboriginal communities, being a transformational leader is not easy (Dokis, 2004). The key to successful relationships is that nurse leaders should not try to change how or what the people in the communities are doing. They should act as facilitators of their own transformation and actively participate in the process of collective transformation that is reflective of a people with their own vision and values.

The Academy of Canadian Executive Nurses states that it becomes important to move away from the traditional style of leadership toward new structures where nurses can see nurses as knowledge workers. Throughout the health care organization, formal leaders must create an environment that allows nurses at all levels to exercise some degree of leadership (Ferguson-Paré, Mitchell, Perkin, & Stevenson, 2002). In today's world, leadership becomes more than influencing the behaviour of others—it is also creating an environment that supports the creativity of its followers (White & Hodgson, 2003; Canadian Nurses Association, 2005).

Scholarly Evidence Supports Transformational Approach

Several research studies support the use of transformational leadership by various professional leaders in the workplace with different types of workers (Fisher, 2005; Arnold, Turner, Barling, Kelloway, & McKee, 2007). For example, Arnold and her researchers investigated the relationship between transformational leadership, the meaning that individuals ascribe to their work, and their psychological well-being. The findings indicated that transformational leadership of supervisors exerts a positive influence on the psychological well-being of workers (Arnold et al., 2007).

Regarding nursing, Gullo and Gerstle (2004) conducted a descriptive study on the impact of middle-level nurse managers' transformational leadership characteristics on hospital registered nurses' sense of empowerment and work satisfaction during hospital restructuring. The findings indicated that the staff registered nurses' sense of empowerment can be enhanced by transformational leadership behaviours perceived to be displayed by the middle-level nurse manager.

Clearly, transformational leadership takes much time and practice, but it is more challenging and effective than other leadership styles (Packard, 2003). Transformational leadership is part of the nurse leader's strategy for improving the performance of team members. Transformational leaders go beyond the exchange relationships to motivate health team members to achieve more than what is considered possible (Bass & Riggio, 2006).

WEBSITES

▓ Canadian Journal of Nursing Leadership

http://www.acen-cjonl.org

The *Canadian Journal of Nursing Leadership* is published by Longwoods Publishing Corporation in Toronto, Ontario. Longwoods publishes academic and scientific research as well as commentary and information related to health sciences and health care. Longwoods' vision is to be the knowledge centre of the health care community—a place where the power of imagination and communication is lived and celebrated, a place where ideas are born, debated, translated, and widely distributed for the benefit of good care, everywhere.

▓ Academy of Canadian Executive Nurses

http://www.acen.ca/

The Academy of Canadian Executive Nurses represents the voice of nursing leadership in Canada. It includes nurse executives in major teaching hospitals, universities, health authorities, government, provincial, and national health-related organizations.

▓ Dorothy Wylie Nursing Leadership Institute

http://www.dwnli.ca/

Participants at previous Institutes are unanimous in their support for the program and the 7-day learning experience. Visit this Website to learn of the valuable nursing leadership opportunities that await you.

REFERENCES

Amendolair, D. (2003). Emotional intelligence: Essential for developing nurse leaders. *Nurse Leader, 1*(6), 25–27.

Arnold, K. A., Turner, N., Barling, J., Kelloway, E. K., & McKee, M. C. (2007). Transformational leadership and psychological well-being: The mediating role of meaningful work. *Journal of Occupational Health Psychology, 12*(3), 193–203.

Barrett, D. J. (2006). *Leadership communication.* Toronto, ON: McGraw-Hill/Irwin.

Bass, B. M., & Riggio, R. E. (2006). *Transformational leadership* (2nd ed.). Mahwah, NJ: Erlbaum.

Bednash, G. (2003). Leadership redefined. *Policy, Politics, & Nursing Practice, 4*(4), 257–258.

Benner, P. (1984). *From novice to expert: Excellence and power in clinical nursing practice.* Menlo Park, CA: Addison-Wesley.

Bolman, L., & Deal, T. (2001). *Leading with soul.* San Francisco: Jossey-Bass.

Boyatzis, R., & McKee, A. (2005). *Resonant leadership: Renewing yourself and connecting with others through mindfulness, hope, and compassion.* Boston: Harvard Business School Press.

Broughton, H. (2001). *Nursing leadership: Unleashing the power.* Ottawa, ON: Canadian Nurses Association.

Buresh, B., & Gordon, S. (2006). *From silence to voice: What nurses know and must communicate to the public* (2nd ed.). Ithaca, NY: ILR Cornell University Press.

Canadian Nurses Association. (2005). Nursing leadership in a changing world. *Nursing Now, 18,* January, 5–6.

Cummings, G., Hayduk, L., & Estabrooks, C. (2005). Mitigating the impact of hospital restructuring on nurses: The responsibility of emotionally intelligent leadership. *Nursing Research, 54*(1), 2–12.

Dokis, L. (2004). Transformational leadership: An imperative for nursing in first nation communities. *The Aboriginal Nurse, 19*(2), 12–13.

Easley, R. (2007). Harmony: A concept analysis. *Journal of Advanced Nursing, 59*(5), 551–556.

Emmerling, R. J., & Goleman, D. (2003). Emotional intelligence: Issues and common misunderstandings. *The Consortium for Research on Emotional Intelligence in Organizations.* Retrieved September 2007 from http://www.eiconsortium.org

Evans, D., & Allen, H. (2002). Emotional intelligence: Its role in training. *Nursing Times, 98*(27), 41–42.

Ferguson-Paré, M., Mitchell, G. J., Perkin, K., & Stevenson, L. (2002). Academy of Canadian executive nurses (ACEN) background paper on leadership. *Canadian Journal of Nursing Leadership, 15*(3), 4–8.

Finkelman, A. W. (2006). *Leadership and management in nursing.* Upper Saddle River, NJ: Pearson Education.

Fisher, E. A. (2005). Facing the challenges of outcomes measurement: The role of transformational leadership. *Administration in Social Work, 29*(4), Online. Retrieved October 2007 from http://www.haworthpress.com/web/ASW

Fletcher, K. (2006). Beyond dualism: Leading out of oppression. *Nursing Forum, 41*(2), 50–59.

Goleman, D. (2006). *Social intelligence: The new science of human relationships.* New York: Bantam Books.

Goleman, D., Boyatzis, R., & McKee, A. (2002). *Primal leadership: Realizing the power of emotional intelligence.* Boston: Harvard Business School Press.

Greco, P., Laschinger, H. K. S., & Wong, C. (2006). Leader empowering behaviours, staff nurse empowerment and work engagement/burnout. *Nursing Leadership, 19*(4), 41–56.

Grossman, S. C., & Valiga, T. M. (2005). *The new leadership challenge: Creating the future of nursing* (2nd ed.). Philadelphia: F. A. Davis.

Gullo, S. R., & Gerstle, D. S. (2004). Transformational leadership and hospital restructuring: A descriptive study. *Policy, Politics, & Nursing Practice, 5*(4), 259–266.

Herbert, R., & Edgar, L. (2004). Emotional intelligence: A primal dimension of nursing leadership? *Nursing Leadership, 17*(4), 56–63.

Johns, C. (2004). Becoming a transformational leader through reflection. *Reflections on Nursing Leadership, 30*(2), 24–26, 38.

Kouzes, J. M., & Posner, B. Z. (1995). *The leadership challenge: How to keep getting extraordinary things done in organizations.* San Francisco: Jossey-Bass, Inc.

Kouzes, J. M., & Posner, B. Z. (2007). *The leadership challenge* (4th ed.). San Francisco: John Wiley & Sons.

Mayer, J. D., & Salovey, P. (1997). What is emotional intelligence? In P. Salovey & D. Sluyter (Eds.), *Emotional development and emotional intelligence: Implications for educators* (pp. 92–117). San Francisco: Jossey-Bass.

McBeth, A. (2003). Commonsense leadership. *Nurse Leader, 1*(3), 26–28.

McGilton, K., Irwin-Robinson, H., Boscart, V., & Spanjevic, L. (2006). Communication enhancement: Nurse and patient satisfaction outcomes in a complex continuing care facility. *Journal of Advanced Nursing, 54*(1), 35–44.

McGuire, E., & Kennerly, S. (2006). Nurse managers as transformational and transactional leaders. *Nursing Economics, 24*(4), 179–185.

Morse, J. M., Bottorff, J., Anderson, G., O'Brien, B., & Solberg, S. (2006). Beyond empathy: Expanding expressions of caring. *Journal of Advanced Nursing, 53*(1), 75–90.

Moss, M. T. (2005). *The emotionally intelligent nurse leader.* San Francisco: Jossey-Bass.

Murphy, L. (2005). Transformational leadership: A cascading chain reaction. *Journal of Nursing Management, 13*, 128–136.

Nahavandi, A. (2003). *The art and science of leadership* (3rd ed.). Upper Saddle River, NJ: Pearson Education, Inc.

Nursing Leadership Development Program, Winnipeg Regional Health Authority. Retrieved October 2007 from http://www.hsc.mb.ca/leadership/default.asp

Packard, T. (2003). The supervisor as transformational leader. In M. J. Austin & K. M. Hopkins (Eds.), *Supervision as collaboration in the human services: Building a learning culture.* Thousand Oaks, CA: Sage.

Pangman, V. C. (2004). Leadership for the future. In L. West (Ed.), *Trends and issues in health care* (3rd ed., pp. 223–241). Toronto, ON: McGraw-Hill Ryerson.

Porter-O'Grady, T. (2003). A different age for leadership: Part II. New rules, new roles. *Journal of Nursing Administration, 33*(3), 173–178.

Porter-O'Grady, T., & Malloch, K. (2007). *Quantum leadership: A resource for health care innovation* (2nd ed.). Toronto, ON: Jones Bartlett Publishers.

Reeves, A. L. (2005). Emotional intelligence: Recognizing and regulating emotions. *American Association of Occupational Health Nurses, 53*(4), 172–176.

Sherwood, G. (2003). Leadership for a healthy work environment: Caring for the human spirit. *Nurse Leader, 1*(5), 36–40.

Shirey, M. R. (2007). Competencies and tips for effective leadership from novice to expert. *Journal of Nursing Administration, 37*(4), 167–170.

Simpson, B., Skelton-Green, J., Scott, J., & O'Brien-Pallas, L. (2002). Building capacity in nursing: Creating a leadership institute. *Canadian Journal of Nursing Leadership, 15*(3), 22–27.

Skelton-Green, J., Simpson, B., & Scott, J. (2007). An integrated approach to change leadership. *Nursing Leadership, 20*(3), Online Exclusive.

Snow, J. L. (2001). Looking beyond nursing for clues to effective leadership. *Journal of Nursing Administration, 31*(9), 440–443.

Taft, S. H. (2006). Emotionally intelligent leadership in nursing and health care organizations. In L. Roussel, R. C. Swansburg, & R. J. Swansburg (Eds.), *Management and leadership for nurse administrators* (4th ed., pp. 28–44). Mississauga, ON: Jones and Bartlett Publishers Canada.

Tourangeau, A. E. (2004). Evaluation study of a leadership development intervention for nurses: Final report to the Change Foundation. Toronto, ON: The Change Foundation. Retrieved October 2007 from http://www.changefoundation.com/

Vanier, J. (2001). *Made for happiness: Discovering the meaning of life with Aristotle.* Toronto, ON: Anansi.

Villeneuve, M., & MacDonald, J. (2006). *Toward 2020: Visions for nursing.* Ottawa, ON: Canadian Nurses Association.

Ward, K. (2002). A vision for tomorrow: Transformational nursing leaders. *Nursing Outlook, 50*, 121–126.

Wheatley, M. J. (2002). *Turning to one another: Simple conversations to restore hope to the future.* San Francisco: Berrett-Koehler Publishers, Inc.

Wheatley, M. J. (2005). *Finding our way: Leadership for an uncertain time.* San Francisco: Berrett-Koehler Publishers, Inc.

White, R., & Hodgson, P. (2003). The newest leadership skills. In M. Goldsmith, V. Govindarahan, B. Kaye, & A. Vicere, *The many facets of leadership* (pp. 181–187). Upper Saddle River, NJ: Prentice Hall.

Winnipeg Regional Health Authority. (2006, April). Nursing leadership development program thread: Critical thinking. Winnipeg, MB: Winnipeg Regional Health Authority, Nursing Leadership Council.

CHAPTER 7

NURSE MANAGER: DEVELOPING AND UTILIZING LEADERSHIP COMPETENCIES IN MANAGEMENT

The profession needs to move toward a model of leadership . . . (wherein) . . . nurse managers lead decisions about structure, process, resources, and the environment in which care is provided.

—Ginette Lemire Rodger, RN, PhD
Past President (2000–2002), Canadian Nurses Association.

From Lemire Rodger, G. (2006). Canadian Nurses Association. In M. McIntyre, E. Thomlinson, & C. McDonald (Eds.), *Realities of Canadian nursing: Professional, practice, and power issues* (2nd ed., pp. 133–151). Philadelphia: Lippincott Williams & Wilkins.

Dr. Lemire Rodger is Vice-President of Professional Practice and Chief Nursing Executive in the Nursing Professional Practice Department at the Ottawa Hospital. Dr. Lemire Rodger has served as practitioner, educator, researcher, and administrator. She holds a Master's Degree in Nursing Administration from Universite de Montreal and a PhD (1995) in Nursing Science from the University of Alberta. In 2004, she was the recipient of Canada's highest nursing honour, the Jeanne Mance Award. Most recently, in recognition of her leadership in strengthening Canada's health system and for her contributions to the nursing profession nationally and internationally, Dr. Lemire Rodger has been named an officer of the Order of Canada, the highest civilian honour for lifetime achievement.

Overview

The need for strong nursing leadership to meet the challenges of the health care delivery system is widely acknowledged. Extensive restructuring within health care has transformed nursing leadership. Increasing demands brought about by expanded and multifaceted responsibilities have dramatically altered nurse manager roles. Today, challenges continually present themselves to nurse managers to work collaboratively with other health care professionals to achieve the vision and purpose developed by their organizations. There is general consensus among nurses and all health professionals that nurse managers must demonstrate outstanding leadership competencies to ensure quality health care for the future.

Leadership and management are different, but they are related and interdependent. Leadership without good management is disorganized. Alternatively, management without leadership is disconnected. Emerging nurse managers need opportunities to establish professional credibility while acquiring leadership competencies.

Nurse managers also need to manage the finances of their cost centres to deliver quality client care, meet staffing needs, and achieve the cost savings that are required to meet the business goals of the organization. Leadership development programs, which are provided at the local, provincial/territorial, and national levels, are an important asset in improving knowledge and ability for nurses in managerial role functions.

Objectives

By critically reflecting upon and processing knowledge throughout this chapter, you will be able to respond effectively to the following objectives:

1. Interpret the meaning of competencies.
2. Compare and contrast the characteristics of leaders and managers.
3. Critique the manager's role in the 21st century.
4. Develop a research hypothesis regarding the importance of relationship management with a cultural group of your interest.
5. Examine the elements of financial management from the nurse manager's point of view.
6. Describe the relevant points of budget development.
7. Differentiate between a capital and operating budget.
8. Critique the information given regarding a few of the costs associated with staffing.
9. Design a supply budget for a unit using a hypothetical inflation rate.
10. Conduct a debate about the importance of the depth of financial knowledge for a nurse manager.

Objectives (continued)

11. Discuss the importance of nursing staffing on client outcomes.
12. Devise a staffing plan whereby the baccalaureate-prepared registered nurses have the highest ratio to other staff nurses.
13. Debate the usage of the evaluation framework for evaluating nursing staff mix decisions on clients, nurses, and health care organizations.
14. Analyze the role of the nurse unit manager for staff nursing decisions.
15. Critique usage of the work measurement tool by staff nurses on a unit.
16. Compare and contrast the benefits and limitations of nurse-to-patient ratios in staffing situations.
17. Describe the importance of leadership development for nurse managers.

Empowerment for Nurse Leaders and Managers

The health care organization continues to experience restructuring issues fueled by increasing consumer expectations and demands for high-quality effective care, advancements in medical and scientific technologies, and a shift in social demographics (Cummings & Estabrooks, 2003; Gallo, 2007). Predictably, these mounting pressures affect not only the roles of health care workers, care providers, and management alike, but also the structures of health care organizations.

Patrick and Laschinger (2006) state that job conditions resulting from restructuring "have disempowered nurse managers and influenced their ability to create positive work environments, mentor potential nurse leaders, and gain satisfaction in the leadership role" (p. 13). These conditions have frustrated nurse managers' ability to facilitate care consistent with the goals inherent in professional standards. In their study of nurse manager job satisfaction, Laschinger, Purdy, and Almost (2007) concluded that those managers who describe their work environment as empowering and who perceive strong organizational support, either by receiving positive feedback or by being recognized for their innovative strategies, feel valued by the organization and report high levels of job satisfaction.

reflective **THINKING** If you were a nurse manager on a busy surgical unit, what structures within the organization would empower you? Reflect on structures other than those cited by Laschinger, Purdy, and Almost (2007).

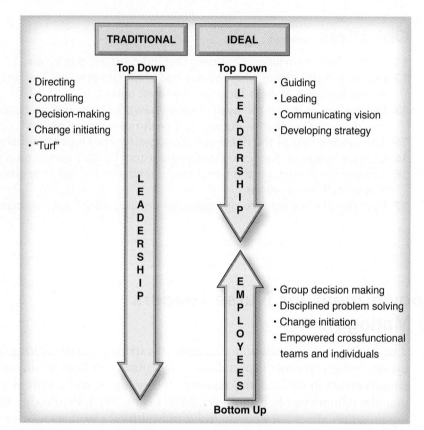

FIGURE 7.1 Becoming a more responsive organization. (Adapted with permission from Gallo, K. [2007]. The new nurse manager: A leadership development program paves the road to success. *Nurse Leader 5*[4], 28–32.)

Restructuring has shifted the organization from the traditional bureaucratic model, which at one time permeated the organization, to an emerging model that is flat, innovative, and flexible. This new model in health care organizations brings a demand for challenging new competencies for nurse leaders who may be shifting from staff nurse to nurse manager (Gallo, 2007). Figure 7.1 outlines leadership skills or competencies in an organization that is responsive to change. The employees are visible and actively involved in the organization.

Leadership in Management

Leadership plays a critical role in management. Finkelman (2006) explains that managers who develop leadership competencies are more effective and are able to manage situations better. That is, a successful manager usually exhibits effective leadership competencies.

Leadership Competencies

Jeans and Rowat (2005) reported on the findings of a study addressing the required competencies of nurse managers and the enablers and barriers affecting the acquisition and maintenance of these competencies. In this report, competencies are defined as skills, knowledge, and personal attributes. Nurse managers are defined as individuals in a first-level management position who manage nurses (and others) who provide direct care. Registered nurses (RNs), licensed practical nurses, and registered psychiatric nurses were included in the study. The main findings are listed in Box 7.1.

reflective **THINKING** Think of a nurse leader you have met or read about and whom you admire. Does this nurse leader exhibit competencies other than those identified in Box 7.1?

The following recommendations, based on the findings of the Jeans and Rowat study, are provided with the aim of improving access to and the quality of client care by strengthening the competencies and clarifying the roles of nurse managers. The recommendations are as follows:

- Health care employers should invest in frontline manager positions. Evidence suggests that a visible, knowledgeable frontline nurse manager can improve the efficiency and quality of client and family care, as well as the morale and motivation of staff.

BOX 7.1 FIRST MINISTERS' ACCORD ON HEALTH CARE RENEWAL, 2003

Altogether, 629 nurses participated in a pan-Canadian multimethod data collection approach to determine the required competencies of nurse managers. Methods used included key informant interviews, a Web-based survey, an analysis of job postings, and 10 focus group discussions. Overwhelmingly similar results through all research methods revealed the following top five competencies for nurse managers. Good nurse managers:

1. Are accountable for professional practice.
2. Communicate well verbally.
3. Build teams.
4. Have good leadership skills.
5. Are skilled at conflict resolution.

Adapted from Jeans, M. E., & Rowat, K. M. (2005). *Proposal to support the strategic plan to implement the Canadian Nursing Advisory Committee Recommendations: Leadership objective C: Competencies required of nurse managers.* Ottawa, ON: Canadian Nurses Association.

■ Employers should provide sufficient clerical and technical support to managers to allow them time to work with staff, clients, and families.

■ Health care employers should provide support for managers and potential managers to access educational programs to strengthen and increase competencies.

■ National and regional mentorship programs should be supported to ensure adequate numbers of qualified managers to sustain the health care delivery system.

■ Local educational programs should be available to support the development of competencies listed in the study.

■ Health care employers and educators should consider interdisciplinary educational programs to teach core health care management/leadership competencies. Competencies such as communication, team-building, and resource management tend to be more generic throughout the professions rather than discipline specific. In fact, several positive outcomes may result from having different health care professionals collaborate for quality care.

These recommendations strive to enable the nurse manager to acquire and sustain the needed competencies. By doing so, increased numbers of nurse managers could be developed, and the capacity and integrity of nursing in the health care system could be improved significantly (Jeans & Rowat, 2005).

In 2006, Canadian nursing leaders participated in a Nursing Leadership, Organization, and Policy Network Day. The intent was to explore workforce issues and to discuss ways to share information and opportunities for collaboration and integration so that nursing challenges could be better addressed. The participants identified the need to develop leadership competencies at all levels and in all groups of nursing positions, such as practitioners and management. Priorities included the need to invest more time and resources in developing clear leadership competencies and expectations at all levels. Another priority was to promote movement between educator, clinician, and manager roles within organizations and provide internships for nurse managers (Canadian Health Services Research Foundation [CHSRF], 2006a).

reflective **THINKING**   If you had been a nurse leader participant at the Nursing Leadership, Organization, and Policy Network Day, what would have been a priority for you regarding the development of leadership competencies?

In Canada, considerable effort is being directed from the staff nurse to the nurse manager level to improve the state of nurse leadership. The momentum must be maintained by governments, professional associations, unions, research institutes, and by employees of health care organizations as well. This collaborative effort is needed to ensure the sharing of information to address current nursing challenges.

Differences Between Managers and Leaders

The key difference between managers and leaders is that *leaders* provide visions and strategies; *managers* implement those visions and strategies. Managers coordinate and staff the organization and handle day-to-day issues, such as budgets (Langton & Robbins, 2007). Although leadership and management are related, most importantly, leadership is not necessarily tied to a position of authority. Each nurse has the responsibility to provide leadership in his or her specific areas of practice, in health care and professional organizations, and in the community (Grossman & Valiga, 2005). The nurse manager's role has developed into a complex dynamic pivotal position within health care organizations. Being a nurse manager has been declared as one of the most challenging of opportunities identified so far in the 21st century. Table 7.1 describes the evolution of the 21st century manager.

Managing Relationships

To be successful, the nurse leader needs to collaborate actively with peers and other health care professionals within the health care organization. As well, the nurse leader must reach outside the health care system to achieve successful outcomes in health care (Gottlieb & Feeley, 2006). For example, the nurse leader could be engaged with community professionals or stakeholders, such as school boards or First Nations band councils. The leader needs to persuade and influence others to move toward a higher level of functioning as members' energy and expertise are united into a cohesive whole (French, 2004).

Empowerment is the key to effective leadership. Empowering staff members with the self-confidence they need is critical to future leadership (Wieck, Prydun, & Walsh, 2002). Although the leader's values are critical, the ability to convey those values to others and achieve their commitment in the organization is equally essential.

> *reflective* **THINKING** What values do you believe are critical for nurse leaders to hold in their belief system so that they are able to build growing relationships with team members?

Establishing quality relationships among team members requires a particular set of interactive skills to encourage others to think critically, solve problems, manage conflict, focus on research-based practice, and obtain positive work outcomes (Porter-O'Grady, 2003). The nurse manager must be a coach, mentor, and a facilitator (Sullivan & Decker, 2005). Most of all, the nurse manager must be a leader who can motivate and inspire staff nurses. Effective leadership behaviours, teamed with clear management roles, are essential to build meaningful and trustworthy connections with team members and to create a quality work effectiveness that

TABLE 7.1 EVOLUTION OF THE 21ST CENTURY MANAGER		
Criteria	**Past Managers**	**Future Managers**
Primary role	Order giver, privileged elite, manipulator, controller	Facilitator, team member, teacher, advocate, sponsor, coach
Learning and knowledge	Periodic learning, narrow specialist	Continuous lifelong learning, generalist with multiple approach specialties
Compensation criteria	Time, effort, rank	Skills, results
Cultural orientation	Monocultural, monolingual	Multicultural, multilingual
Primary source of influence	Formal authority	Knowledge (technical and interpersonal)
View of people	Potential problem	Primary resource
Primary communication pattern	Vertical	Multidirectional
Decision-making style	Limited input for individual decisions	Broad-based input for joint decisions
Ethical considerations	Afterthought	Forethought
Nature of interpersonal relationships	Competitive (win-lose)	Cooperative (win-win)
Handling of power and key information	Hoard and restrict access	Share and broaden access
Approach to change	Resist	Facilitate

Adapted with permission from Kreitner, R., Kinicki, A., & Cole, N. (2007). *Fundamentals of Organizational Behaviour: Key Concepts, Skills, and Best Practices* (2nd Canadian ed., p. 6). Toronto, ON: McGraw-Hill Ryerson.

maintains a sustainable impact on quality client care. This strong partnership between nurse manager and team members is critical for an understanding of the issues that are important for staff nurses (Ferguson-Paré, 2003; Rogers, 2005). Several reports have identified the importance of nurse managers in retaining nursing staff (Kerfoot, 2000; Fletcher, 2001; Upenieks, 2003). For example, nurse managers play an integral role in creating and maintaining a high-quality health care work environment, and always nurse managers model the way for staff nurses (Shirey, 2006).

Research Identifies Supportive Behaviours

In an American study conducted by Kramer and her researchers, staff nurses identified a list of supportive role behaviours of nurse managers (Kramer et al., 2007). The nine most supportive role behaviours are identified in Box 7.2. Beyond supportive role behaviours, supporting structures and programs were identified by managers and leaders and included the following: "support from the top," peer group support, educational programs and training sessions, a "lived" culture, secretarial or administrative assistant support, private office space, and computer classes and seminars (Kramer et al., 2007).

Implications for Nurse Managers

Nurse administrators are learning from exit interviews with nursing staff who leave a position that nurse management behaviours and leadership styles directly

---

BOX 7.2 SUPPORTIVE NURSE MANAGER ROLE BEHAVIOURS

More than 2,000 U.S. staff nurses completed the Nurse Manager Support Scale. Responses were supported by semi-structured interviews and focus groups to identify the following nine *most supportive* role behaviours of nurse managers. A good nurse manager:

1. Is approachable and safe.
2. Cares.
3. "Walks the talk."
4. Motivates development of self-confidence.
5. Gives genuine feedback.
6. Provides adequate and competent staffing.
7. "Watches our back."
8. Promotes group cohesion and teamwork.
9. Resolves conflicts constructively.

Adapted from Kramer, M., Maguire, P., Schmalenberg, C., Brewer, B., Burke, R., Chmielewski, L., et al. (2007). Nurse manager support: What is it? Structures and practices that support it. *Nursing Administration Quarterly, 31*(4), 325–340.

affect job satisfaction and the desire either to stay or leave the organization (VanOyen Force, 2005). Subtle behaviours, such as caring, being friendly, and wanting to know how staff members are feeling, are tremendously important. The maintenance of a healthy work environment by nurse managers is critical for staff nurse retention.

> *reflective* **THINKING**   What does the notion of a healthy work environment mean to you?

Managing Finances

The costs of health care services are escalating dramatically each year. Consequently, the pressures to control costs are much greater in today's health care environment than they were a few years ago. The increasing complexity of the health care system requires nurse managers to plan systematically how organizational funds will be obtained, allocated, used, and controlled. The nurse manager has the primary responsibility to set goals and implement plans for the efficient use of human, material, and structural resources to meet the desired outcomes. In essence, nurse managers are expected to have extensive knowledge about the components of financial management and be able to manage the fiscal resources associated with their unit of responsibility (Finkler, Kovner, & Jones, 2007). A glossary of basic financial terminology is presented in Box 7.3.

> *reflective* **THINKING**   In examining the literature on financial management, you read that the economic success of a health care organization depends on those who are involved with service delivery. What specific aspects of your nursing strategies can effectively contribute to the economic success of the organization where you are practicing nursing?

Definition: Business Plan and Funding

Financial management comprises an overall business plan and a systematic process for funding essential activities for health care organizations and regions. Hibberd, Doody, and Hennessey (2006) state, "The plan must be based on strategic directions established by the province and must provide a seamless continuum of health services" (p. 694). The plan, which is similar in most health care organizations, must ensure that core health services are available, accessible, and affordable.

BOX 7.3 BASIC FINANCIAL TERMINOLOGY

Revenue—Income generated through various means, such as government grants, personal and corporate donations to the organization, and parking fees.

Budget—A detailed financial plan of the proposed expenditures for a given period of time found in most health care organizations.

Operating budget—A financial plan for the day-to-day activities of the organization, including income (revenue, if any) and expenses encountered through daily operation.

Capital budget—A financial plan related to the purchase of major capital items such as equipment.

Statistical budget—A statistical statement to accompany the operating budget, it is compiled and summarized based on the previous year's operation, and its purpose is to help in the formulation of projections for the next fiscal year.

Variance—The difference between budgeted and actual amounts spent to achieve a service or activity.

Variance analysis—A comparison of actual results to the budget, followed by an examination to determine why variances occurred.

Cost centre—An organizational unit for which costs can be identified and managed (a patient care unit, for example).

Elements of Financial Management

According to Baker and Baker (2006), the four major elements of financial management are as follows:

1. *Planning:* It is imperative that data is gathered from the environment. Assessment includes obtaining an inventory of current health programs and services offered in the region. The health care needs of the population must also be considered (Yoder-Wise, 2007). Next, the objectives and goals compiled must be reassessed in light of the organization's mission statement. Human (staffing), material (supplies), and structural (equipment) resources are prioritized and taken into consideration for developing the budget. The budget becomes a tool for planning and controlling financial resources (Hibberd, Doody, & Hennessey, 2006).

2. *Controlling:* Controlling involves the assurance that the plan and strategies that have been developed are being followed as formulated. It is critical, prior to implementation, to recognize which strategies are financially sound. Next, reports of actual performance compared with the projected budget are reviewed. The difference between the performance and the budget allocated is the variance. Variances can be positive (budget surplus) or negative (budget deficit) (Yoder-Wise, 2007). The variance analysis, which is the comparison of actual results as compared with the budget, followed by investigation to determine why variances occurred, is the major control process (Finkler, Kovner, & Jones, 2007).

3. *Organizing/directing:* This element relates to the nurse manager's role in using human, material, and structural resources to best advantage. As an example of human resource management, nurse managers who establish a staffing plan can then assess the degree to which it is in compliance with safe client care on a daily, weekly, or monthly basis (Baker & Baker, 2006). Consultations with the human resource department, nursing administration, medical staff, maintenance, and housekeeping can be a valuable asset to carry out functions of planning and controlling.

4. *Decision making:* For each of these elements, the processes of analysis and evaluation are critical. Feedback is obtained regularly so that activities can be adjusted to maintain efficient operations (Yoder-Wise, 2007). It is important to select the best alternative so that objectives and goals are met.

These elements present a framework by which essential activities on the unit can be controlled by the nurse manager. Box 7.4 presents an overview of the elements. Due to spiralling health care expenditures, nurse managers must expect to find ways to manage, or reduce, costs while maintaining, or enhancing, the quality of health care and services (Baker & Baker, 2006).

---

reflective **THINKING** Assess a personal budget you have set for a 2-week period to determine the variance. What do you conclude when you compare the actual results with the 2-week budget?

BOX 7.4 ELEMENTS OF FINANCIAL MANAGEMENT

Planning
- Assess the health care needs of the environment.
- Establish objectives and goals.
- Prioritize resources.
- Develop a budget.

Controlling
- Follow established strategies.
- Review variance reports.

Organizing and Directing
Use resources to best advantage.

Decision Making
Analyze and evaluate each element to select the best alternative.

Adapted from Baker, J. J., & Baker, R. W. (2006). *Health care finance: Basic tools for financial managers* (2nd ed.). Toronto, ON: Jones & Bartlett.

Processing a Budget: Definition and Types

Nurse managers are designated to prepare a budget for their cost centre. They are held accountable for the costs incurred and have the responsibility to control these costs. Generally, a budget is a realistic detailed financial plan that provides formal quantitative expressions of proposed expenditures for a given time period (Finkler, Kovner, & Jones, 2007). Budgets usually follow a predictable annual pattern and are prepared for the fiscal year, which typically begins April 1 and ends March 31. Budgets begin with direct communication from Provincial Health Departments announcing guidelines by which Regional Health Authorities (RHAs) must prepare their budgets. Within the RHA, the budget process is delegated to the finance director, who identifies and interacts with the managers responsible for the various cost centres. Budgets are based on a combination of past activity and current and future trends (Hibberd, Doody, & Hennessey, 2006). The budget for an entire organization is known as a master budget. The budgets prepared at each cost centre by nurse managers become integral parts of the master budget.

To develop their budget, nurse managers must clearly define their objectives, then identify and list the essential activities and resources needed to meet those objectives. As a planning tool, the budget enables managers to determine expenditures, establish priorities, and implement better decisions in the process of providing specific services (Sullivan & Decker, 2005). The budget types that are most familiar to nurse managers include capital and operating budgets.

Capital Budgets

Capital budgets include plans for the costs of major purchases (Danna, 2006). They deal with cost outlays, such as maintenance, renovation, improvements, and remodelling. Usually, the capital equipment budget includes items that cost more than $1,000 or have an expected lifespan longer than 3 to 5 years (Hibberd, Doody, & Hennessey, 2006).

Most frequently, nurse managers of cost centres are involved in preparing capital equipment budgets. For example, they might receive requests from other professional health team members for new equipment. Some of these requests are considered essential for safe operation or for specialized service for a client (Sullivan & Decker, 2005). Generally speaking, the request for new equipment should be accompanied with as much information as possible, especially regarding the importance and urgency of its purchase.

Operating Budgets

The *operating budget* is the financial plan for the daily activities of a cost centre. It consists of statements of revenue and expenses (Yoder-Wise, 2007). Revenue consists mainly of grants from the provincial or territorial government. Meanwhile, *direct expenses* include the costs of providing service; *indirect expenses* are for items such as phones that are not directly related to patient care (Haviley, 2003). Examples of direct expenses include the cost of staffing and supplies, such as drugs and oxygen and medical and surgical items (Hibberd, Doody, & Hennessey, 2006). Another example of direct expenses associated with patient care in a cost centre is salaries. Box 7.5 highlights some staffing costs based on bed allocation, numbers of client days, and average hours of nursing care.

The accounting guidelines for developing operating budgets were drawn up through the collaborative efforts of the federal, provincial/territorial, and health care associations. The management information systems (MIS) standards (formerly MIS guidelines) are followed by most health care organizations. They provide a standardized framework for the collection and reporting of daily financial and statistical data on the operations of health service organizations across the continuum of care. The functions of MIS specify what data to collect to facilitate more informed management decisions (Canadian Institute for Health Information, 2007). Workload measurement systems (WMS) are key components of the MIS standards for determining nursing resource intensity. Because of the many ways to measure nursing workload, the MIS standards provide a framework for collecting and reporting nursing workload data, thereby enabling nurse managers to compare information as needed (Canadian Nurses Association [CNA], 2003).

According to the MIS standards, supplies are divided into various categories, such as drugs, medical and surgical supplies, laundry and linen, and printing and office supplies. Supplies usually represent about 20% of the total operating budget (Hibberd, Doody, & Hennessey, 2006). The nurse manager should carefully review all actual costs incurred during the previous year and adjust those amounts affected by such factors as workload changes and inflation. Changes may be influenced by patient acuity, bed closures, and new physicians. A new physician can affect a change in the cost centre simply by admitting clients who require a higher level of care.

Such a change in the intensity of care will undoubtedly result in increased usage of more costly drugs and higher demands for medical–surgical supplies. For example, if all other factors, such as occupancy rate and the number of beds, remain constant, then the nurse manager must make an adjustment only for inflation. If the inflation rate is estimated at 4.5% and the actual cost of the previous year was $324,000, the projected costs for the budget year's supplies would be $338,580 ($324,000 × 1.045). Table 7.2 highlights an allocation of cost supplies with an estimated rate of inflation of 4.5%.

Implications for Nurse Managers

According to Barker, Sullivan, and Emery (2006), significant pressure to decrease overall health care expenditures will continue to prevail in health care

| BOX 7.5 | STAFFING BUDGET FOR A 20-BED SURGICAL UNIT IN A MANITOBA HEALTH CARE CENTRE |

Prerequisites

Occupancy rate (OR) is ratio of occupied beds (patient days) to the total no. of beds on the unit

$$OR = \frac{\text{actual no. of occupied beds}}{\text{total no. of beds on the unit}}$$

Potential (P) for the number of client days possible on the unit is the number of beds multiplied by no. of days in the year

$$P = \text{no. of beds} \times \text{no. of days in year}$$
$$= 20 \times 365$$
$$= 7{,}300 \text{ client days}$$

Anticipated changes during next fiscal year

Assume patient population and surgical programs remain unchanged

Patient activity, acuity, and bed usage

During the previous fiscal year, the actual no. of patient days was 6,900.

$$ADO = \frac{6{,}900}{365} = 18.9 \text{ occupied beds per day}$$

Average daily occupancy (ADO) is the number of patient days divided by 365, and ADO (%) is patient days in the year divided by no. of beds × 365.

$$ADO\ (\%) = \frac{6{,}900}{20 \times 365} = \frac{6{,}900}{7{,}300}$$
$$= 0.945 = 94.5\%$$

Determination of the number of full time equivalents (FTEs) required

Institutions carefully determine the number of hours of service that each patient should receive. For this example, that figure has been set at 5.25 hours per 24-hr period.

No. of FTEs =
$$\frac{\text{no. of beds occupied} \times \text{hrs of care per patient per 24 hr} \times 365}{\text{No. of earned hrs per FTE*}}$$

$$= \frac{18.4 \times 5.25 \times 365}{2{,}015}$$

$$= \frac{35259}{2{,}015} = 17.49 \text{ or } 17.5$$

(box continues on page 180)

BOX 7.5   STAFFING BUDGET FOR A 20-BED SURGICAL UNIT IN A MANITOBA HEALTH CARE CENTRE (continued)

Average staffing pattern	Assume staff mix on staff is: BNs = 75% and RNs = 25% Parameters: ■ Must provide 5.25 hours of direct care to 20 patients ■ Must adhere to the negotiated salary from a collective agreement	The 17.5 FTEs needed would consist of: BNs: $0.75 \times 17.5 = 13.125$ or 13 1/8 RNs: $0.25 \times 17.5 = 4.375$ or 4 3/8 No. shifts/day = $(5.25 \times 20) \div 7.75$ = $105 \div 7.75$ = 13.55 shifts/day
Salary needs	BNs @ $36.04/hr RNs @ $33.54/hr	13.125 BNs required $\times$ $36.04/hr $\times$ 2,015 hrs/yr. = $13.125 \times \$36.04 \times 2,015 =$ $ 953,145.37 4.375 RNs required $\times$ $33.54/hr $\times$ 2,015 hrs/yr = $4.375 \times 33.54 \times 2,015 =$ $ 295, 676.06 Total budgetary needs for salaries† $1,248,821.14

*The Manitoba Nurses Union has stated that the regular hours of work for full-time nurses will be 7.75 hours per day and 2,015 hours per year (Manitoba Nurses Union, 2004, Article 1401).

†The full complement of FTEs calculated above has not made allowance for relief staff used during vacations and staff illness.

BN, Bachelor of Nursing degree; RN, registered nurse.

TABLE 7.2   SUPPLY COSTS WITH INFLATION AT 4.5%

Supplies	Expenditures ($) in Year 2009	Estimated Expenditures ($) in Year 2010
Drugs	175,000	182,875
Medical surgical supplies	130,000	135,850
Printing and office supplies	19,000	19,855
Totals	324,000	338,580

> ### Reflections on Leadership Practice
>
> *Y*ou have been hired as a nurse manager for a medical unit. In reviewing the budget, you notice that the medical supplies have been in excess of the budget by 25% during the last 2 months. You decide to ask for staff input into ways of decreasing the use of such supplies. What steps might you take to proceed in this process of cost containment?

organizations as a result of spiralling health care costs. It is important that nurse managers have a basic working knowledge of the elements of financial management and the development of a budget. Rising health costs, cost-management efforts, and increasing accountability together serve as a strong impetus for nurse managers to learn the fundamentals of the budgeting process (Danna, 2006). When nurse managers undertake budgetary accountability, they dramatically increase their responsibility realm in the areas of predicting, planning, and presenting budgets to management.

Managing Staff

Hospital restructuring has resulted in significant organizational changes. The move toward cost-effectiveness has created dramatic changes in the work environment. Changes include reductions both in management and in nursing staff (O'Brien-Pallas, Thomson, Alksnis, & Bruce, 2001). As a result, nurses voice concerns about unmanageable workloads and an inability to provide quality care in accord with personal and professional standards (O'Brien-Pallas & Baumann, 2000). Nurse staffing decisions, it has been realized, do make a critical difference to clients and their families in health outcomes.

Nursing Staffing and Client Outcomes

According to Dechant (2006), nurse staffing is the process used to determine the acceptable number and skill mix of nurses and personnel needed to meet the care needs of clients and their families in various health care settings. During the last decade, a significant number of studies has concentrated on the relationship between nurse staff levels and client outcomes and safety (Tourangeau et al., 2006; MacPhee, Ellis, & Sanchez McCutcheon, 2006; McGillis Hall, Doran, & Pink, 2004; Needleman, Buerhaus, Mattke, Stewart, & Zelevinsky, 2002). After synthesizing the findings, a prevalent conclusion emerged: staffing plans should maximize the proportion of RNs in their staff mix. Spilsbury and Meyer (2001) reviewed the literature that addressed the connection between nursing staff and quality of care. They found strong evidence to support the claim that care by RNs makes a quality difference to client outcomes. However, due to insufficient evidence on a related matter, the authors were unable to draw conclusions regarding the most effective staff mix.

> **reflective THINKING**   What do you think are some of the benefits available to clients as a result of a high proportion of RNs in the staff mix on a surgical unit?

A report by the Canadian Health Service Research Foundation (CHSRF), *Staffing for Safety: A Synthesis of the Evidence on Nursing Staffing and Patient Safety*, focused on the state of evidence regarding the relationship between nurse staffing and client safety. The synthesis integrated the findings of the 2005 research report *Evaluation of Patient Safety and Nurse Staffing* compiled by Sanchez McCutcheon et al. (2006) with the results of a February 2006 decision-maker roundtable hosted by the CHSRF (2006b). The five recommendations in this synthesis are aimed at encouraging evidence-informed decision making around nurse staffing issues. One recommendation states that patients should be cared for by experienced nurses. Experience can be viewed as the number of years a nurse has been in practice, the particular expertise the nurse has acquired, or the familiarity a nurse has, either in a particular care setting, or with a specific client population. Another recommendation urged that patients should be cared for by highly educated nurses and that employers should strive to have as many baccalaureate-prepared RNs as possible on their staff.

Nursing Staffing and Staff/Organizational Outcomes

Studies of nursing staffing influences on staff outcomes have been conducted. Rogers, Hwang, Scott, Aiken, and Dinges (2004) examined the work patterns of hospital staff nurses and endeavoured to determine whether a relationship exists between hours worked and the frequency of errors. They found that the likelihood of making errors increased as the number of hours worked increased. In particular, the odds of making an error were three times higher when RNs worked shifts 12.5 hours or longer.

In another study, O'Brien-Pallas et al. (2004) found that units with productivity/utilization levels exceeding 80% had high nurse absenteeism and low nurse job satisfaction. Units with productivity/utilization levels exceeding 83% had nurses who had a high intent to leave.

In an international sample of hospitals, Aiken, Clarke, and Sloane (2002) examined the effects of nurse staffing and organizational support for nursing care on nurses' job dissatisfaction, nurse burnout, and quality of client care as reported by RNs. One of their principal findings was that in all five jurisdictions, 38.3% to 48.1% of RNs reported job dissatisfaction, and 32.9% to 54.2% stated they experienced burnout. Another finding dealing with staffing and organizations was that in hospitals with lower staffing and weak organizational support, RNs were three times more likely to report low-quality care than RNs in hospitals with higher staffing and strong organizational support. McGillis Hall et al. (2001) concluded that a higher proportion of regulated nursing staff was associated with higher nurse job satisfaction. Regarding organizations, Estabrooks, Midodzi, Cummings, Ricker, and Giovannetti (2005) found that health care organizations with higher proportions of baccalaureate-prepared nurses were associated with lower 30-day patient mortality rates (patients dying within 30 days of hospital admission).

> *reflective* **THINKING** Review the staffing plan on your unit. What is the staff mix? What do you think should remain the same or be changed regarding staffing patterns?

Evaluation Framework for Nursing Staff Mix

The national associations of the regulated nurses groups (CNA, Canadian Practical Nurses Association, Canadian Council of Practical Nurse Regulators, and the Registered Psychiatric Nurses of Canada) have formed a strong collaboration to advocate for the evaluation of nursing staff mix decisions on clients, nurses, and the health care organization (CNA, 2005a). The evaluation framework is based on the examination of relevant literature pertaining to staff mix decisions and their outcomes. Three of the principles that guide this framework are as follows:

- Client and family, nurse, and system outcomes are central to the evaluation of nursing staff mix decisions.
- Evaluation framework recognizes and respects the value and contribution of each regulated nursing group.
- Evaluation of the impact of nursing staff mix decisions is complex and requires a comprehensive and systematic approach using all components of this framework. (CNA, 2005b).

This evaluation collaborative framework is available on the CNA's Website (www.cna-aiic.ca).

> *reflective* **THINKING** After reviewing the evaluation framework on the CNA's Website, describe how this framework can promote client safety.

Implications for Nurse Managers

According to the CNA (2005a), health care providers, policymakers, administrators, educators, researchers, regulators, and employers must work together to ensure that Canadians receive safe and effective care. Nurse leaders can do much, both individually and collectively, to ensure that nursing staff-mix decisions are made in the best interest of nurses, clients, and families. Nurses should use evidence-based documents, such as the CNA position statement, to assess their work environments and advocate for constructive change (MacPhee, Ellis, & Sanchez McCutcheon, 2006). Research indicates that one of the issues central to ensuring the best client outcomes is to determine the right mix of care providers for the client population (CNA, 2004).

McGillis Hall, Doran, and Pink (2004) state that efforts must be made by unit managers to balance both the experience level and the mix of nursing staff to ensure that quality client outcomes are not compromised in efforts to reduce costs. In making staffing decisions, nurse managers must ensure that staffing is adequately matched to the needs of clients and their families. The importance of nurse management practices that actually increase nurses' professional autonomy must be emphasized. Such practices include shared governance, continuous learning, promotion and advancement, and flexible scheduling. These practices promote a culture of respect and collaboration, and they support nurses who engage in making decisions that influence client care (Apker, Zabava Ford, & Fox, 2003).

In regard to staffing initiatives, several evidence-based staffing initiatives have been recommended by the Canadian Federation of Nurses Unions in their report *Taking Steps Forward: Retaining and Valuing Experienced Nurses* (Wortsman & Janowitz, 2006). A few of these recommendations focus on respect and recognition for nursing, flexible scheduling, work arrangements, and workplace practices.

According to MacPhee, Ellis, and Sanchez McCutcheon (2006), nurse staffing initiatives should be linked to effective leadership. Doran et al. (2004) examined the relationship between leadership, span of control, and outcomes as measured by job satisfaction, client satisfaction, and unit turnover. They concluded that transformational leadership style was a significant predictor of nurses' job satisfaction and unit turnover. Transformational leaders provide staff with encouragement, open communication, positive feedback, support, and individual consideration. Nurse managers who use the transformational leadership style generate work environments characterized by teamwork and fewer interpersonal conflicts. These findings on the effect of transformational leadership style correspond with the evidence reported by other investigators (Bakker, Killmer, Siegriest, & Schaufeli, 2000; Stordeur, D'Hoore, & Vandenberghe, 2001).

reflective **THINKING** Assume you are a nurse manager using a transformational leadership style on a palliative care unit and an angry family comes to see you, stating that their mother is not receiving the care she needs. How would handle the situation?

A study by McGillis Hall et al. (2006) explored nurse staffing decision-making processes, supports in place for nurses, nurse's workload being experienced, and perceptions of nursing care and outcomes in Canada. Four key themes emerged (see Box 7.6). Controversial issues in the area of nursing WMSs are ongoing in health care organizations. Hadley, Graham, and Flannery (2004) used a pan-Canadian approach to compile a report called *Assess Use, Compliance and Efficacy Nursing Workload Measurement Tools*. Findings from the survey focus

---

BOX 7.6 KEY THEMES: POLICY AND PRACTICE RELATED TO CANADIAN NURSING WORKLOADS

Staffing Principles and Framework

Managers and nurse leaders should use existing resources (principles and frameworks that exist when making staff decisions in relation to the context of quality patient care) to test the effectiveness of nurse staffing decisions in their institutions in relation to patients, system, and nurse outcomes.

Nursing Workload Measurement System

It is apparent that problems exist with the reliability, validity, and utility of the nursing Workload Measurement System. Managers must take a leadership role in the next steps in nursing workload measurement. These steps include clarifying a commitment to the measurement of nursing workload in Canada and determining what data should be collected and for what purpose.

Standardized Nurse-to-Patient Ratios

Solid evidence to support the effectiveness of standardized ratios as a mechanism to provide frontline nurses with protection from high workloads and an opportunity to quantify nursing care does not yet exist. However, it is important for nursing leadership organizations and policy makers to monitor this area closely and remain current on any new information that emerges and to be proactive in the debate.

Uptake of the Evidence on Nurse Staffing

Despite a number of research syntheses that have identified the need for implementing effective mechanisms for nurse staffing, little or no policy or practice action has been taken. Nurse staffing is one of the few areas in health care in Canada where evidence is ignored in decision making. A knowledge translation strategy that outlines the importance of evidence on nurse staffing models needs to be developed by nurse leaders in collaboration with practitioners, stakeholders, and policy makers. This strategy must be clearly linked to patient safety and outcomes.

Adapted from McGillis Hall, L., Pink, L., Lalonde, M., Tomblin Murphy, G., O'Brien-Pallas, L., Spence Laschinger, H. K., et al. (2006). Decision making for nurse staffing: Canadian perspectives. *Policy, Politics, & Nursing Practice*, 7(4), 261–269.

groups and key informants were consistent with the information gathered through the literature review.

Participants repeatedly reported dissatisfaction with the WMS tool. It is timely that nurse managers do examine the required steps in nursing workload measurement to be certain the tool is understood by staff nurses and that they be given time to input the data. The WMS helps nurse managers decide where to allocate nurses on the unit (CNA, 2003). Nurse-to-patient ratios have been a contentious, but valid, issue for many nurses and nurse managers. The extensive amounts of attention and discussion that have arisen have resulted in the possibility of mandatory nurse-to-patient ratios. Ellis and Clements (2006) state that there may be benefits to nurse-to-patient ratios, but it must be noted that current evidence for their effectiveness is inconclusive.

As a matter of interest, the State of California has legislated specific numerical licensed nurse-to-patient ratios in acute care hospitals. Upenieks, Akhavan, Kotlerman, Esser, and Ngo (2007) conducted a study to examine the relative amounts of time allocated to workload activities among RNs to thoroughly understand the implications of the California regulatory staffing ratios on nursing units. They concluded that it is easier to mandate prescribed ratios and consider staffing situations optimal because the "numbers" are being met. However, the process of care needs to be examined and data gathered in situations where processes may not be optimally supporting the staff and/or clients. Based on the data obtained, improvements can then be made to ensure safe and quality client care. In Canada, nurse managers must continue to dialogue and try to determine whether nurse-to-patient ratios would, in fact, be an effective means to improve client safety.

reflective **THINKING** You are to go to an administrative meeting in a few hours to discuss the benefits and disadvantages of nurse-to-patient ratios. Comment briefly on what specifically you see as a benefit and what you see as a disadvantage.

Challenges for Nurse Managers

Some observers point to a serious problem arising with nurse managers. Currently, intense job-related demands often result in stress, affecting job performance and personal well-being. Nurse managers are caught between the work expectations of senior management and the personal and professional desires of nursing staff (Laschinger, Almost, Purdy, & Kim, 2004). For instance, nurse managers are expected to do more with fewer resources while maintaining quality standards and, at the same time, encourage staff to remain in the organization

(Judkins, Massey, & Huff, 2006). Nurse managers play an essential role in providing leadership for managing change, cultural integration, morale, and staff performance. According to Morash, Brintnell, and Lemire Rodger (2005), nurse managers play a critical role in the delivery of health care, particularly within nursing services. Technology, research, and innovation can improve working processes and working conditions. In fact, good working conditions are essential to attracting and retaining highly qualified staff (Sanchez McCutcheon et al., 2006). Support for the professional practice of nurse managers should be a stated priority in health care organizations (Laschinger, Purdy, & Almost, 2007).

reflective **THINKING** In what ways can nurse managers see technology improving the nursing workload? The nursing shortage?

Leadership Development for Managers

The need for nurses to take strong positions on health care and societal issues and to provide effective leadership within organizations and the profession is essential. Clearly, leadership is essential for management effectiveness (Scoble & Russell, 2003). Leadership development should not be left to chance, but it should be recognized as an area of study. That is, the acquisition of knowledge, competencies, and attitudes associated with leadership must be given front and centre attention at the basic level (French, 2004). Meanwhile, at the graduate level, all students should acquire advanced preparation in leadership and management specific to their area of interest. Gallo (2007) states that health care organizations should provide learning environments sufficiently well appointed to complement formal postgraduate education. For example, the concept of action learning is an exciting and valuable approach to individual and organizational development for nurse managers. It promotes a learning environment in which the new nurse manager has the opportunity to work in a team and apply knowledge and skills acquired from internal experts and formal education to confront substantive organizational challenges.

Leadership Issue

Examine the leadership development program that is operational in the facility where you are in clinical practice. What are the benefits of this model? In what ways will the program facilitate the development of your leadership competencies?

Today, most health care organizations have some type of leadership or management development program. These programs must continue to be strategic organizational endeavours designed to develop highly competent nurse managers with strong leadership competencies. Development is needed, for example, in core management areas, particularly human resource management skills such as budgeting, staffing, and staff development (Loo & Thorpe, 2003). These competencies need to be harnessed and promoted to the utmost so that nurse managers can be as successful as possible in their multidimensional roles. Grohar-Murray and Dicroce (2003) state that given the increase in diverse and complex nursing care, coupled with the myriad social and professional factors—the nurse manager role is, and will continue to be, the most challenging role in any industry.

WEBSITES

■ The Management Information System (MIS) Standards

http://secure.cihi.ca/cihiweb/dispPage.jsp?cw_page=mis_e

The MIS Standards provide a standardized framework for collecting and reporting financial and statistical data on the day-to-day operations of health service organizations.

■ Quality Management

http://www.intelex.com/

Intelex's Quality Management Software is a 100% Web-based highly configurable quality management system that helps organizations track, analyze, and report on quality management initiatives, including product defect tracking, supplier management, and corporate objectives and activities.

■ Canadian Health Services Research Foundation (CHSRF)

http://www.chsrf.ca/

The CHSRF supports the evidence-informed management of Canada's health care system by facilitating knowledge transfer and exchange—bridging the gap between research and health care management and policy.

REFERENCES

Aiken, L. H., Clarke, S. P., & Sloane, D. M. (2002). Nurse staffing: Inadequate nurse staffing and poor organizational support affect patient safety globally. *International Journal for Quality in Health Care, 14*(1), 5–13.

Apker, J., Zabava Ford, W., & Fox, D. (2003). Predicting nurses' organizational and professional identification: The effect of nursing roles, professional autonomy, and supportive communication. *Nursing Economics, 21*(5), 226–233.

Barker, A. M., Sullivan, D. T., & Emery, M. J. (2006). *Leadership competencies for clinical managers: The renaissance of transformational leadership.* Toronto, ON: Jones and Bartlett.

Baker, J. J., & Baker, R. W. (2006). *Health care finance: Basic tools for non-financial managers* (2nd ed.). Toronto, ON: Jones and Bartlett.

Bakker, B., Killmer, C., Siegriest, J., & Schaufeli, W. (2000). Effort-reward imbalance and burnout among nurses. *Journal of Advanced Nursing, 31*(4), 884–891.

Canadian Health Services Research Foundation. (2006a). *Looking forward, working together: Priorities for nursing leadership in Canada.* Ottawa, ON: CHSRF. Retrieved November 2007 from http://www.chsrf.ca

Canadian Health Services Research Foundation. (2006b). *Staffing for safety: A synthesis of the evidence on nurse staffing and patient safety.* Ottawa, ON: CHSRF. Retrieved November 2007 from http://www.chsrf.ca

Canadian Institute for Health Information. (2007). *MIS Standards, 2006.* Ottawa, ON: CIHI. Retrieved November 2007 from http://secure.cihi.ca/

Canadian Nurses Association. (2003). Measuring nurses' workload. *Nursing Now, 15,* March, 1–4.

Canadian Nurses Association. (2004). *Nurse staff mix: A literature review.* Ottawa, ON: Author.

Canadian Nurses Association. (2005a). Nursing staff mix: A key link to patient safety. *Nursing Now, 19,* January, 1–5.

Canadian Nurses Association. (2005b). *Evaluation Framework to determine the impact of nursing staff mix decisions*. Ottawa, ON: Author.

Cummings, G., & Estabrooks, C. A. (2003). The effects of hospital restructuring that included lay-offs on individual nurses who remained employed: A systematic review of impact. *International Journal of Sociology and Social Policy, 23*(8/9), 8–53.

Danna, D. (2006). Principles of budgeting. In L. Roussel, R. C. Swansburg, & R. J. Swansburg (Eds.), *Management and leadership for nurse administrators* (4th ed., pp. 272–307). Toronto, ON: Jones and Bartlett.

Dechant, G. M. (2006). Human resource allocation: Staffing and scheduling. In J. M. Hibberd, & D. L. Smith (Eds.), *Nursing leadership and management in Canada* (3rd ed., pp. 625–647). Toronto, ON: Elsevier Mosby.

Doran, D., Sanchez McCutcheon, A., Evans, M., MacMillan, K., McGillis, L., Pringle, D., et al. (2004). *Impact of the manager's span of control on leadership and performance*. Ottawa, ON: Canadian Health Services Research Foundation. Retrieved November 2007 from http://www.chsrf.ca

Ellis, J., & Clements, D. (2006). Nurse staffing and patient safety: Ratios and beyond. *Healthcare Quarterly, 9*(3), 18–20.

Estabrooks, C. A., Midodzi, W. K., Cummings, G. G., Ricker, K. L., & Giovannetti, P. (2005). The impact of hospital nursing characteristics on 30-day mortality. *Nursing Research, 54*(2), 74–84.

Ferguson-Paré, M. (2003). What is leadership in nursing administration? *Nursing Leadership, 16*(1), 35–37.

Finkelman, A. W. (2006). *Leadership and management in nursing*, Upper Saddle River, NJ: Pearson Prentice Hall.

Finkler, S. A., Kovner, C. T., & Bland Jones, C. (2007). *Financial management for nurse managers and executives* (3rd ed.). St. Louis, MO: Saunders Elsevier.

Fletcher, C. (2001). Hospital RNs' job satisfactions and dissatisfactions. *Journal of Nursing Administration, 31*(6), 324–331.

French, S. (2004). Challenges to developing and providing nursing leadership. *Nursing Leadership, 17*(4), 37–40.

Gallo, K. (2007). The new nurse manager: A leadership development program paves the road to success. *Nurse Leader, 5*(4), 28–32.

Gottlieb, L. N., Feeley, N., & Dalton, C. (2006). *The collaborative partnership approach to care: A delicate balance*. Toronto, ON: Elsevier Canada.

Grohar-Murray, M. E., & DiCroce, H. R. (2003). *Leadership and management in nursing* (3rd ed.). Upper Saddle River, NJ: Pearson Education.

Grossman, S.C., & Valiga, T.M. (2005). *The new leadership challenge: Creating the future of nursing* (2nd ed.). Philadelphia: F. A. Davis.

Hadley, F., Graham, K., & Flannery, M. (2004). *Workforce management objective A: Workload measurement tools*. Ottawa, ON: Canadian Nurses Association. Retrieved November 2007 from http://www.cna-nurses.ca/

Haviley, C. (2003). Budget concepts for patient care. In P. Kelly-Heidenthal (Ed.), *Nursing leadership & management* (pp. 217–237). New York: Thomson Delmar Learning.

Hibberd, J. M., Doody, L. M., & Hennessey, M. (2006). Business planning and budget preparation. In J. M. Hibberd & D. L. Smith (Eds.), *Nursing leadership and management in Canada* (3rd ed., pp. 691–714). Toronto, ON: Elsevier Canada.

Jeans, M. E., & Rowat, K. M. (2005). *Proposal to support the strategic plan to implement the Canadian Nursing Advisory Committee Recommendations: Leadership objective competencies required of nurse managers*. Ottawa, ON: Canadian Nurses Association.

Judkins, S., Massey, C., & Huff, B. (2006). Hardiness, stress, and use of ill-time among nurse managers: Is there a connection? *Nursing Economics, 24*(4), 187–192.

Kerfoot, K. (2000). On leadership: The leader as a retention specialist. *Nursing Economics 18*(4), 216–218.

Kramer, M., Maguire, P., Schmalenberg, C., Brewer, B., Burke, R., Chmielewski, L., et al. (2007). Nurse manager support: What is it? Structures and practices that support it. *Nursing Administration Quarterly, 31*(4), 325–340.

Langton, N., & Robbins, S. P. (2007). *Fundamentals of organizational behaviour* (3rd Canadian ed.). Toronto, ON: Pearson Education Canada.

Laschinger, H. K. S., Almost, J., Purdy, N., & Kim, J. (2004). Predictors of nurse managers' health in Canadian restructured healthcare settings. *Nursing Leadership, 17*(4), 88–105.

Laschinger, H. K. S., Purdy, N., & Almost, J. (2007). The impact of leader-member exchange quality, empowerment, and core self-evaluation on nurse manager's job satisfaction. *Journal of Nursing Administration, 37*(5), 221–229.

Lemire Rodger, G. (2006). Canadian nurses association. In M. McIntyre, E. Thomlinson, & C. McDonald (Eds.), *Realities of Canadian nursing: Professional, practice, and power issues* (2nd ed., pp. 133–151). Philadelphia: Lippincott Williams & Wilkins.

Loo, R., & Thorpe, K. (2003). A Delphi study forecasting management training and development for first-line nurse managers. *Journal of Management Development, 22*(9), 824–834.

MacPhee, M., Ellis, J., & Sanchez McCutcheon, A. (2006). Nurse staffing and patient safety. *Canadian Nurse, 102*(8), 19–23.

Manitoba Nurses Union. (2007). *Nurse salaries: Central salary scale.* Winnipeg: MNU. Retrieved November 2007 from http://www.nursesunion.mb.ca/

McGillis Hall, L., Doran, D., & Pink, G. H. (2004). Nurse staffing models, nursing hours, and patient safety outcomes. *Journal of Nursing Administration, 34*(1), 41–45.

McGillis Hall, L., Irvine Doran, D., Baker, G. R., Pink, G. H., Sidani, S., O'Brien-Pallas, L., et al. (2001). *A study of the impact of nursing staff mix models and organizational change strategies on patient, system and nurse outcomes: A summary report of the nursing staff mix outcomes study.* Toronto, ON: Faculty of Nursing, University of Toronto.

McGillis Hall, L., Pink, L., Lalonde, M., Tomblin Murphy, G., O'Brien-Pallas, L., Spence Laschinger, H. K., et al. (2006). Decision making for nurse staffing: Canadian perspectives. *Policy, Politics, & Nursing Practice, 7*(4), 261–269.

Morash, R., Brintnell, J., & Lemire Rodger, G. (2005). A span of control tool for clinical managers. *Nursing Research, 18*(3), 83–89.

Needleman, J., Buerhaus, P., Mattke, S., Stewart, M., & Zelevinsky, K. (2002). Nurse-staffing levels and the quality of care in hospitals. *New England Journal of Medicine, 346*(22), 1715–1722.

O'Brien-Pallas, L., & Baumann, A. (2000). Towards evidence based policy decisions: A case study of nursing human resources in Ontario, Canada. *Nursing Inquiry, 7*(4), 248–257.

O'Brien-Pallas, L., Irvine Doran, D., Murray, M., Cockerill, R., Sidani, S., Laurie Shaw, B., et al. (2002). Evaluation of a client care delivery model, part 2: Variability in nursing utilization in community home nursing. *Nursing Economics, 20*(1), 13–21, 36.

O'Brien-Pallas, L., Thomson, D., Alksnis, C, & Bruce, S. (2001). The economic impact of nurse staffing decisions: Time to turn down another road? *Hospital Quarterly, 4*(3), 42–50.

Patrick, A., & Laschinger, H. K. S. (2006). The effect of structural empowerment and perceived organizational support on middle level nurse managers' role satisfaction. *Journal of Nursing Management, 14*(1), 13–22.

Porter-O'Grady, T. (2003). A different age for leadership, part 1: New context, new content. *Journal of Nursing Administration, 33*(2), 105–110.

Rogers, A. E., Hwang, W.-T., Scott, L. D., Aiken, L. H., & Dinges, D. F. (2004). The working hours of hospital staff nurses and patient safety. *Health Affairs, 23*(4), 202–212.

Rogers, L. G. (2005). Why trust matters: The nurse manager-staff nurse relationship. *Journal of Nursing Administration 35*(10), 421–423.

Sanchez McCutcheon, A., MacPhee, M., Davidson, J. M., Doyle-Waters., Mason, S., & Winslow, W. (2005). *Evaluation of patient safety and nurse staffing*, Ottawa, ON: Canadian Health Services Research Foundation.

Scoble, K. B., & Russell, G. (2003). Vision 2020, Part 1: Profile of the future nurse leader. *Journal of Nursing Administration, 33*(6), 324–330.

Shirey, M. R. (2006). Stress and coping in nurse managers: Two decades of research. *Nursing Economics, 24*(4), 193–203, 211.

Spilsbury, K., & Meyer, J. (2001). Defining the nurse contribution to patient outcome: Lessons from a review of the literature examining nurse outcomes, skill mix and changing roles. *Journal of Clinical Nursing, 10*, 3–14.

Stordeur, S., D'Hoore, W., & Vandenberghe, C. (2001). Leadership, organizational stress, and emotional exhaustion among hospital nursing staff. *Journal of Advanced Nursing, 35*(4), 533–542.

Sullivan, E. J., & Decker, P. J. (2005). *Effective leadership & management in nursing* (6th ed.). Upper Saddle River, NJ: Pearson Education.

Tourangeau, A., Doran, D., Pringle, D., O'Brien-Pallas, L., McGillis Hall, L., Tu, J. V., et al. (2006). *Nurse staffing and work environments: Relationships with hospital-level outcomes.* Ottawa, ON: Canadian Health Services Research Foundation. Retrieved November 2007 from http://www.chsrf.ca

Upenieks, V. (2003). Nurse leaders' perception of what comprises successful leadership in today's acute inpatient environment. *Nursing Administration Quarterly, 27*(2), 140–153.

Upenieks, V., Akhavan, J., Kotlerman, J., Esser, J., & Ngo, M. J. (2007). Value-added care: A new way of assessing nursing staffing ratios and workload variability. *Journal of Nursing Administration, 37*(5), 243–252.

VanOyen Force, M. (2005). The relationship between effective nurse managers and nursing retention. *Journal of Nursing Administration 35*(7/8), 336–341.

Wieck, K. L., Prydun, M., & Walsh, T. (2002). What the emerging workforce wants in its leaders. *Journal of Nursing Scholarship, 34*(3), 283–288.

Wortsman, A., & Janowitz, S. (2006). *Taking steps forward: Retaining and valuing experienced nurses.* Ottawa, ON: Canadian Federation of Nurses.

Yoder-Wise, P. S. (2007). *Leading and managing in nursing* (4th ed.). St. Louis, MO: Mosby Elsevier.

8

PROFESSIONALISM AND THE ROLE OF THE NURSE LEADER: ETHICAL PRACTICE AND KNOWLEDGE UTILIZATION

We need formal and informal leadership in ethics throughout every facet of our profession. And we need leadership that can support the ethical practice of our colleagues in other disciplines.

—**Dr. Janet Storch,** RN, BScN, MHSA, PhD, DSc (Hon), CHE

Janet Storch has been involved in bioethics, health ethics, and administrative, organizational, and research ethics since the mid-1970s. She served as President of the Canadian Bioethics Society in 1991 to 1992 and as member and President of the National Council on Ethics in Human Research from 1994 to 2002. She is a Professor Emeritus at the University of Victoria, where she served as Director of the School of Nursing and where she continues an active research program in nursing and health care ethics. She chaired the University of Victoria Human Research Ethics Committee from 2002 to 2005 and was a member of the Vancouver Island Health Authority during those same years. Before her appointment at University of Victoria in 1996, she was Dean of Nursing at the University of Calgary, and before 1990, she was Professor and Director of the Master in Health Administration Program at the University of Alberta. Her academic training includes a BScN, an MHSA, and a PhD in Sociology, as well as a certificate from her studies at the Kennedy Institute of Ethics in Washington, DC. Dr. Storch continues active service on several local clinical ethics committees and serves on the British Columbia Ministry of Health committee to develop clinical ethics resources and on other provincial and national committees, including two committees of Health Canada. She was scholar in residence at the Canadian Nurses Association (CNA) in 2001 to 2002 and continues to work with CNA in reviewing and revising the Code of Ethics for Registered Nurses, as well as in developing research ethics guidelines for registered nurses.

Overview

Nursing has undergone many significant changes and faced many challenges during the past few decades in its quest for professionalism in Canada. Social scientists and nursing leaders have worked for more than half a century to define what constitutes a profession. Several professional characteristics have evolved over the years and are attributed to the nursing profession. One essential characteristic of professional leadership is the Code of Ethics. Today, nurses are confronted with intricate issues and frequently with ethical dilemmas.

Another component of professionalism is knowledge utilization in practice environments. Nurse leaders need to empower nurses to remain abreast of the scholarly literature and to apply in their practice the evidence presented in the literature. Only by understanding and exploring the issues of professionalism will nurse leaders know how to support effective nursing practice and meet the complex challenges now and in the future.

Objectives

By critically reflecting upon and processing knowledge throughout this chapter, you will be able to respond effectively to the following objectives:

1. Defend nursing as a profession.
2. Examine the nurse leader's role in the profession of nursing.
3. Evaluate the characteristics of a profession.
4. Analyze the Code of Ethics as it applies to nursing practice.
5. Examine the standards of practice in different provinces and territories.
6. Illustrate the importance of examining personal, professional, and organizational values in nursing practice.
7. Defend the importance of knowledge utilization in nursing.
8. Critique the concept of advocacy.
9. Identify an issue pertinent to nursing, and analyze the issue using the given framework.
10. Prepare a position statement about the issue and use one of the strategies to either defend or refute the issue.
11. Debate about the importance of the Privacy Act.

Professionalism in Nursing

Ross-Kerr (2003) states that "the *raison d'être* of any profession is found in the contribution it makes to society" (p. 30). Over the years, nurses and nursing have made dramatic impacts on the delivery of health care in Canada (Clarke & Wearing, 2001). The history of nursing in Canada began when a few nuns arrived in Quebec from France to provide nursing care to a few local people. Years later, today's nurse has specialized knowledge and is responsive to change in clients and their families within the scope of practice in a vast variety of settings (Ross-Kerr, 2003).

Today's nurse is making dramatic contributions to the health and well-being of individuals, families, and communities through the continuing development and application of knowledge utilization. The concept of knowledge utilization (also called evidence-based practice) is an essential component of current nursing practice in the health care delivery system (Edgar et al., 2006).

Nurse Leaders

Nurse leaders are contributing to the profession and society through their leadership competencies in clinical, educational, research, and management practice. Nurse leaders participate as well in the arenas of politics and policy, where they have been able to enhance the participation of nurses in decisions about national health care (Wynd, 2003). For example, in 2001, nurse representatives from the CNA were front and centre, presenting the views of the nursing profession to both the Commission on the Future of Health Care in Canada (Romanow Commission), and the Senate Committee on Science and Social Affairs and Technology (Kirby Committee) (CNA, 2001a). The nurses' message in their presentation was strong, focusing on the recruitment and retention of nurses and other health care providers for the sustainability of the health care system. At the same time, they established that the primary health care approach was the most effective model for health care delivery.

Influence of Aboriginal Nurse Leaders

An affiliate group of CNA, the Aboriginal Nurses Association of Canada (ANAC), is the only Aboriginal professional nursing organization in Canada. The nurse leaders and members in that organization are convinced that they can empower people to make a positive difference in Aboriginal communities. They encourage the Aboriginal people to consider a nursing career and join other skilled professionals in Aboriginal communities to share a vision of healing to improve health and wellness in Aboriginal people (ANAC, 2004). Further insights into the ANAC plan can be found on the ANAC Website (see Websites at the end of this chapter).

reflective **THINKING** After considering the ANAC publications, evaluate the publication *A Guide for Health Care Professionals Working with Aboriginal Peoples*. What insight can you, as a nurse leader, gain from this publication?

Florence Nightingale

The beginning of professional nursing can be traced to 19th century England to the school founded by Florence Nightingale (Butts, 2008). Her vision of trained nurses and her model of nursing education influenced the development of professional nursing. In her writings, health emerged as the central concept for nursing. She believed that nurses should spend their time caring for patients, not doing manual work. Moreover, she was convinced that nurses must continue to learn through their lifetime and not become stagnant. Florence Nightingale believed that nurses should be intelligent and use their intelligence to improve conditions for the patient. And possibly most profoundly, she urged that nursing leaders should have social standing. She had a vision of what nursing could be and should be (Ellis & Hartley, 2008). She considered ethical conduct in nursing to be largely dependent on character, and she believed that ethical conduct in potential nurses embraced such attributes as honesty, kindness, and truthfulness (Lamb, 2004). She began a movement, which is now called modern nursing. Since the days of Florence Nightingale, women and men who have entered nursing are motivated to provide care to individuals as well as to society as a whole (Killeen, 2001).

reflective **THINKING** In what ways does knowledge about Florence Nightingale help you as a nurse leader appreciate the heritage of the profession of nursing?

Characteristics of a Profession

Initially, many social scientists and nurse leaders debated on whether nursing is an occupation or a profession. As the growth of nursing as a profession continued amid phenomenal changes in the nature and scope of nursing, the debate seemed less relevant. Today, nursing is making enormous strides and gaining global recognition as a profession (Kozier et al., 2000; Oweis, 2005; Zabalegui et al., 2006; Karadağ, Hisar, & Elbaş, 2007). The criteria, qualities, and behaviours of a profession are cited in Box 8.1.

BOX 8.1   QUALITIES OF A PROFESSION

1. A profession uses in its practice a well-defined and well-organized body of knowledge that is intellectual in nature and describes its phenomena of concern.
2. A profession constantly enlarges the body of knowledge it uses and subsequently imposes on its members the life-long obligation to remain current in order to "do no harm."
3. A profession entrusts the education of its practitioners to institutions of higher education.
4. A profession applies its body of knowledge in practical services that are vital to human welfare and [that are] especially suited to the tradition of seasoned practitioners shaping the skills of newcomers to the role.
5. A profession functions autonomously (with authority) in formulating professional policy and in monitoring its practice and practitioners.
6. A profession is guided by a code of ethics that regulates the relationship between professional and client.
7. A profession is distinguished by the presence of a specific culture, norms, and values that are common among its members.
8. A profession has a clear standard of educational preparation for entry to practice.
9. A profession attracts individuals of intellectual and personal qualities who exalt service above personal gain and who recognize their chosen occupation as a life's work.
10. A profession strives to compensate its practitioners by providing freedom of action, opportunity for continuous professional growth, and economic security.

Adapted from Joel, L., & Kelly, L. Y. (2002). *The nursing experience: Trends, challenges, and transitions* (4th ed., pp. 16–17). New York: McGraw-Hill.

According to one Canadian nurse leader (Lemire Rodger, 2006), a profession is recognized by several characteristics that have evolved over the years. They most frequently include the following:

- Specialized body of knowledge
- Code of ethics
- Competent application of knowledge
- Standards of practice
- Self-regulation
- Tradition of public service
- Autonomy
- Accountability
- Professional association

The following characteristics of the profession are described within the Canadian context using Dr. Ginette Lemire Rodger's outline as a guide.

Codes of Ethics

Codes of ethics serve many useful functions for a professional group. A code provides guidance in terms of ethical principles for members of the profession (Storch & Nield, 2003). Ethics codes, in an applied context such as health care, are intended to establish a set of standards as a structure for the regulation and enhancement of ethical behaviour (Hadjistavropoulos, Malloy, Douaud, & Smythe, 2002). The practice of nursing by registered nurses is guided by the CNA *Code of Ethics for Registered Nurses* (CNA, 2008a). At CNA, the Code is considered a fundamental document for the CNA and for the profession of nursing.

The *Code of Ethics for Registered Nurses* has numerous professional functions as well. It provides guidance for decision making concerning ethical matters, it serves as a means for self-reflection and self-evaluation regarding ethical nursing practice, and it provides a basis for peer-review initiatives. The code also serves as an ethical foundation from which nurses can advocate for quality work environments that support the delivery of safe, compassionate, competent, and ethical care (CNA, 2008a). It is structured around eight primary values. Box 8.2 cites the values, which are central to ethical nursing practice.

Nurses place a high value on the human dignity and worth of others. The nursing profession expects integrity of its nurses. That is, nurses are to be truthful and provide care based on the ethical framework that is accepted within the profession (Kozier et al., 2000). Because nursing in Canada is by law a provincial responsibility, each province and territory must specify a code of ethics for nurses (Ross-Kerr, 2006). A statutory requirement within the act regulating the nursing profession mandates that nurses must uphold ethical standards. In fact, many provinces and territories use the CNA Code of Ethics (Registered Nurses Association of the Northwest Territories and Nunavut, 2006; Wood, 2003).

Ethical codes change gradually as the needs and values of society change. Storch (2007) states that CNA revises its codes every few years to address the changing social values and conditions that challenge nurses. It is critical that the code meets the needs of nurses in their everyday practice. Some of the factors that prompt the code to be revised include the increasing use of technology, changing ways in nursing practice, and moving care into the communities. The CNA has been revising the 2002 Code of Ethics, and the final version was released in June 2008. When the draft code was released in January 2007, it was circulated widely throughout the nursing community in Canada and other professional groups, both nationally and internationally. Nurses provided input by studying and responding to this code.

Of the several important new guidelines included in the revised code, one promotes emergency preparedness during pandemics and disasters; another

BOX 8.2 — CANADIAN NURSES ASSOCIATION CODE OF ETHICS FOR REGISTERED NURSES

The Canadian Nurses Association (CNA) Code of Ethics for Registered Nurses, 2008 Centennial Edition, outlines the values that guide Canadian nursing practice. Each value is accompanied by an itemized list of ethical responsibilities. For a detailed presentation of the complete Code of Ethics for Registered Nurses, the reader is directed to the complete CNA document available at the CNA Website. CNA believes the following seven values are central to nursing practice.

1. Safe, Compassionate, Competent, and Ethical care
Nurses value the ability to provide safe, compassionate, competent, and ethical care that allows them to fulfill their ethical and professional obligations to the people they serve with other members of the health care team. Nurses must strive to build relationships through meaningful communication.

2. Health and Well-Being
Nurses value health promotion and well-being and assisting persons to achieve their optimum level of health in situations of normal health, illness, injury, disability, or at the end of life. Nurses advocate for the use of the least restrictive measures possible for those in their care.

3. Informed Decision Making
Nurses respect and promote the autonomy of capable persons and help them to express their health needs and values and also to obtain desired information and services so they can make informed decisions. If a person is incapable of consent, the nurse respects the law on capacity assessment and substitutes decision making in his or her jurisdiction.

4. Dignity
Nurses recognize and respect the inherent worth of each person and advocate for respectful treatment of all persons. Nurses maintain appropriate professional boundaries with clients.

5. Privacy and Confidentiality
Nurses recognize the importance of privacy and confidentiality and safeguard personal, family, and community information obtained in the context of a professional relationship. Nurses must ensure that the information is shared outside the health care team only with the person's informed consent, or as may be legally required, or where the failure to disclose would cause significant harm.

(box continues on page 200)

> ### BOX 8.2 CANADIAN NURSES ASSOCIATION CODE OF ETHICS FOR REGISTERED NURSES (continued)
>
> **6. Justice**
> Nurses uphold principles of justice by safeguarding human rights, equity, and fairness and by promoting the public good.
>
> **7. Accountability**
> Nurses are answerable for their practice, and they act in a manner consistent with their professional responsibilities and standards of practice. Nurses must maintain their fitness to practice.
>
> ---
>
> Adapted and reproduced courtesy of Canadian Nurses Association. (2008). *Code of ethics for registered nurses* (2008 centennial ed.). Ottawa, ON: Author.

intends that clients' needs for privacy and confidentiality be assured and, as well, that client safety needs be met. Another aspect of the code focuses on how societal issues affect health and well-being. This means that nurses endeavour to maintain awareness of aspects of social justice that affect health and well-being and advocate for change. According to Storch (2007), it is critical that the new version of the code characterizes nursing at its best, while it provides guidance for strengthening ethical practice in nursing. However, unless nurses choose to act in accordance with the code, values, and standards, the code remains only abstract ideas. It is only when nurses act upon and follow the code explicitly that the guidelines become fully meaningful as lived reality (Pilkington, 2004).

The 2008 Code of Ethics is organized into two parts, as follows:

1. The first part describes the core responsibilities central to ethical nursing practice. Nurses in all settings of practice bear the ethical responsibilities that are identified under each of the seven primary nursing values. These responsibilities apply to nurses' interactions with individuals, families, groups, populations, communities, and society as well as nursing students, colleagues, other health care professionals, and the public.
2. The second part endeavours to address broad aspects of social justice that are associated with health and well-being and are part of ethical nursing practice. These aspects relate to the need for change in systems and societal structures in order to create greater equity for all. This part of the code contains 13 statements entitled "ethical endeavours," which are intended to guide nurses in their practice.

Practice environments have a significant influence on nurses' ability to be successful in upholding ethics in their practice. Nurses must recognize that they are moral agents in providing care. Nurses in all facets of the profession must reflect on their practice, not only on the quality of their interactions with others, but on the resources they need to maintain their own well-being (CNA, 2008b).

reflective **THINKING** After first examining the current version of the CNA Code of Ethics and then thinking about your own clinical practice, what changes would you like to see in the code? Explain.

Professional Regulation

The regulation of registered nurses in Canada, which is considered key to the nursing profession, is bound on the principle of self-regulation in the interest of public health and safety (CNA, 2001a). Self-regulation is based on the belief that the profession has the special knowledge necessary to set standards of practice and to evaluate the conduct of its members through peer review. Nurses are bound by the ethical values of the profession to base their nursing practice on current and relevant knowledge. Nurses are also bound by the same ethical values to demonstrate respect for the well-being, autonomy, and dignity of clients receiving care (CNA, 2001a).

In Canada, the authority to regulate the nursing profession comes from legislation enacted by provincial or territorial governments. The legislature permits the professional associations, or colleges, to establish the rules and regulations that uphold professional nursing practice. That is, each province and territory has legislation that grants authority to a nursing regulatory body (Brunke, 2006). These regulatory bodies are accountable to the public for enlisting competent, ethical, and safe nursing care. They also grant memberships to registrants, ensure standards of professional practice, investigate complaints, and discipline members accordingly (Shapiro & Durbin, 2006). Nursing regulatory bodies work together with the CNA to develop national frameworks for regulatory matters, such as:

- Using the registered nurse title.
- Setting standards of professional practice.
- Developing codes of ethics, professional discipline, and nursing telepractice.
- Approving educational programs and continuing competence for registrants (Brunke, 2006).

Nursing regulatory bodies in Canada have worked together for many years to facilitate nurses who wish to move across provincial/territorial borders without compromising the quality of practice. A mutual recognition agreement has been approved that sets out commonly held registration/licensure principles throughout Canada. In most cases, a nurse, who is registered and in good standing in one jurisdiction, can easily move to and work in another jurisdiction (CNA, 2001b).

The College and Association of Registered Nurses of Alberta (CARNA) is the regulatory and professional body for registered nurses. However, the Health Professions Act (2000) and the Registered Nurses Profession Regulation (2005) set out the responsibilities of CARNA. CARNA achieves these responsibilities through a variety of regulatory processes, such as registration and licensure (CARNA, 2006). The College of Nurses of Ontario (CNO) regulates the profession of nursing. Under the Regulated Health Profession Act, CNO and all other health colleges must follow certain guidelines for their respective professions. One guideline for CNO is to establish the standards of practice with which members must comply (CNO, 2005a).

In British Columbia, the Health Professions Act provides a common regulatory structure for the governance of health professions and gives the College of Registered Nurses of British Columbia its mandate and power (College of Registered Nurses of British Columbia, 2006). The Health Professions Act provides new definitions, requirements, and expectations for professional scope of practice, registration, continuing competence, and the disciplinary process. When this new Act was being initiated, Clarke and Wearing (2001) stated that the Act must ensure that the scope of practice for registered nurses reflects the reality of nursing practice today. It is also expected that the Act will promote flexibility for the evolution of nursing practice to meet changing health care needs.

A recent Conference Board of Canada report called *Achieving Public Protection Through Collaborative Self-Regulation: Reflections for a New Paradigm* explores health profession legislation and regulation (Conference Board of Canada, 2007). The objective of the report is to identify key issues in regulation and to reflect views on the future of regulation for the health professional in Canada. A highlight of the report was that regulators have an important role to play in supporting collaborative practice through developing partnerships among regulators, educators, governments, and the public. This report advises policymakers and regulators about the future role that legislation and regulation could, and should, play in enhancing collaborative practice and improving human resources in health management (CNA, 2007).

reflective **THINKING**   Examine the article "Regulatory and medico-legal barriers to interprofessional practice" by Lahey and Currie (2005) (see References). What needed changes, if any, do you see in the present principle of self-regulation for interdisciplinary teams?

Standards of Practice

One of the characteristics of a self-regulating profession is the development of standards of practice that serve as objective guidelines for nurses to implement and provide care. Such standards evolve and become established based on research and clinical evidence (Ross-Kerr, 2006). These guidelines assure clients and families that they are receiving the best possible care. Each professional organization is responsible for developing standards for practice in their particular province and territory (CNA, 2008b). Table 8.1 outlines the standards of care and indicators developed by the CNO. It is the responsibility of all registered nurses to understand the standards of practice and to apply them to their own practice regardless of their roles or practice settings.

(text continues on page 206)

Leadership Issue

*R*eview the *Standards of Practice for Registered Nurses* in your own province or territory. Compare those Standards of Practice to the ones used by the CNO. Which standards are the same and which standards are different? What are the implications of having different standards?

TABLE 8.1 | STANDARDS OF PROFESSIONAL PRACTICE

Standard and Description	Indicators	
	A Nurse Demonstrates the Standard by:	A Nurse–Administrator Demonstrates the Standard by:
Accountability *Each nurse is accountable to the public and is responsible for ensuring that her/his practice and conduct meets legislative requirements and the standards of the profession.* Nurses are responsible for their actions and the consequences of those actions. Part of this accountability includes conducting themselves in ways that promote respect for the profession.	▪ Advocating for clients, the profession, and the health care system. ▪ Ensuring practice is consistent with standards of practice, guidelines, and legislation. ▪ Maintaining competence and refraining from performing activities for which she/he is not competent. ▪ Taking responsibility for errors when they occur and taking appropriate action to maintain client safety.	▪ Creating an environment that encourages ongoing learning.
Continuing Competence *Each nurse maintains and continually improves her/his*	▪ Assuming responsibility for her/his own professional	

(table continues on page 204)

TABLE 8.1	STANDARDS OF PROFESSIONAL PRACTICE (continued)	
Standard and Description	**Indicators**	
	A Nurse Demonstrates the Standard by:	A Nurse–Administrator Demonstrates the Standard by:

competence by participating in the College of Nurses of Ontario's Quality Assurance (QA) Program. Competence is the nurse's ability to use knowledge, skill, attitudes, and values to perform in a given role, situation, and practice setting. Continuing competence ensures that the nurse can perform in a changing health environment. It also contributes to quality nursing practice and increases the public's confidence in the nursing profession.	development and for sharing knowledge with others. ▪ Engaging in a learning process to enhance her/his practice. ▪ Providing colleagues with feedback that encourages professional growth. ▪ Advocating for quality practice improvements in the workplace.	
Ethics *Each nurse understands, upholds, and promotes the values and beliefs described in the College's* Ethics *practice standard.* Ethical nursing care means promoting the values of client well-being, respecting client choice, assuring privacy and confidentiality, respecting sanctity and quality of life, maintaining commitments, respecting truthfulness, and ensuring fairness in the use of resources. It also includes acting with integrity, honesty, and professionalism with the client and other health team members.	▪ Identifying ethical issues and communicating them to the health team. ▪ Identifying options to resolve ethical issues. ▪ Evaluating the effectiveness of the actions taken to resolve ethical issues. ▪ Identifying personal values and ensuring they do not conflict with professional practice.	
Knowledge *Through basic education and continuing learning, each nurse possesses knowledge relevant to her/his professional practice.* RNs and RPNs study from the same body of nursing knowledge. RPNs study for a shorter period of time,	▪ Providing evidence-based rationale for all decisions. ▪ Being informed about the various nursing roles and their relationships to one another and to the health care delivery system.	▪ Using relevant leadership and management principles.

Standard and Description	Indicators	
	A Nurse Demonstrates the Standard by:	A Nurse–Administrator Demonstrates the Standard by:
resulting in a more focused or basic foundation of knowledge in clinical practice. RNs study for a longer period of time for a greater breadth and depth of knowledge in clinical practice, decision making, critical thinking, research utilization, and leadership in both the health care delivery systems and resource management.	• Understanding the legislation and standards relevant to nursing and the practice area • Obtaining knowledge of the cultural backgrounds related to the health needs encountered.	
Knowledge Application *Each nurse continually improves the application of professional knowledge.* The quality of professional nursing practice reflects nurses' application of knowledge. Nurses apply knowledge to practice using nursing frameworks, theories, and/or processes.	• Assessing the client situation using a theory, framework, or evidence-based tool. • Identifying/recognizing abnormal or unexpected client responses and taking action. • Managing multiple nursing interventions simultaneously. • Evaluating the outcome of interventions and modifying the plan. • Evaluating and integrating research findings into professional service and practice. • Evaluating theoretical and research-based approaches for application to practice.	
Leadership *Each nurse demonstrates her/his leadership by providing, facilitating, and promoting the best possible care/service to the public.* Leadership requires self-knowledge (understanding one's beliefs and values and being aware of how one's behaviour affects others), respect, trust, integrity, shared vision, learning, participation, interpersonal communication skills, and the ability to be a change	• Role-modelling professional values, beliefs, and attributes. • Collaborating with clients and the health team to provide professional practice that respects the rights of clients. • Acting as a role model and mentor to less experienced nurses and students. • Participating in nursing associations, committees, or interest groups.	• Involving nursing staff in decisions that affect their practice.

(table continues on page 206)

TABLE 8.1	STANDARDS OF PROFESSIONAL PRACTICE (continued)	
Standard and Description	**Indicators**	
	A Nurse Demonstrates the Standard by:	**A Nurse–Administrator Demonstrates the Standard by:**
facilitator. All nurses have opportunities for leadership.	▪ Providing leadership through formal and informal roles (e.g., team leader, charge nurse).	
Relationships *Each nurse establishes and maintains respectful, collaborative, therapeutic, and professional relationships.* Relationships include therapeutic nurse–client relationships and professional relationships with colleagues, health team members, and employers.	▪ Demonstrating respect, empathy, and interest for clients. ▪ Maintaining boundaries between professional, therapeutic relationships and nonprofessional, personal relationships. ▪ Ensuring that personal needs are met outside of therapeutic nurse–client relationships.	▪ Promoting a philosophy of client-centred care and collaborative relationships.
Professional Relationships *Professional relationships are based on trust and respect and result in improved client care.*	▪ Role-modelling positive collegial relationships ▪ Demonstrating knowledge of, and respect for, each other's roles, knowledge, expertise, and unique contribution to the team. ▪ Demonstrating effective conflict-resolution skills.	▪ Valuing and acknowledging nursing expertise and contributions to the health care of clients.

Note: This table of standards represents a broad description of a representative sample of the expectations of nurses. These standards were prepared by the College of Nurses of Ontario, but the general indicators and standards are relevant to all nurses in Canada.
Adapted from College of Nurses of Ontario. (2005). *Professional Standards (Revised 2002),* Toronto, ON: Author.

According to Ross-Kerr (2006), the guiding principles that lead to the most appropriate courses of action in certain standard practice situations are known as *best practices* or *clinical practice guidelines.* These guidelines are built on a foundation of biological, statistical, clinical, and population health science. The best practice guidelines differ from the much more general nursing practice standards in that they apply to specific clinical nursing practice situations. Nurses need best practice guidelines to improve outcomes for clients and to make nursing practice more effective and efficient. Recent studies indicate that practice guidelines have definitely improved the health care of clients (CNA, 2004b). Some of the ways a nurse leader can make practice guidelines more captivating to nurses are as follows:

- Support the guideline with transformational leadership along with a work environment that embraces change.
- Present evidence that is consistent with what nurses comprehend from clinical experiences and client preferences.
- Introduce change(s) appropriately with accountability for success shared equally among guideline developers, implementers, users, and evaluators (CNA, 2004b).

Quality Assurance Measures

Quality assurance programs are measures designed to ensure that standards of practice are maintained and that they adhere to high-quality outcomes for clients and families (Ross-Kerr, 2006). *Continuous quality improvement* uses tools and techniques to create a systematic approach to problem analysis, resolution, and evaluation. However, Sidani, Doran, and Mitchell (2004) state that a theory-driven approach is a strategy to determine whether the quality of nursing practice yields its expected outcomes to clients, groups, and communities. The development of such an approach should encompass the many relevant factors, such as characteristics of clients, professional characteristics, type of interventions, and the nature and timing of outcomes resulting from care received.

The main proposition of the theory-driven approach is that these factors influence outcomes. A realistic and comprehensive evaluation requires the evaluator to attend to the various elements inherent in everyday nursing practice. To determine which processes of nursing care actually attain favourable outcomes is essential to evaluate fully the contribution of nursing within the health care system. On the other hand, recognizing processes that are ineffective in achieving desired outcomes is necessary for refining the standards of care, whether the refinement be in streamlining services or in improving the quality and safety of services. Even though this strategy may require certain modifications in research methods and data analysis, the sound knowledge base obtained can guide quality improvement further and provide appropriate designs for nursing care delivery models and any necessary changes in policy.

reflective **THINKING** In considering the factors that influence the delivery and effectiveness of care, can you think of other factors, beyond the ones given, that might affect care and that need to be considered when evaluating nursing practice?

Specialized Knowledge and Evidenced-Based Practice

Of all the various characteristics of nursing, one that demands a particular status of professional importance is that of specialized knowledge. The current trend in providing education for professionals has shifted toward programs in colleges and universities. The Canadian Association of Schools of Nursing and CNA believe that the baccalaureate degree is the level of education required for entry to practice (CNA, 2004a). It is the baccalaureate educational program for nurses that provides the beginning of specialized knowledge.

A valuable professional companion to specialized knowledge for nurses is that of evidence-based nursing within practice settings. Evidence-based nursing is the accepted standard for providing professional care to clients (Thurston & King, 2005). Nursing in Canada is continuing to establish a well-defined body of knowledge and expertise that will facilitate evidence-based nursing within practice settings. The CNA, in its *Position Statement: Evidence-Based Decision-Making and Nursing Practice* (CNA, 2002), states that evidence-based decision making is essential to optimize outcomes for clients and families, improve clinical practice, achieve cost-effective nursing care, and ensure transparency and accountability in decision making. Evidence-based nursing practice recognizes the importance of intuition and sound judgment, but at the same time, also incorporates the components of current best research evidence on which clinical practice guidelines are based. These are essential to improve clinical outcomes of clients (Rycroft-Malone et al., 2004).

reflective **THINKING**   What are the benefits of evidenced-based nursing practice in a wellness centre?

Leading Within the Scope of Professionalism

Findings of the following research studies indicate the importance of the nurse leader's role in enhancing professional nursing practice. To empower nurses, the nurse leader should consider the implementation of transformational leadership, which commits individuals to action. In fact, in transformational leadership, both the leader and the follower raise one another to higher levels of performance (Grohar-Murray & DiCroce, 2003).

Ethical Practice

A study by Varcoe et al. (2004) explored, from the perspective of nurses, the meaning of ethics and the enactment of ethical practice in nursing. Varcoe et al. found that nurses described ethics in their practice as both a way of being and a process of enactment. Nurses described how they developed a growing awareness of themselves as moral agents. They described a process burdened with personal and professional struggles as they sought to sustain their identity as moral agents. It was the identification of themselves as a moral agent that emerged as the key to the development of ethical practice. Enacting ethical practice involved working in the spaces "in between" various members, such as family, clients, staff, and managers, while they worked through the process of encountering tensions and conflicts in values, making choices, and choosing their responses.

In summary, nurses in this study described ethical practice as *relational* and *highly contextual*. These nurses mourned the lack of support and leadership in nursing practice. It is important for nurse leaders to realize that personal values may conflict with the values promoted by the Code of Ethics and by the employing health care organization. Nurse leaders must remain mindful of the need to take into consideration that resources for ethical nursing practice include the importance of being receptive and responsive to the needs of practising nurses. They must also be cognizant that individual values are strong indicators of professional performance. Because there may be potential for conflict between individual and organizational values, it is important for nurse leaders to be especially attentive to identifying various options they might implement to resolve these differences.

---

reflective **THINKING**   Reflect on which organizational or professional values in your work or academic setting are in conflict with your own personal values. As a nurse leader, how do you address those conflicts?

Storch, Rodney, Pauly, Brown, and Starzomski (2002) studied the meaning of ethics for nurses providing direct care for clients. The implications of their findings were directed toward nurse leaders. They concluded that nurse leaders are moral agents. Nurse leaders need moral courage to be self-reflective, to identify their own moral distress, and to act so that their nursing staff can be moral agents. Moral distress arises when inconsistency exists between one's beliefs and one's actions. Nurse leaders need to use their competencies as a positive force to promote, provide, and sustain quality practice environments for competent, safe, and ethical practice. Nurse managers play a pivotal role in ensuring that health care organizations enable basic nursing values to be realized. They may be called

Reflections on Leadership Practice

You have been a staff nurse at a small hospital in a rural community for 3 years now, and you are getting to know a considerable number of people in the town of 2,000 people. You are a member of one of the four churches in town, and you have enjoyed singing in the church choir for several months. You ice curl in winter and play slow-pitch baseball in the summer. The hospital where you work has a developing interdisciplinary health care team, and you enjoy a good professional and social relationship with most members of the health care team.

One Saturday night, at about 2300 hours, you and the three other nurses on duty are startled by a commotion in the entrance of the hospital. Someone is calling your name, asking you to "Please come to the door." When you arrive at the door you recognize two young men and two young women whom you met as opposing players on one of the baseball teams, all of whom you and your teammates came to know somewhat over drinks after two or three games. One young man appears to have a broken arm and his face is cut and bleeding. The other young man is holding his head and ribs and appears highly agitated. The young women are both dishevelled and have some cuts. You suspect they have some injuries from broken glass.

You believe you can detect alcohol on their breath. They confide in you that they have had a car accident with the car of one of the young men's parents, which they were using without permission. They ask you not to notify the local police, nor their parents. Because their car went into the ditch near the hospital, they were able to walk to the hospital. They knew you often work weekends, and they hoped that you would be able to "fix them up."

You are quite confident at knowing what to do to treat their injuries. However, their requests to not call the police nor notify their parents are giving you some uncertainty. What will you do about that?

1. To follow the Code of Ethics, what are your responsibilities to parents, police, and the rest of the interdisciplinary health care team in this situation?
2. What relevance does the age of any or all of the young people have in such a case?
3. What do you do about the question of alcohol consumption while you are with the injured and frightened people, both at the door and inside the unit?

As a nurse leader, what are your options toward the young people who know and trust you, to the other nurses on duty, and to the health care team?

---

upon to challenge the organization and health care system to higher moral decision making (Kellen, Oberle, Girard, & Falkenberg, 2004).

According to Hardingham (2004), nurse leaders need to work to build strong moral community. They need to work with their nursing colleagues, professional associations, and other members of the health care team to achieve a quality professional practice environment that will support moral integrity and decision making. Figure 8.1 outlines the CNA model of a quality professional

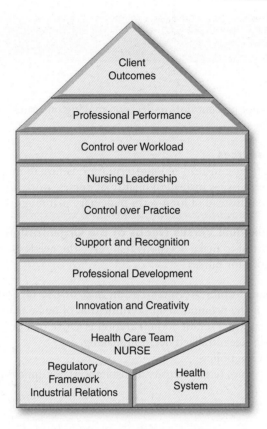

FIGURE 8.1 Canadian Nurses Association model of a quality professional practice environment.

practice environment. The model identifies six attributes of a healthy workplace. The quality professional practice environment is a primary value that is central to ethical nursing practice and plays an important role in decreasing moral or ethical distress (CNA, 2003a). Nurse leaders must strive, as their fundamental responsibility, to provide adequate staff to meet the requirements for nursing care and to promote practice environments where safe care can be maintained.

In a study conducted by Gaudine and Beaton (2002), ethical conflicts were examined in the workplace as experienced by nurse managers. Four themes emerged, as did various factors that would mitigate nurse managers' ethical conflicts within hospitals (Box 8.3). It was concluded that nursing leadership and management courses should cover ethical issues faced by nurse managers and the ways direct-care nurses can influence decision making. It was also stated that policymakers must ensure that organizational structures facilitate open and collaborative communication between nurse managers and administrators. In an

BOX 8.3 NURSE MANAGERS' ETHICAL CONFLICTS WITH HOSPITALS AND POSSIBLE MITIGATORS

Ethical Conflicts
Voicelessness
- Nurse managers not present during decision making on issues that affect nursing
- Nursing not valued

Allocation of Resources
- Spending on acute care instead of long-term care; failure to invest in staff development; focus on short-term issues instead of quality of nurses' work life
- Crisis management instead of long-term budgetary planning

Rights of the Individual Versus Needs of the Organization
Nurse manager forced to make decisions that serve the needs of the organization but have negative implications for nurses

Unjust Practices of Senior Administration and/or the Organization
- Unfair policies for the promotion and termination of nurse managers
- Failure to act even when senior administration is aware of a problem
- Centralized versus decentralized decision making
- Punitive absenteeism policy
- Hospital's stated values (e.g., integrity, consultation) not upheld by administration and board

Mitigating Factors
Support
- Support from other nurse managers, hospital administrators, physicians, hospital ethics committee, staff nurses, family, public
- Internal strength gained from knowing that one is morally right
- Internal strength gained from knowing that one is following the Canadian Nurses Association's Code of Ethics

Problem Solving and Growth
- Problem solving with other nurse managers, hospital administrators, physicians, hospital ethics committee, staff nurses
- Learning to separate personal values from professional responsibilities
- Developing and presenting a proposal to senior administrators

Refocusing
- Hoping that the next generation of (better-educated) nurses will improve nursing
- Focusing on one's own goals and on what one can do
- Focusing on the high quality of care that nurses provide
- Dwelling on the positive when senior administration begins to address a problem

Adapted from Gaudine, A. P., & Beaton, M. R. (2002). Employed to go against one's values: Nurse managers' accounts of ethical conflict with their organizations. *Canadian Journal of Nursing Research*, 34(2), 17–34.

earlier study by Oberle and Tenove (2000) that explored ethical issues in public health nursing, similar outcomes regarding nurse leadership emerged. That is, nurse leaders need to provide more support for nurses, and they need to engage in cooperative and supportive dialogue with administrative leaders.

> reflective **THINKING** As a nurse leader, what do believe that you need to know, or understand, from the nurses in the community before you can provide support to them?

Evidence-Based Practice

Paramonczyk (2005) studied the perceptions of barriers to research implementation in a sample of 25 Canadian nursing professionals. Although nurses have a professional responsibility to keep up with current research literature, Paramonczyk found that nurses claim they do not have time at work to read research material. In addition, administration, physicians, and other staff were unsupportive and uncooperative regarding research implementation. That is, for this sample, the work setting did not appear to foster a culture of research-related activities. The results of the Paramonczyk study may represent a widespread common situation encountered by nurses in Canada.

> reflective **THINKING** What options are available to nurse leaders who encounter the situation revealed in the Paramonczyk study?

According to Penz and Bassendowski (2006), clinical nurse issues must be addressed to promote evidence-based practice. A few of these issues include the following:

- Time factors
- Access to information and resources
- Nurses' research knowledge and skills
- Current nursing culture

It follows that nurse managers are faced with the need to encourage nurses to access current best evidence and to supply relevant literature and compile it in one place on the unit. The nurse manager can facilitate the understanding of what benefits occur when knowledge utilization is practiced.

In a theoretical article which begins by outlining the results of a study the researchers conducted on the competencies of first-line managers, the benefits and barriers of evidence-based nursing practice (EBNP) in the workplace are described. The discussion then proceeds to nurse leaders and EBNP (Udod & Care, 2004). Table 8.2 outlines the researcher's description of the role of nursing

TABLE 8.2	LEADER'S ROLE IN PROMOTING EVIDENCE-BASED NURSING PRACTICE (EBNP)	
The Individual	**The Organization**	**The Environment**
Role modelling EBNP: Leaders must demonstrate commitment by role modelling and "championing" EBNP.	Change and EBNP: Understanding the culture of the organization and the organization's history related to change are essential to developing, implementing, and sustaining EBNP.	Human resources as a commodity: Organizations are quickly realizing that human health resources are a necessary commodity in making a difference to patient outcomes and cost efficiency. Nurse leaders need to foster relationships that work collaboratively with staff nurses, as they will be the primary users of evidence-based practice.
Creating network opportunities: Nurses can search for and share evidence in a collaborative atmosphere. Forming collaborative networks, such as journal clubs, can provide highly relevant and concise information.	Client outcomes: Nurse leaders can encourage nurses to begin addressing practice issues that lead to variations in outcomes, or are questioned by other nurses in their practice. For evaluation, demonstrate whether change was appropriate, effective, and efficient.	Establishing a questioning culture: Nurses should ask questions related to their practice (e.g., Is there evidence to substantiate their clinical activities?). A shift is required to establish a culture that supports EBNP— and it needs to begin with the leadership and permeate all levels of the organization.
Shared leadership: The concept of shared leadership is gaining support within the discipline of nursing and fits well with the notion of evidence-based practice. If staff nurses are to use research, they should be active participants in decision-making processes affecting their practice.	Training and development: The nurse leader acts as a facilitator of EBNP by advocating for resources for staff nurses. Comprehensive training programs that focus on what EBNP is, stating the reasons for the practice, and educating nurses how to critically appraise research are integral elements to sustaining the change. Nurses require adequate access to computers and the library.	Learning organization: To be an evidence-based organization, the entire organization must focus on learning. Nurse leaders can promote nurturing links between front-line practice and academia, encourage conference attendance and educational leaves, and establish "lunch and learn" sessions. Nurse leaders must be stewards for knowledge building in the organization.
Psycho-social support: If EBNP is to be sustained, nurses must be supported	Rewards and recognition: Aligning clinical advancement recognition rewards and with	

The Individual	The Organization	The Environment
both in word and action by their nurse leaders. Visible support creates the capacity for change by encouraging and enabling nurses to perform desired competencies.	the expectation of conducting and disseminating research, as in academia, will demonstrate that the organization supports the practice. Rewarding and recognizing nurses who take an active role in solving clinical problems sets a positive tone for motivating others.	

Note: It is reality, according to Udod and Care (2004), that the individual, the organization, and the environment all pose significant barriers to evidence-based practice. Strategies are needed to overcome these barriers. A multifaceted and synergistic approach directed toward the role of the leader for each level is suggested. From Udod, S. A., & Care, W. D. (2004). Setting the climate for evidence-based nursing practice: What is the leader's role? *Nursing Leadership, 17*(4), 64–75.

leaders in promoting EBNP in their health care settings. Nurse leaders play a significant role when they integrate knowledge utilization into practice. Udod and Care (2004) claim that by linking the individual, organization, and environment, evidence-based practice will progress.

Nurse Leaders Taking Action

Nurse leaders have earned the responsibility and have accepted accountability for their professional actions. For a manager to formulate an approach, much consideration must be given to ethical guidelines rooted in professional, organizational, and personal values. McIntyre, Thomlinson, and McDonald (2006)

Reflections on Leadership Practice

*R*ecently you attended a leadership conference where a presentation on evidence-based practice caught your professional interest. The presenter identified an information-skills approach (Snowball, 2005). This approach entails formulating questions, searching databases, critically analyzing knowledge in scholarly articles and research reports to identify the best evidence, using that knowledge, and evaluating client change.

As a nurse manager on a palliative care unit, what steps will you use to implement an information-skills approach for your health team?

state that the issues into which professional organizations have pledged their support include the following:

- Acting as advocates for clients and families
- Responding to issues that directly affect the health of Canadians
- Lobbying for positive change in the health care system
- Improving the visibility and image of nursing

Advocacy

An examination of the nursing literature reveals several different interpretations of what advocacy is. The meaning of advocacy stems from a traditional paternalistic view to a more contemporary consumer-centric and empowering perspective (Hellwig, Yam, & DiGiulio, 2003). In a philosophical analysis of advocacy in nursing, Grace (2001) asserts that advocacy stems from the profession's purpose and promise to society to engage in practice with the following intention to improve health at the levels of the individual, health care system, and society generally. Spenceley, Reutter, and Allen (2006) state that such an idea of advocacy enlarges the professional assessment of obstacles to achieving health and also increases the possibility that answers to underlying problems can be discovered.

MacDonald (2007) analyzed themes from accounts of nurses' experiences with advocacy. The purpose of this analysis was to expand the understanding of advocacy in nursing practice. The author came to realize that the nature and context of relationships play significant roles in influencing the enactment of advocacy and that the application of advocacy in nursing practice is complex. Because advocacy is universally considered a moral obligation in nursing practice, the advancement of knowledge about its nature is critical to nursing practice across multiple contexts and cultures.

In another study, by Schwartz (2007), the question posed was "What are the perceptions of advocacy from the nurse case manager's perspectives?" The data analysis indicated that the work of nurse managers should be carefully examined to enhance the understanding of the specific knowledge and behaviours, as well as the general environment that supports or hinders client advocacy. Schwartz (2007) advocates that knowledge of ethics is helpful, but the skills of negotiation and communication are most important. In view of these findings, it would seem to be beneficial for nurse leaders themselves to conduct research studies to examine the specific roles, behaviours, and skills that support advocacy.

reflective **THINKING** As a nurse leader, have you ever advocated for a client and/or the client's family? What was the result? Would you act the same way again or differently?

Political Action

Politics refers to the process of attempting to influence decision makers to implement changes to advance the lives of clients and their families, communities, and populations (CNA, 2000). To be politically active, nurse leaders must be able to examine, articulate, and develop strategies to act on an issue that is critical in health care. It is pertinent that the nurse leader has all the relevant facts necessary about the issue. Some issues call for a particular framework or an approach to analysis; others benefit from more than one approach. McIntyre, Thomlinson, and McDonald (2006) outline a framework for the articulation and analysis of issues. The steps in the framework follow:

- Identify the issue of interest and articulate it clearly (ask yourself whether or not it is a nursing issue).
- Define your own assumptions, values, and beliefs about the issue (what strikes you about this issue as a nurse? As a person?).
- Proceed with the *historical, ethical and legal, social and cultural, political,* and *economic* analysis of the issue. (*Historical*—how did the issue come into being? *Ethical and legal*—how does the professional code affect this issue? *Social and cultural*—how does this issue affect society? What values of the dominant culture influence this issue? *Political*—who benefits from this issue staying the same or changing? *Economic*—what are the benefits or handicaps of this issue?)
- List barriers to the resolution of the issue. (What prevents the issue from being resolved?)
- Explore actions for resolution of the issue. (What are the strategies for resolving the issue?)

It is through this process of analysis that the nurse leader learns what the specific issue entails, whom it will benefit, who might be left out, and what costs are involved. After analyzing the issue, it is essential to follow the appropriate steps either to maintain the status quo or to create change. Sullivan (2004) has developed a series of steps to follow in the political action process. These steps are delineated in Box 8.4.

CNA (2000) has issued a list of strategies that have been found to be effective for political action. These strategies include networking with colleagues, lobbying politicians, creating public support, involving those directly affected, speaking from lived experience, using the media, taking a multifaceted approach, and whistle blowing. Other steps could be letter writing, developing resolutions, and forming coalitions. A position paper may be developed as a preliminary step to clearly identify the issue, take a position on the issue, provide evidence for your position, and present strategies to resolve it. An outline of how to write a position statement is provided in Box 8.5. It is important to remember that being

---

BOX 8.4   STEPS IN POLITICAL ACTION

- Determine what is wanted:
  - Decide whether to change an existing policy or create a new one.
  - Consider what research about the issue might be necessary.
- Learn about the players and what they want:
  - Think about what the stakeholders want.
- Gather supporters and form coalitions:
  - Enlist allies and know that there is power in numbers.
- Be prepared to respond to opponents:
  - Be assertive and clearly express the intention of the group.
- Explain the benefits to the decision makers you want to influence:
  - Express the beneficial aspects of the approach.

Adapted from Sullivan, E. J. (2004). *Becoming influential: A guide for nurses.* Upper Saddle River, NJ: Pearson Education.

politically active can, at times, be somewhat discouraging and frustrating. An open mind, a positive attitude, and well-articulated knowledge about the issue can be most helpful.

It is extremely beneficial when nurse leaders collaborate with their own health team, the organization, and the stakeholders to promote the political advancement of the nursing profession. A united front is much more politically

---

BOX 8.5   WRITING A PERSONAL POSITION STATEMENT

Given all the information you have gained in your research, determine how you feel about the issue. What is the specific problem? How does the issue or problem affect you as a nurse leader, your health team members, and your organization?
Use the following format to organize your ideas and write your notes.

Position Statement Format
In a position statement, you will choose a side of the argument, an issue, or position and defend it with specific evidence.
Step 1. Identify the problem(s):

_____

_____

Step 2. Choose your side and explain your opinion in two or three sentences. For instance, will a proposed change solve the problem or not? Why do you feel this way? This will provide the basis of your thesis or opening statement.

My position (am I for or against?)
Explanation (because?)

Step 3. Providing evidence to support your ideas. Your position can be based on personal opinion, but it must be supported with specific evidence and examples from your research. Use at least three pieces of evidence to indicate a good understanding of the topic and your opinion and why your position is valid.

My Idea or Reason	**Supported by or based on (Evidence)**
My Idea or Reason	**Supported by or based on (Evidence)**
My Idea or Reason	**Supported by or based on (Evidence)**

Step 4. If there is a problem to be solved, **provide a possible solution** and explain why you think your solution can work.

Solution to the problem:
Why I think it can work:

Step 5. Write a conclusion. Sum up your opinion and examples about the issue to make your point a final time. Use the space below for your notes or first attempt.

_____

_____

From WAMC Northeast Public Radio. (2008). Youth Media Project: Student Town Meetings—Writing a personal position statement. Retrieved January 2008 from http://www.wamcstudenttownmeetings.org

powerful than a fragmented appeal. Today, nurse leaders are showing insightful expertise and determination in understanding and following the political processes while implementing the skills involved to influence others and to exercise increasing control over issues that are important in health care. Nurses do have direct experience and a thorough knowledge of the health care needs of individuals, families, and communities. One important aspect of being politically active is conducting public policy research and influencing the formation of public policy for health promotion (Sullivan, 2004).

Today, nurse leaders are confronted with numerous opportunities by which they can use their political action skills to acquire resources to improve client and family care, increase the profession's ability to improve health, and enhance their communities (Racher, 2008).

reflective **THINKING**   What issue, as a nurse leader, is important for you today to analyse? After your analysis, what strategy will you use to set about to resolve the issue?

Privacy Act

Nurse leaders face a number of privacy issues in their daily professional practice. As well as using the Code of Ethics in their professional practice, it is important for nurses to understand that they have a responsibility to protect privacy, obtain informed consent, follow set policies on health care, as well as question policies that are not reflective of current ethical standards of practice and relevant legislation (CNA, 2003b). It is critical for nurse leaders and nurses to vocalize their support and concerns about policy discussions. Box 8.6 outlines a set of strategies that nurses can follow to ensure privacy in professional practice. Nursing as a profession is ideal to facilitate and promote public education, dialogue, and debate about privacy issues in all areas of health care.

Today, in a dynamic area of health care where conditions change rapidly, the acquisition of relevant knowledge and effective skills is essential for nurse leaders. Power and empowerment are gained as nurse leaders continue to increase the visibility of the nursing profession. Nurse leaders believe that in the coming years, the professional nursing movement will accelerate in quality and depth to provide health services to an increasingly diverse and complex population in Canada.

BOX 8.6 STRATEGIES FOR NURSES TO ENSURE PRIVACY IN PROFESSIONAL PRACTICE

Nurses can do a great deal to participate in, and shape, public policy concerning privacy and to ensure adequate respect for privacy in professional practice, including the following:

- Furthering education in privacy issues and the values and concepts by means of which to analyze them
- Furthering knowledge of law, professional codes, and institutional policy concerning privacy, particularly as it applies to one's professional practice
- Furthering sensitivity to privacy, particularly bearing in mind that much privacy infringement is due not to a values conflict, but to inadvertence or carelessness, such as discussing details about a patient on a crowded elevator
- Fostering research about privacy issues and their impact on patients, families, and communities
- Participating, individually and collectively, in public policy debate and information
- Participating in the formation and review of institutional policies and practices
- Participating in the design of the health information system to ensure that privacy concerns are adequately addressed
- Educating patients, families, and communities about their privacy rights and limitations to those rights

Courtesy of Canadian Nurses Association. (2003). *Ethics in practice: Ethical distress in health care environments*. Ottawa, ON: Author.

WEBSITES

■ Canadian Association for the History of Nursing (CAHN)

http://www.cahn-achn.ca/
The mission of CAHN is to promote interest in the history of nursing and to develop scholarship in the field. CAHN is a charitable organization founded in 1987 and is an affiliate group of the Canadian Nurses Association.

■ Aboriginal Nurses Association of Canada

http://www.anac.on.ca
The Aboriginal Nurses Association of Canada is a nongovernmental, nonprofit organization that was established out of the recognition that Aboriginal people's health needs can best be met and understood by health professionals of a similar cultural background. An affiliate group of the Canadian Nurses Association, it is the only Aboriginal professional nursing organization in Canada.

■ Florence Nightingale Museum

http://www.florence-nightingale.co.uk/
Florence Nightingale was a legend in her lifetime, but the Crimean War years, which made her famous, were just 2 out of a life of 90 years.

■ Canadian Association of Schools of Nursing (CASN)

http://www.casn.ca
CASN/ACESI (Association Canadienne des Ecoles de Sciences Infirmières) is the national voice for nursing education and nursing research and represents nursing programs in Canada.

■ The Canadian Nurses Protective Society (CNPS)

http://www.cnps.ca
The CNPS is a nonprofit society owned and operated by nurses, for nurses. CNPS offers legal liability protection related to nursing practice to eligible registered nurses by providing information, education, and financial and legal assistance.

■ Department of Justice Canada

http://laws.justice.gc.ca
This is the online source of consolidated Acts and regulations of Canada. The site provides links to consolidated statutes, including the Criminal Code of Canada and the Privacy Act.

REFERENCES

Aboriginal Nurses Association of Canada. (2004). Aboriginal Nurses Association of Canada. Ottawa, ON: ANAC. Retrieved January 2008 from http://www.anac.on.ca/
Brunke, L. (2006). Canadian provincial and territorial professional associations and colleges. In M. McIntyre, E. Thomlinson, & C. McDonald (Eds.), *Realities of Canadian nursing:*

Professional, practice and power issues (2nd ed., pp. 152–168). Philadelphia: Lippincott Williams & Wilkins.

Butts, J.B. (2008). Ethics in professional nursing practice. In J. B. Butts & K. L. Rich (Eds.), *Nursing ethics: Across the curriculum and into practice* (2nd ed., pp. 81–117). Toronto, ON: Jones and Bartlett.

Canadian Nurses Association. (2000). *Nursing is a political act – the bigger picture*. Ottawa, ON: Author.

Canadian Nurses Association. (2001a). *Canadian Nurses Association annual report*. Ottawa, ON: Author.

Canadian Nurses Association. (2001b). *Self-regulation: Safeguarding the privilege*. Ottawa, ON: Author.

Canadian Nurses Association. (2002). *Position statement: Evidence-based decision-making and nursing practice*. Ottawa, ON: Author.

Canadian Nurses Association. (2003a). *Ethical distress in health care environments*. Ottawa, ON: Author.

Canadian Nurses Association. (2003b). *Privacy and health information: Challenges for nurses and for the nursing profession*. Ottawa, ON: Author.

Canadian Nurses Association. (2004a). *Joint position statement: Educational preparation for entry to practice*. Ottawa, ON: Author.

Canadian Nurses Association. (2004b). *Making best practice guidelines a reality*. Ottawa, ON: Author.

Canadian Nurses Association. (2007). *Looking out, looking around, looking forward*. Ottawa, ON: Author.

Canadian Nurses Association. (2008a). *Code of ethics for registered nurses* (2008 centennial ed.). Ottawa, ON: Author.

Canadian Nurses Association. (2008b). *Nursing practice*. Standards and best practices. Ottawa, ON: Author.

Clarke, H. F., & Wearing, J. (2001). Regulation of registered nursing: The Canadian perspective. *Reflections on Nursing Leadership, 27*(4), 26–35.

College of Nurses of Ontario. (2005a). *Professional standards*. Ottawa, ON: Author.

College of Nurses of Ontario. (2005b). *What is CNO? Self-regulation*. Ontario, ON: Author.

College of Registered Nurses of British Columbia. (2006). *Overview of health professions act, nurses (registered) and nurse practitioners regulation, and CRNBC bylaws*. Vancouver, BC: Author.

Conference Board of Canada. (2007). *Achieving public protection through collaborative self-regulation: Reflections for a new paradigm*. Ottawa, ON: Author.

Edgar, L., Herbert, R., Lambert, S., MacDonald, J., Dubois, S., & Latimer, M. (2006). The joint venture model of knowledge utilization: A guide for change in nursing. *Nursing Leadership, 19*(2), 41–55.

Ellis, J. R., & Hartley, C. L. (2008). *Nursing in today's world: Trends, issues and management* (9th ed.). Philadelphia: Lippincott Williams & Wilkins.

Gaudine, A. P., & Beaton, M. R. (2002). Employed to go against one's values: Nurse managers' accounts of ethical conflict with their organizations. *Canadian Journal of Nursing Research, 34*(2), 17–34.

Grace, P. J. (2001). Advocacy: Widening the scope of accountability. *Nursing Philosophy, 2*, 151–162.

Grohar-Murray, M. E., & DiCroce, H. R. (2003). *Leadership and management in nursing* (3rd ed.). Upper Saddle River, NJ: Pearson Education.

Hadjistavropoulos, T., Malloy, D. C., Douaud, P., & Smythe, W. E. (2002). Ethical orientation, functional linguistics, and the codes of ethics of the Canadian Nurses Association and the Canadian Medical Association. *Canadian Journal of Nursing Research, 34*(2), 35–51.

Hardingham, L. B. (2004). Integrity and moral residue: Nurses as participants in a moral community. *Nursing Philosophy, 5*, 127–134.

Hellwig, S. D., Yam, M., & DiGiulio, M. (2003). Nurse case managers' perceptions of advocacy: A phenomenological inquiry. *Lippincott's Case Management, 8*(2), 53–65.

Joel, L., & Kelly, L. Y. (2002). *The nursing experience: Trends, challenges, and transitions* (4th ed., pp. 16–17). New York: McGraw-Hill.

Karadağ, A., Hisar, F., & Elbaş, N. O. (2007). The level of professionalism among nurses in Turkey. *Journal of Nursing Scholarship, 39*(4), 371–374.

Kellen, J. C., Oberle, K., Girard, F., & Falkenberg, L. (2004). Exploring ethical perspectives of nurses and nurse managers. *Nursing Leadership, 17*(1), 78–87.

Killeen, M. L. (2001). Socialization to professional nursing. In J. L. Creasia & B. Parker (Eds.), *Conceptual foundations: The bridge to professional nursing practice* (3rd ed., pp. 45–94). St. Louis, MO: Mosby.

Kozier, B., Erb, G., Burke, K., Bouchal, D. S. R., & Hirst, S. P. (2000). *Fundamentals of nursing: The nature of nursing practice in Canada* (Canadian ed.). Upper Saddle River, NJ: Prentice-Hall.

Lahey, W., & Currie, R. (2005). Regulatory and medico-legal barriers to interprofessional practice. *Journal of Interprofessional Care, May Supplement 1*, 197–223.

Lamb, M. (2004). A historical perspective on nursing and nursing ethics. In J. L. Storch, P. Rodney, & R. Starzomski (Eds.), *Toward a moral horizon: Nursing ethics for leadership and practice* (pp. 20–41). Toronto, ON: Pearson.

Lemire Rodger, G., (2006). Canadian Nurses Association. In M. McIntyre, E. Thomlinson, & C. McDonald (Eds.), *Realities of Canadian nursing: Professional, practice, and power issues* (2nd ed., pp.134–151). Philadelphia: Lippincott Williams & Wilkins.

MacDonald, H. (2007). Relational ethics and advocacy in nursing: Literature review. *Journal of Advanced Nursing, 57*(2), 119–126.

McIntyre, M., Thomlinson, E., & McDonald, C. (2006). Nursing issues: A call to political action. In M. McIntyre, E. Thomlinson, & C. McDonald (Eds.), *Realities of Canadian nursing: Professional, practice, and power issues* (2nd ed., pp. 3–28). Philadelphia: Lippincott Williams & Wilkins.

Oberle, K., & Tenove, S. (2000). Ethical issues in public health nursing. *Nursing Ethics, 7*(5), 425–438.

Oweis, A.I. (2005). Bringing the professional challenges for nursing in Jordan to light. *International Journal of Nursing Practice, 11*, 244–249.

Paramonczyk, A. (2005). Barriers to implementing research in clinical practice. *Canadian Nurse, 101*(3), 12–15.

Penz, K. L., & Bassendowski, S. L. (2006). Evidence-based nursing in clinical practice: Implications for nurse educators. *The Journal of Continuing Education in Nursing, 37*(6), 250–256.

Pilkington, F. B. (2004). Exploring ethical implications for acting faithfully in professional relationships. *Nursing Science Quarterly, 17*(1), 27–32.

Racher, F. E. (2008). Ethics for community practice. In A. R. Vollman, E. T. Anderson & J. McFarlane (Eds.), *Canadian community as partner: Theory and multidisciplinary practice* (2nd ed., pp. 26–47). Philadelphia: Lippincott Williams & Wilkins.

Registered Nurses Association of the Northwest Territories and Nunavut. (2006). *Standards of nursing practice for registered nurses*. Yellowknife, NT: Author.

Ross-Kerr, J. C. (2003). Professionalization in Canadian nursing. In J. C. Ross-Kerr & M. J. Wood (Eds.), *Canadian nursing: Issues and perspectives* (4th ed., pp. 30–38). Toronto, ON: Elsevier Science Canada.

Ross-Kerr, J. C. (2006). The development of nursing practice in Canada. In P. A. Potter, A. G. Perry, J. C. Ross-Kerr, & M. J. Wood (Eds.), *Canadian fundamentals of nursing* (3rd ed., pp. 35–50). Toronto, ON: Elsevier Canada.

Rycroft-Malone, J., Seers, K., Titchen, A., Harvey, G., Kitson, A., & McCormack, B. (2004). What counts as evidence in evidence-based practice? *Journal of Advanced Nursing, 47*, 81–90.

Schwartz, L. (2002). Is there an advocate in the house? The role of health care professionals in patient advocacy. *Journal of Medical Ethics, 28*, 37–40.

Shapiro, C., & Durbin, C. (2006). Legal implications in nursing practice. In P. A. Potter, A. G. Perry, J. C. Ross-Kerr, & M. J. Wood (Eds.), *Canadian fundamentals of nursing* (3rd ed., pp. 112–124). Toronto, ON: Elsevier Canada.

Sidani, S., Doran, D. M., & Mitchell, P. H. (2004). A theory-driven approach to evaluating quality of nursing care. *Journal of Nursing Scholarship, 36*(1), 60–65.

Snowball, R. (2005). Finding the evidence: An information skills approach. In M. Dawes, P. T. Davies, A. M. Gray, J. Mant, K. Seers, & R. Snowball (Eds.), *Evidence-based practice: A primer for health care professionals* (2nd ed., pp. 17–38). London: Elsevier Limited.

Spenceley, S. M., Reutter, L., & Allen, M. N. (2006). The road less traveled: Nursing advocacy at the policy level. *Policy, Politics, & Nursing Practice, 7*(3), 180–194.

Storch, J. L. (2004). Nursing Ethics: A Developmental Moral Terrain. In J. L. Storch, P. Rodney, & R. Starzomski (Eds.), *Toward a moral horizon: Nursing ethics for leadership and practice*. Toronto, ON: Pearson Education Canada.

Storch, J. L. (2007). Enduring values in changing times: The CNA codes of ethics. *The Canadian Nurse, 103*(4), 29–33.

Storch, J. L., & Nield, S. (2003). Keeping codes current: An ethics program to support nursing practice. *Nursing Leadership Forum, 7*(3), 103–108.

Storch, J. L., Rodney, P., Pauly, B., Brown, H., & Starzomski, R. (2002). Listening to nurses' moral voices: Building a quality health care environment. *Canadian Journal of Nursing Leadership, 15*(4), 7–16.

Sullivan, E. J. (2004). *Becoming influential: A guide for nurses.* Upper Saddle River, NJ: Pearson Education.

Thurston, N. E., & King, K. M. (2005). Implementing evidence-based practice: Walking the talk. *Journal of Vascular Nursing, 23*(2), 54–60.

Udod, S. A., & Care, W. D. (2004). Setting the climate for evidence-based nursing practice: What is the leader's role? *Nursing Leadership, 17*(4), 64–75.

Varcoe, C., Doane, G., Pauly, B., Rodney, P., Storch, J. L., Mahoney, K., McPherson, G., Brown, H., & Starzomski, R. (2004). Ethical practice in nursing: Working the in-betweens. *Journal of Advanced Nursing, 45*(3), 316–325.

Wood, M. J. (2003). Ethical issues and dilemmas in nursing practice. In J. C. Ross-Kerr & M. J. Wood (Eds.), *Canadian nursing: Issues and perspectives* (4th ed., pp. 210–228). Toronto, ON: Elsevier Science Canada.

Wynd, C. A. (2003). Current factors contributing to professionalism in nursing. *Journal of Professional Nursing, 19*(5), 251–261.

Zabalegui, A., Macia, L., Marquez, J., Ricoma, R., Nuin, C., Mariscal, I., et al. (2006). Changes in nursing education in the European Union. *Journal of Nursing Scholarship, 38*(2), 114–118.

TODAY'S HEALTH CARE TEAM AND THE ROLE OF THE NURSE LEADER

The leader's primary role is to build a real and sustaining sense of a team.

—Kathy Malloch and Tim Porter-O'Grady

Kathy Malloch is president of Kathy Malloch Consulting Services, vice-president of Arizona State Board of Nursing, and faculty associate in the College of Nursing, Arizona State University, Tempe, AZ. Tim Porter-O'Grady is senior partner of Tim Porter-O'Grady Associates, Inc., Atlanta, GA, and associate professor at Emory University, Atlanta, GA.

Overview

As the Canadian health care delivery system continues to increase in complexity, the role of the nursing leader will entail the increasing challenge of working in teams with other health care professionals and providers to optimize the delivery of primary health care.

Objectives

By critically reflecting upon and processing knowledge throughout this chapter, you will be able to respond effectively to the following objectives:

1. Examine the concepts of teams from your perspective in a health care delivery system.
2. Apply several leadership strategies that you, as a nurse leader, could initiate to work with the challenges that confront teams.
3. Analyze the dynamics of team work in various settings.
4. Evaluate the effectiveness of team members' roles in delivering quality health care.
5. Assess how the use of research results on team work would have clinical relevance on your health care setting.
6. Determine how a framework of important characteristics drawn from the different definitions of teams can assist you to understand the functioning of teams.
7. Using the list of team-building attributes provided in the text, specify the steps you would initiate as a nurse leader to build an effective functioning team.
8. Illustrate the advantages and disadvantages of a team performance model to facilitate team effectiveness.
9. Critique the important characteristics of different types of teams.
10. Illustrate the effectiveness of collaboration in an interprofessional team on client care and the family.
11. After studying a few research reports (to be found in the Reference section of this chapter) on the importance of interdisciplinary teams for improving client health outcomes, propose a research study to determine the effectiveness of either a real, or hypothetical, interdisciplinary team on client outcomes.
12. Examine the relevance of intercollaborative education to promote collaborative patient-centered practice.

Teams

A broad agreement exists that health care teams are necessary in various health care settings (Health Canada, 2005; Shortel et al., 2004). However, the implementation of a team approach comes with particular challenges because of the various perspectives that different members from each discipline bring (Pesut, Baker, Elliott, & Johnson, 2000).

Definitions

To comprehend the process of teamwork, it is first necessary to define what a team is. A few of the definitions of team provided recently by scholarly authors are shown in Table 9.1.

Characteristics

Through the analysis and synthesis of the definitions presented, Box 9.1 provides the three predominant characteristics that seem to prevail among effective teams. These characteristics provide a framework that the nurse leader can use in teamwork. First, the nurse must be aware that a set of consistent team-related characteristics exists. Second, the nurse needs to use effective collaborative skills to facilitate team members to recognize theses characteristics. Third, the reciprocal interaction will allow team members to reflect upon and internalize their own personal meaning of these characteristics to comprehend the essence of teamwork. Cowley, Bliss, Mathew, and McVey (2002) argue that this type of interchange of reciprocal interaction facilitates the development of a common language among

TABLE 9.1	DEFINITIONS OF TEAM
Author(s)	**Definition**
Yoder-Wise (2007)	A team is a number of persons associated together in specific work or activity. (p. 342)
Finkelman (2006)	A team is a specific number of consistent people working together who have a common purpose and work toward common goals. (p. 202)
Lemieux-Charles & McGuire (2006)	Team is a multidimensional construct, and team structures and processes can vary widely according to membership, scope of work, tasks, and interactions. (p. 202)
Dessler & Starke (2004)	A team is a group of people who work together and share a common work objective. (p.265)

BOX 9.1 PREVALENT CHARACTERISTICS ACROSS TEAMS

- Number of individuals working and interacting together
- Common purpose and goal
- Specific tasks

---

team members. Each member needs to develop a set of realistic expectations of contributions from each member of the team. Even though differences will undoubtedly exist among the team members, those differences should be harnessed to strengthen the team and to lead to the establishment of problem-solving strategies. Furthermore, open communication and supportive interpersonal relationships tend to promote positive attitudes toward the work environment. Such attitudes frequently lead to job satisfaction, improved job performance, and an observable increase in retention (Amos, Hu, & Herrick, 2005).

The feeling among team members that each member is working toward the success of the team and the achievement of the team goals promotes an important sense of personal accomplishment (Hall, 2005). Furthermore, the team as a whole needs to feel that it has meaningful work to accomplish and is responsible for the outcome of its work. The team also needs to receive feedback about the results of its accomplishments (Lawler, 2003). It is a key leadership responsibility that the nurse communicates effectively with the team members. Interacting positively encourages the members to remain focused and be accountable as they continue their professional growth and commit themselves to the process and task.

> *reflective* **THINKING** Think for a moment about how a team differs from a group. What does a team need to exhibit to enable it to qualify as an effective functioning team?

Teams and Health Care Reform

In Canada, one of the key features of primary health reform involves providing effective and comprehensive health care services to clients, families, and communities through the effective implementation of teams of health professionals and providers. These teams interact and deliver quality health care to achieve desired outcomes (Health Canada, 2005; Doran, 2005). The characteristics of the individual team members can vary in accord with the particular needs of the clients, families, and communities they serve.

A final determinant of a primary health team's composition can be based partially upon the priorities of the provinces and territories. A growing consensus exists that a mix of physicians, nurses, and other professionals working as partners tends to result in better health, improved access to health services, more efficient uses of resources, and greater satisfaction of care for clients and their families. Canada's health care teams are well positioned to implement a proactive approach to health issues and to focus on health promotion and illness, as well as on injury prevention (Health Canada, 2005).

Challenges

With the challenges of restructuring and an increased emphasis on performance improvement, health care teams are experiencing new and challenging opportunities as professional expectations for such teams change and evolve. For example, teams are expected to use new technologies and information systems to communicate and document their activities. In fact, quality interaction systems and procedures that operate across teams, as well as within teams, are instrumental in restructuring and performance (Zeiss, 2002).

Health care administrators look toward their teams in the organization to manage increasingly growing numbers of clients who present ever-changing diverse cultural needs and increasingly complex health problems. Administrators expect professional team members to collaborate more efficiently and more effectively as the added pressures resulting from reorganized and restructured health care organizations, cost containment, health care knowledge, and related variables reinforce the need for quality performance (Heinemann, 2002).

Nurse leaders must be ready to respond to changing economic conditions, consolidations, and unit closures within hospital settings. They must become more aware of changes in health care delivery strategies within the community. As discussed in chapter 5, as complexity theory suggests, anticipating and responding to accelerated "white-water" change becomes a challenge in complex situations (Sullivan & Decker, 2005). Furthermore, learning to recognize when team members are overwhelmed and knowing how to intervene to improve the situation is essential. Focusing on the team, connecting, and building team members' relationships are considered a premiere leadership strategy. The aim is to develop a group of individuals into a cohesive whole in which the members share goals, expectations, and behavioural norms. At the same time, the team members are responsible for recognizing individual differences and the unique contribution of each member (Barker, Sullivan, & Emery, 2006). Leaders must be able to use skills and tools to develop and promote best practices and methods to the success of the team and organization (Contino, 2004). See Box 9.2 for ways to enhance leadership and team skills.

BOX 9.2 LEADERSHIP AND TEAM ENHANCEMENT SKILLS KIT

- Establish rapport with team members.
- Assess team profile.
- Assess boundaries, expectations, and standards of team members.
- Promote climate for positive interactions.
- Discover knowledge and expertise of team members.
- Inform team members of own knowledge and expertise.
- Collaborate with team members on issues of clients and families.
- Develop together goals and a plan of care.
- Implement and evaluate plan of care.
- Evaluate team effectiveness.

> *reflective* **THINKING** In what ways can the nurse leader inspire colleagues to invest their positive energies within the team?

Teamwork

Heinemann (2002) argues that the team approach to health care involves health care professionals working together, especially when issues, needs, and problems are complex, chronic, and overlapping. These influences become especially relevant when the solution requires input from a variety of diverse perspectives. In fact, feedback from health professionals with different value systems, knowledge bases, and skill levels may actually be required for a healthy outcome.

Looking at a hypothetical scenario may best exemplify the team approach. For example, an elderly client who has had a hip replacement needs, first of all, a nurse to assess and dress the wound, administer medications, provide emotional and spiritual support to the client and family, and to evaluate the effectiveness of care. That client also needs a physiotherapist to plan and implement physical exercise to restore mobility, a dietician to plan menus to promote healing following the Canada Food Guide, a physician to continue the hip replacement treatment, and a social worker who may help coordinate home care as needed. When all professionals become involved in the care of a client, effective teamwork is essential.

In the complex health arena, the team approach improves the quality of care and services to clients and their families through a team-generated care plan (Villeneuve & MacDonald, 2006). However, a critical assumption underlying the rationale for the team approach is that the team itself is well functioning (Heinemann, 2002). Box 9.3 delineates the composition of a health care team.

BOX 9.3   HEALTH CARE TEAM MEMBERS

Many disciplines convene in an effective health care team. Among team members are the following:
- Client, the client's family, and significant others
- Nurse
- Physician
- Pharmacist
- Social worker
- Physiotherapist
- Dietician
- Occupational therapist
- Pastoral counselor

> reflective **THINKING**   In your estimation, if you are the team leader, what behaviours will you observe in your team members that suggest the team is functioning well? What may be a few behaviours of a poorly functioning team?

The ability to understand teamwork in health care, find methods to assess its functioning, and effectively intervene to promote effective teamwork has already become increasingly important as a research agenda. Doran (2005) claims that assessing teamwork among nurses and other members of the health care profession is a relatively new phenomenon that needs to be addressed through research.

> reflective **THINKING**   What research methods would you propose to study the effectiveness of team work?

Types of Teams

Teamwork has become a common approach for effective practice and the organization of services delivery in health care (Temkin-Greener, Gross, Kunitz, & Mukamel, 2004). In examining the literature on teamwork, it becomes apparent that various definitions (Table 9.2) are cited to qualify teams and the interactions that take place in team environments (D'Amour, Ferrada-Videla, San Martin Rodriguez, & Beaulieu, 2005).

TABLE 9.2	CHARACTERISTICS OF DIFFERENT TYPES OF TEAMS	
Multidisciplinary Teams	**Interdisciplinary Teams**	**Transdisciplinary Teams**
• Several professionals work on same project, either independently or in parallel	• Greater collaboration among team members	• Consensus-seeking professional practice with an opening up of professional territories
• Interactions are limited or transient	• Common goal • Common decision-making process	• Boundaries become blurred, or vanish
D'Amour, Ferrada-Videla, San Martin Rodriguez, and Beaulieu (2005) Paul and Peterson (2001)	D'Amour, Ferrada-Videla, San Martin Rodriguez, and Beaulieu (2005) Paul and Peterson (2001)	D'Amour, Ferrada-Videla, San Martin Rodriguez, and Beaulieu (2005) Stepans, Thompson, and Buchanan (2002)

Temkin-Greener, Gross, Kunitz, and Mukamel (2004) claim that the interdisciplinary type of team is the most developed. Often in the literature, however, the terms *interdisciplinary* and *interprofessional* appear to be used interchangeably. Both terms refer to the team as a *group of health care professionals* who engage in planned interdependent collaboration with a common goal and decision-making process to deliver primary health care services (Bailey, Jones, & Way, 2006; D'Amour, Ferrada-Videla, San Martin Rodriguez, & Beaulieu, 2005; Health Council of Canada, 2005). According to Amundson (2005), crucial members of the team are the clients and their families, which raises the question of whether the clients and their families are being sufficiently included in the study of health care teams.

Interprofessional approaches to client care are believed to have the potential for improving professional relationships, increasing efficiency and coordination of services, and ultimately promoting health outcomes for clients (Cullen, Fraser, & Symonds, 2003; Reeves & Freeth, 2002). The key aspect here is that as the role of interprofessional teamwork evolves, a model of shared leadership is suggested (McCallin, 2003). Such a concept requires development not only in nursing, but also in all health-related disciplines.

reflective **THINKING** | What is your understanding of shared leadership?

Process of Building Teams

The value of team building cannot be underestimated. Providing safe and effective health care to clients and their families involves teams of health care providers interacting and delivering care to achieve desired outcomes (Doran, 2005). For teams to be productive, they must perform efficiently and interact effectively (Amos, Hu, & Herrick, 2005). The members' perceptions about teamwork, in addition to attitudes, may influence individual and overall team performance (Malone & McPherson, 2004). The successful functioning of the team is dependent upon its members, as well as on its leadership (Yoder-Wise, 2007). The leader's role is to establish clear objectives to allow team members to be productive in an organized way. Team organization is not easy, and it requires tremendous self-discipline.

> *reflective* **THINKING**   Compile a list of strategies that would make a team function effectively.

Current Thinking on Team Building

An examination of current literature on team building indicates that management and health care experts focus on strategies and skills that are deemed valuable for enhancing a well-functioning team. For example, Druskat and Wolff (2001) claim that building an underlying foundation for an effective functioning team is necessary. Three components that they advocate are a sense of mutual trust among members, a sense of team identity, and a sense of team efficacy. Team efficacy means that the team performs well and its members are creative in their method of working together. The authors state that when these conditions are absent, the team will not be as effective as possible, because the members will choose to hold back rather than engage fully. The leader's ability to collaborate effectively with team members becomes increasingly important to the team's success.

LaFasto and Larsen (2001) conducted extensive research on team members' assessments of each other, as well as on work relationships in organizations. Their analysis led them to conclude that key behaviours and conditions are necessary for effective relationships within teams. One of the key behaviours is a unified commitment of all members to the work of the team. The second key behaviour is the ability to share information, perceptions, and feedback openly to facilitate understanding. The third key behaviour is the willingness to display basic respect for others' points of view. In addition, they emphasize the importance of effective team leadership behaviours, such as focusing on the goal, ensuring a collaborative climate, building confidence, demonstrating sufficient technical know-how, setting priorities, and managing performance. These behaviours promote team success because they enable the team to focus on goal achievement and to develop a form of discipline that includes a commitment to remain productive (Smith, Meyer, & Wylie, 2006).

Kreitner, Kinicki, and Cole (2007) argue that the goal of team building is to create teams with high-performance levels demonstrating the following eight attributes:

1. *Participative leadership*—developing interdependency by empowering, freeing up, and contributing to others
2. *Shared responsibility*—creating an environment whereby all team members feel as responsible as the leader does for the performance of the work unit
3. *Aligned on purpose*—having a common goal about the existence of the team and its function
4. *Strong communication*—establishing a climate of trust and open, honest dialogue among all team members
5. *Future-focused*—viewing change as an opportunity for growth, both personally and professionally
6. *Focused on task*—attending and keeping meetings focused on results
7. *Creative talents*—applying each member's creativity and talents
8. *Rapid response*—identifying and acting on possibilities

According to the authors, these eight attributes are salient and combine many of today's progressive ideas on team building. A few other attributes that they include are participation, empowerment, service ethic, active listening, trust, and envisioning. It behooves the leader to be patient and diligent as it may take some time for a high-performance team to develop (Kreitner, Kinicki, & Cole, 2007).

In health care organizations, Grohar-Murray and DiCroce (2003) claim that team building brings a fundamental change in the structure of work. Open communication and supportive interpersonal relationships, integral to building a cohesive team, have been consistently linked with positive attitudes toward the work environment (Amos, Hu, & Herrick, 2005).

DiMeglio et al. (2005) conducted a study to determine the impact of team-building interventions on group cohesion, nurse satisfaction, and turnover rates. They concluded that a few unit-based strategies, such as communication, active collaborative rounds, and facilitation of critical thinking skills, improved group cohesion, and nurse satisfaction and reduced turnover rates.

Brown et al. (2003) assert that effective communication is critical to a team's success. Effective communication focuses on "connecting the dots"—how plans, actions, and decisions are linked, first to team members, and second, to the overall functioning of the team. Communication is fundamental to the team-building process (Coyne, 2005). Mulkins, Eng, and Verhoef (2005) claim that in team building, it is critically important for each member to believe that his or her contributions are respected and appreciated. In addition, team building requires that members be accepting and respectful toward different philosophies of team members and to demonstrate a commitment to work through these differences.

Reid Ponte et al. (2003) argues that the ability to collaborate effectively involves the following: sharing information, working together to brainstorm, deliberating possible solutions, and remaining open to suggestions given by others. These facilitative behaviours are vital to team building, and the leader must be aware of them to foster collaboration and collegiality among the team members.

Another important strategy to build effective teams is that of conflict resolution. Porter-O'Grady (2004a) states that conflict in teams delivering complex health care is due to the diversity of players who energize creativity and innovation as well as a variety of human expressions. All conflict is normative and is fundamental to the human experience (Porter-O'Grady, 2004b). In fact, conflict is requisite of all human interaction. Conflict is dynamic, not static. If not resolved, conflict continues to deepen and expand in a profound way. It is important for the leader not only to anticipate the embedded elements of conflict but also to facilitate the exploration of barriers and work collaboratively early to manage conflict (Outhwaite, 2003).

---

reflective **THINKING**   You are called to a unit to resolve a conflict between two team members. They are speaking loudly at each other in the hallway. Outline a plan to deal with this conflict.

Team members with experiential backgrounds that are decidedly different from those of the team members can place special demands upon a team. Cultural differences can create substantial obstacles to effective teamwork (Brett, Behfar, & Kern, 2006). For team members, to adapt to a new culture involves overcoming several obstacles and setbacks. Leaders who intervene early and set norms, who structure social interaction, and who work to involve all members on the team can unify the team to function cohesively (Brett, Behfar, & Kern, 2006). Figure 9.1 pictures the team-building process leading to effectiveness.

Team Performance Model: Domains, Dimensions, and Elements

One model of team performance that has particular significance for nurse leaders was developed by Heinemann and Zeiss (2002). They claim that their model of team performance—comprising domains, related dimensions, and elements—

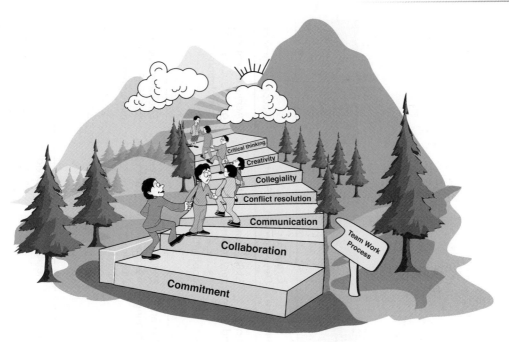

FIGURE 9.1 Teamwork process.

relates particularly well to current changes in the health care system, and as well to the growth and evolution of the health care team.

So that the nurse leader may begin applying this model of team performance, a brief presentation of the four domains is provided in Table 9.3. The two dimensions that occur under each of the domains are described briefly. Finally, a few of the important elements under each of the dimensions are discussed. A detailed insight into the application of the model is contained in the original work of Heinemann and Zeiss (see References).

Structure

Two types of structure are significant with regard to team performance: the structure of the organization in which the team is working and the structure of the team itself. The *organizational dimension* depicts how the structure is designed. Recently, the traditional organizational structure of health care organizations has given way to a more integrative care line structure. This new structure uses a team approach for developing and accomplishing goals. The team is understood, appreciated, and used effectively. For example, more collaboration among team members is occurring and less dependence is required on top management. The mission and goals of the organization are clear. In fact, in many teams, self-management is the goal within the more integrative care line structure.

(text continues on page 240)

TABLE 9.3 TEAM PERFORMANCE MODEL: DOMAINS, DIMENSIONS, AND ELEMENTS

Structure		Context		Process	Growth/Development	Productivity	
Organizational	Team	Organizational	Team	Interdependence		Strategies	Accomplishments
Mission, goals, and direction	Mission, purpose, and direction	Managerial modelling of, and support for, the team approach	Attitudes toward teams and teamwork	Utilization of resources and team members	Skills, mastery, maintenance, and application	Action plans	Achievement of goals/successful completion of tasks
Team fit within organization	Fit between organizational, team, and individual goals	Change, flexibility, and innovation	Being oneself and getting to know others	Participation and workload sharing	Utilization of feedback/learning from mistakes	Patient care plans	Effective leadership/self management
Allocation of authority and responsibility within teams	Roles and responsibilities	Trust, confidence, respect, and value	Caring, warm, and accepting climate	Giving and receiving feedback	Flexibility	Individual development plans	Positive outcomes related to patients and trainees

Mechanisms for communication and decision making	Norms, values, expectations, and standards	Commitment, cohesion, and loyalty	Trust, confidence, respect, and value	Collaboration	Creativity, uniqueness, innovation, and risk-taking	Use of technology	Impact on organization
Objective recognition and rewards for teamwork and to teams	Boundaries and permeability	Motivation and morale	Climate permits free expression	Cooperation, coordination, and efficiency		Marketing	
		Satisfaction/security with job and working relationships	Commitment to team, members, and teamwork	Power and leadership sharing		Time management	
				Decision making	Problem solving	Self-monitoring and evaluation	

From Heineman, G. D., & Zeiss, A. M. (Eds.) (2002). *Team performance in health care: Assessment and development.* New York: Kluwer Academic/Plenum Publishers. Copyright 2002 by Kluwer Academic. Adapted with permission.

Meanwhile the dimension of *team* almost always evolves slowly. At first, in newly developed teams, a lack of mission, purpose, and role clarity results in feelings of awkwardness within the team. However, as the team develops over time, members come to have shared understanding of the team's mission, goals, and objectives. The members interact and participate more equally in the team's tasks as they become familiar with boundaries and with their permeability.

Context

Context refers to how it "feels" to work in a certain organization. *Context* is the particular milieu, climate, or environmental affect in which the team is embedded within the organization. The *organizational* and *team dimensions* deeply affect the team members and, in turn, the functioning of the team.

In regard to the organizational dimension, many managers in organizations are highly effective at setting an atmosphere for collaboration and respect among members. In doing so, they engender feelings of empowerment. Elements such as motivation, commitment, loyalty, and morale flourish in such an environment. On the other hand, without the establishment of these elements, a climate of rippling mistrust can develop among the team members. Mistrust, in turn, can lead to dissatisfaction with the work situation, and in extreme cases, eventual departure from the organization can result.

The dimension of team is also a critical component. It refers to the affect and atmosphere among team members—their perceptions and feelings regarding the socioemotional climate in which they work. Several aspects influence the team dimension. One, for example, is the different styles in which team members relate to one another. Another significant aspect is the set of interpersonal skills demonstrated by the team leader. These skills can be energizing and constructive or deflating and destructive. As the team develops, the members begin to work together more comfortably. They begin to participate with one another more democratically, and they come to share more effectively in the team's tasks in a more equal and supportive manner.

Process

Process refers to the series of progressive and integrated activities that teams use to accomplish their tasks. Within the process domain, the dimension of *interdependence* is the key to interprofessional and interdisciplinary team work. Interdependence does not come naturally to team members. As the team matures, however, members of successful teams begin to learn from one another and become increasingly successful at accepting the role or perspective of the other. When this maturity occurs, communication and collaboration across professional disciplines become more natural and satisfyingly productive. A few major elements of interdependence include the use of the team's resources and team members' skills and abilities to accomplish tasks, share the workload, and problem solve effectively.

The other dimension within the process domain refers to *growth and development*, which is the ability of the team members to grow and mature so that they come to function effectively within the team. The leader is influential in creating the conditions that allow members to use feedback and to learn from mistakes, be creative, be innovative, and learn to take risks. The more open and democratic the leader is, the greater the ability of the team and its members to grow and improve over time. The members learn and become better health care providers, as well as more skilful team members. As a result, they improve the functioning of the team.

Productivity

Productivity includes the strategies teams use to be productive in their actual accomplishments. In the *strategy dimension* of the productivity domain, the key assertion is that teams must diligently document action plans, client care plans, and individual development plans. Time management is one particular strategy to which teams must be accountable in order to be productive. Team members must use available technology to collect, store, manage, analyze, and present information documenting their productivity.

The other dimension of productivity is *accomplishment*. The achievement of both task-oriented and process goals is necessary if the team is to perform successfully in the organization. Task-oriented goals are related to the team's mission and purpose, whereas process goals are related to how effectively the team members work together to accomplish the tasks. Effective team meetings and connected relationships with other teams in the organization and with clients are important requisites of the team. Good working relationships across teams throughout the organization enhance the quality health care and client service, each of which contributes to satisfaction among all who are involved. Positive outcomes regarding clients' health status are major objectives of clinical teams. Examples include maintaining quality of life, increasing health promotion strategies, ensuring death with dignity, and supporting the family throughout the duration of the client's involvement with the team. Most importantly, teams that contribute to positive outcomes should continue to receive support and resources from management (Heinemann & Zeiss, 2002).

Assessing Team Performance

Effective teams, composed of members committed to working together toward a shared goal of providing cost-effective, improved health care, are essential in the health care delivery organization (Yoder-Wise, 2007). On the basis of that premise, it becomes imperative to assess team performance in health care because it can impact directly, or indirectly, on the quality of health care provided to the client and their family (Heinemann, 2002). Key elements in assessing team performance are education and data collection (Heinemann & Zeiss, 2002). Team members must learn how to evaluate objectively the team's performance. In educational workshops, role playing exercises are often helpful in having the team members identify their strengths and weaknesses and evaluate their own processes and outcomes.

Quantitative data collection tools can be introduced to evaluate the effectiveness of the team members working together. Tools such as Likert scales and survey questionnaires can be used to measure team performances. The objective data gathered enable the team leader to assess further and evaluate team member effectiveness. Decisions can then be made by the leader, based on both the leader's subjective observations and the objective data obtained from the tools, about how to encourage the team to proceed.

When team members actively and cooperatively participate in decision-making processes about what factors/behaviours are to be assessed, and how the information will be used, they are likely to engage more productively and enjoyably in the process and provide reliable and accurate information. Team performance can also be monitored by using qualitative strategies, such as focus groups and personal interviews. For example, following focus groups, some teams may schedule meetings to identify the team's strengths and weaknesses and to examine ways to improve the team's performance. The main aspect is that the model of team performance can help teams improve their own self-monitoring and evaluation in order to achieve high standards of performance (Heineman, 2002).

The effective adaptation of the framework of the Heinemann Model, with its clearly delineated domains, dimensions, and elements, can assist the nurse leader in assessing team functioning and performance.

reflective **THINKING**   What do you think are the main components to consider in assessing team performance in the clinical area?

Leadership Issue

Reflect on the health team in the clinical area where you work or study. To improve the functioning of the team, as a leader, what steps will you take to apply the Team Performance Model? What would you do to assess the performance of this team?

Leadership and Collaboration

The need for partnerships among health care professionals is increasing as complex health care needs, trends, and issues proliferate (see Reflections on Leadership Practice). Nurses are vital contributors to these alliances and partnerships (Boswell Cannon, 2005). Collaboration is a complex process that requires intentional knowledge sharing and a joint responsibility for client care (Lindeke & Sieckert, 2005). Nurses recognize and comprehend the value of collaboration, both within the nursing profession and with other health care professionals and community leaders (Daiski, 2004). Essentially, collaboration and teamwork are synonymous concepts (Doran, 2005). Successful collaboration includes interacting, networking, coordinating of care, joint decision-making skills, and visioning—all of which are important aspects of leadership, especially while relationships between team members are being developed (Lemire Rodger, 2006; Villeneuve & MacDonald, 2006; Boswell & Cannon, 2005). Effective collaboration within nursing and other health care professionals is necessary to achieve high-quality outcomes in an interdependent health care delivery system that continues to grow in complexity and importance (Gardner, 2005).

An important element of collaboration is effective leadership. Wesorick (2002) claims that leaders need the ability to transform practice cultures to achieve the desired health outcomes. Leaders must be willing to take the time to investigate and deliberate about issues. They need to become knowledgeable about various strategies to achieve success in the team. Leaders also need to remain enthusiastic, politically active, and visibly aware of the goals of the organization for the outcomes to be successful (Wagner, 2004). It is important that

Reflections on Leadership Practice

*Y*our aging aunt resides in a personal care home where you know that an interprofessional team is in place. When you arrive to visit your aunt before lunch, you meet the dietician, who informs you that your aunt has not been eating well. Therefore, she has prepared an extra snack for your aunt to take on her afternoon outdoor outing. As you enter your aunt's room, she tearfully informs you that the occupational therapist had told everyone at breakfast time they would be going outside for a picnic today. However, when her assigned nurse assisted her with her AM care in mid-morning, she said that none of the residents would be going out because the nurse unit manager said the weather was too cold and the risk of flu was high.

What suggestions do you have for the nurse unit manager on how this situation was handled? How could this event have been better managed?

leaders be fully engaged with team members—reinforcing them even for small successes. Laying a firm foundation of leadership and membership for the collaborative efforts can be time-consuming, but in the long run, the effort is invaluable to the success of the venture (Boswell & Cannon, 2005).

> reflective **THINKING**   Outline a plan you as a leader would implement to develop effective collaboration in a team.

Research on Effectiveness of Health Care Teams

The use of health care teams has increased in the health care delivery system. Consequently, a new trend has occurred toward examining the importance of teams for improving client outcomes (Lemieux-Charles & McGuire, 2006). The findings of several studies indicate two main thrusts: the importance of team process and the role of perceived team effectiveness in improving quality care.

In their literature review, Lemieux-Charles and McGuire (2006) used an Integrated Team Effectiveness Model to summarize research findings and to identify gaps in the literature on health care team effectiveness. The analysis suggests that the type and diversity of clinical expertise involved in team decision making accounts largely for improvement in client care and organizational effectiveness. In fact, collaboration, participation, conflict resolution, and cohesion are the elements that are most likely to influence staff satisfaction and perceived team effectiveness.

In the study conducted by Shortell et al. (2004), data were obtained from 40 teams participating in the national evaluation of the Improving Chronic Care Program. The findings suggest the importance of developing effective teams for improving the quality of care for clients with chronic illness. The researchers identified three major factors that might influence perceived team effectiveness. First is the organization's culture. A group culture that emphasizes teamwork and supports participation facilitates team decision making and goal agreement. Second is the organization's commitment to quality improvement. An organization's commitment to client satisfaction and related dimensions is more likely to provide the teams with sufficient education, support, resources, and recognition to enable the teams to be effective. Third, the question of whether or not the team has a "champion" was examined—that is, the presence of a team member, a nurse, or a physician who would act as a specific facilitator of change in the process of team effectiveness.

Other studies indicated that multidisciplinary interventions can improve health outcomes of clients (Bellomo et al. 2004; Caplan, Williams, Daly, & Abraham, 2004; Chin et al., 2004). One Canadian study, however, indicated that inpatient interdisciplinary care did not result in significantly better outcomes in elderly clients with hip fractures (Naglie et al., 2002).

This brief review indicates that evidence of considerable interest and activity in studying perceived team effectiveness is appearing in the literature. However, more studies are needed to comprehend how health care teams affect organizational and clinical effectiveness. These studies should exemplify multiple research designs and methods, as well as more rigorous conceptualization of team dimensions, traits, and processes, and outcomes (Lemieux-Charles & McGuire, 2006). Finally, further Canadian studies are needed to examine the impact of interdisciplinary interventions on quality of care delivered to clients and their families.

> *reflective* **THINKING**   As a nurse leader, what steps would you take to initiate a research study in your team of the effectiveness of care for childhood obesity?

Interprofessional Education

In Canada, many articles have been commissioned by Health Canada to be written about interprofessional policy, practice, and education (Barr, 2005). In fact, D'Amour and Oandasan (2005) developed a framework that is now being used by Health Canada to advance Interprofessional Education for Collaborative Patient-Centred Practice.

According to Herbert (2005), collaborative patient-centred practice is a practice orientation, a way that health care professionals work together with their clients. The Interprofessional Education for Collaborative Patient-Centred Practice is an initiative, sponsored by Health Canada, designed to facilitate and to support the implementation of an approach to interprofessional education for collaborative patient-centred practice across all health sectors. One of the specific objectives is to increase the number of health professionals trained for patient-centred interprofessional team practice at the level of entry to practice, graduate education, and continuing education (Hebert, 2005). This initiative led Health Canada to place calls for proposals for interprofessional learning projects. Dr. Ruby Grymonpre (principal investigator) and her team and Dr. Judy Anderson, both from the University of Manitoba, successfully received funding. The University of Manitoba now has two interprofessional education initiatives running simultaneously, which helps strengthen the interprofessional care initiative established across Canada (Riverview Health Centre, 2006).

Gilbert (2005) argues that the implementation of interprofessional education is needed to reflect the holistic process of facilitating trust among professionals. To develop collaborative skills, students in the various health-related fields need opportunities to spend time together and to learn and to work together in constructive and meaningful ways (Hall, 2005). It is anticipated that the projects that have been initiated at the University of Manitoba will inspire administration and professors across the nation to adapt curricula to promote interprofessional education.

reflective **THINKING**   What benefits do you think you will achieve in being part of the interprofessional educational project at your university?

WEBSITES

■ **Health Canada. Health Care System, Highlights (2008)**

http://www.hc-sc.gc.ca/hcs-sss/news-nouvelles-eng.php
This section of the health care system area will alert you to new health issues that have been added from time to time.

■ **Health Council of Canada, Health Care in Canada, Clearing the Road to Quality (2006)**

http://www.healthcouncilcanada.ca/docs/rpts/2006/2006_AnnualReport.pdf
The First Ministers' Health Accord of 2003 and the 10-Year Plan to Strengthen Health Care in 2004 moved from debating health care renewal to delivering it. In the process, the Health Council of Canada was uniquely charged with tracking that renewal and reporting its progress to Canadians. This site provides a report of that progress, including interprofessional primary health care teams.

■ **The Public Health Agency of Canada**

http://www.phac-aspc.gc.ca/
The creation of the Public Health Agency of Canada in December, 2006 marked the beginning of a new approach to federal leadership and collaboration with provinces and territories on efforts to renew the public health system in Canada and support a sustainable health care system. This site provides many links to Canadian health care developments, as well as the latest health care news and advisories/warnings.

REFERENCES

Amos, M. A., Hu, J., & Herrick, C. A. (2005). The impact of team building on communication and job satisfaction of nursing staff. *Journal for Nurses in Staff Development 21*(1), 10–16.

Amundson, S. (2005). The impact of relational norms on the effectiveness of health and human service teams. *The Health Care Manager, 24*(3), 216–224.

Bailey, P., Jones, L., & Way, D. (2006). Family physicians/nurse practitioner: Stories of collaboration. *Journal of Advanced Nursing, 53*(4), 381–391.

Barker, A. M., Taylor Sullivan, D., & Emery, M. J. (2006). *Leadership competencies for clinical managers: The renaissance of transformational leadership.* Toronto, ON: Jones and Bartlett.

Barr, H. (2005, May). Canada as a case study. *Journal of Interprofessional Care,* (Suppl. 1), 5–7.

Bellomo, R., Goldsmith, D., Uchino, S., Buckmaster, J., Hart, G., Opdam, H., et al. (2004). Prospective controlled trial of effect of medical emergency team on postoperative morbidity and mortality rates. *Critical Care Medicine, 32*(4), 916–921.

Boswell, C., & Cannon, S. (2005). New horizons for collaborative partnerships. *Online Journal of Issues in Nursing, 10*(1), manuscript 2. Retrieved January 2007 from http://www.nursingworld.org/ojin/

Brett, J., Behfar, K., & Kern, M. (2006). Managing multicultural teams. *Harvard Business Review, 84*(11), 84–91.

Brown, M., Ohlinger, J., Rusk, C., Delmore, P., & Ittmann, P. (2003). Implementing potentially better practices for multidisciplinary team building: Creating a neonatal intensive care unit culture of collaboration. *Pediatrics, 111*(4), 482–488.

Caplan, G., Williams, A., Daly, B., & Abraham, K. (2004). A randomized, controlled trial of comprehensive geriatric assessment and multidisciplinary intervention after discharge of elderly from the emergency department–The DEED II study. *Journal of the American Geriatric Society, 52*, 1417–1423.

Chin, M., Cook, S., Drum, M., Jin, L., Guillen, M., Humikowski, C., et al. (2004). Improving diabetes care in Midwest community health centers with the health disparities collaborative. *Diabetes Care, 27*(1), 2–8.

Contino, D. S. (2004). Leadership competencies: Knowledge, skills, and aptitudes nurses need to lead organizations effectively. *Critical Care Nurse, 24*(3), 52–64.

Cowley, S., Bliss, J., Mathew, A., & McVey, G. (2002). Effective interagency and interprofessional working: Facilitators and barriers. *International Journal of Palliative Nursing, 8*(1), 30–39.

Coyne, C. (2005). Strength in numbers: How team building is improving care in a variety of practice settings. *PT—Magazine of Physical Therapy, 13*(6), 40–51.

Cullen, L., Fraser, D., & Symonds, I. (2003). Strategies for interprofessional education: The interprofessional Team Objective Structured Clinical Examination for midwifery and medical students. *Nurse Education Today, 23*(6), 427–433.

D'Amour, D., & Oandasan, I. (2005, May). Interprofessionality as the field of interprofessional practice and interprofessional education: An emerging concept. *Journal of Interprofessional Care*, (Suppl. 1), 8–20.

D'Amour, D., Ferrada-Videla, M., San Martin Rodriguez, L., & Beaulieu, M.-D. (2005, May). The conceptual basis for interprofessional collaboration: Core concepts and theoretical frameworks. *Journal of Interprofessional Care*, (Suppl. 1), 116–131.

Daiski, I. (2004). Changing nurses' dis-empowering relationship patterns. *Journal of Advanced Nursing, 48*(1), 43–50.

Dessler, G., & Starke, F. A. (2004). *Management: Principles and practices for tomorrow's leaders.* Toronto, ON: Pearson Prentice Hall.

DiMeglio, K., Padula, C., Piatek, C., Korber, S., Barrett, A., Ducharme, M., et al. (2005). Group cohesion and nurse satisfaction: Examination of a team-building approach. *Journal of Nursing Administration, 35*(3), 110–120

Doran, D. (2005). Teamwork—nursing and the multidisciplinary team. In L. McGillis Hall (Ed.), *Quality work environments for nurse and patient safety* (p. 39). Toronto, ON: Jones and Bartlett.

Druskat, V., & Wolff, S. (2001). Building the emotional intelligence of groups. *Harvard Business Review, 79*(3), 81–91.

Finkelman, A. W. (2006). *Leadership and management in nursing.* Upper Saddle River, NJ: Pearson Prentice Hall.

Gardner, D. (2005, January). Ten lessons in collaboration. *Online Journal of Issues in Nursing, 10*(1), manuscript 1. Retrieved January 2007 from http://www.nursingworld.org/ojin/

Gilbert, J. (2005). Inter-professional education for collaborative, patient-centred practice. *Nursing Leadership, 18*(2), 32–38.

Grohar-Murray, M., & DiCroce, H. (2003). *Leadership and management in nursing* (3rd ed.). Upper Saddle River, NJ: Prentice Hall.

Hall, P. (2005, May). Interprofessional teamwork: Professional cultures as barriers. *Journal of Interprofessional Care*, (Suppl. 1), 188–196.

Health Canada, Health Care System Delivery. (2005). Retrieved January 14, 2007, from http://www.hc-sc.gc.ca/hcs-sss/delivery-prestation/index-eng.php

Health Council of Canada. (2005). *Healthcare renewal in Canada: Clearing the road to quality. Annual report to Canadians 2005.* Toronto, ON: Health Council of Canada.

Heinemann, G. D. (2002). Teams in health care settings. In G. D. Heinemann & A. M. Zeiss (Eds.), *Team performance in health care* (p. 3). New York: Kluwer Academic/Plenum Publishers.

Herbert, C. (2005, May). Changing the culture: Interprofessional education for collaborative patient-centred practice in Canada. *Journal of Interprofessional Care* (Suppl. 1), 1–4.

Kreitner, R., Kinicki, A., & Cole, N. (2007). *Fundamentals of organizational behaviour* (2nd Canadian ed.). Toronto, ON: McGraw-Hill Ryerson.

LaFasto, F., & Larsen, C. (2001). *When teams work best: 6,000 team members and leaders tell what it takes to succeed.* Thousand Oaks, CA: Sage Publications.

Lawler, E. (2003). *Treat people right! How organizations and individuals can propel each other into a virtuous spiral of success.* San Francisco: Jossey-Bass.

Lemieux-Charles, L., & McGuire, W. L. (2006). What do we know about health care team effectiveness? A review of the literature. *Medical Care Research and Review, 63*(3), 263–300.

Lemire Rodger, G. (2006). Leadership challenges and directions. In J. M. Hibberd & D. L. Smith (Eds.), *Nursing leadership and management in Canada* (3rd ed., pp. 497–513). Toronto, ON: Elsevier Mosby.

Lindeke, L., & Sieckert, A. (2005). Nurse-physician workplace collaboration. *Online Journal of Issues in Nursing, 10*(1), manuscript 4. Retrieved January 2007 from http://www.nursingworld.org/ojin/

Malloch, K., & Porter-O'Grady, T. (2005). *The quantum leader: Applications for the new world of work* (p. 23). Toronto, ON: Jones and Bartlett.

Malone, D. M., & McPherson, J. (2004). Community- and hospital-based early intervention team members' attitudes and perceptions of teamwork. *International Journal of Disability, Development and Education, 51*(1), 99–116.

McCallin, A. (2003). Interdisciplinary team leadership: A revisionist approach for an old problem? *Journal of Nursing Management 11*(6), 364–370.

Mulkins, A., Eng, J., & Verhoef, M. (2005). Working towards a model of integrative health care: Critical elements for an effective team. *Complementary Therapies in Medicine, 13*, 115–122.

Naglie, G., Tansey, C., Kirkland, J., Ogilvie-Harris, D., Detsky, A., Etchells, E., et al. (2002). Interdisciplinary inpatient care for elderly people with hip fracture: A randomized controlled trial. *Canadian Medical Association Journal, 167*(1), 25–32.

Outhwaite, S. (2003). The importance of leadership in the development of an integrated team. *Journal of Nursing Management, 11*, 371–376.

Paul, S., & Peterson, C. (2001). Interprofessional collaboration: Issues for practice and research. *Occupational Therapy in Health Care, 15*, 1–12.

Pesut, B., Baker, S., Elliott, B., & Johnson, J. (2000). Leadership through interdisciplinary teams: A case study of an acute pain service. *Canadian Journal of Nursing Leadership, 13*(4), 5–10.

Porter-O'Grady, T. (2004a). Embracing conflict: Building a healthy community. *Health Care Management Review, 29*(3), 181–187.

Porter-O'Grady, T. (2004b). Constructing a conflict resolution program for health care. *Health Care Management Review, 29*(4), 278–283.

Reeves, S., & Freeth, D. (2002). The London training ward: An innovative interprofessional learning initiative. *Journal of Interprofessional Care, 16*(1), 45–52.

Reid Ponte, P., Branowicki, P., Somerville, J., Anderson, D., Ives Erickson, J., Kruger, N., et al. (2003). Collaboration among nurse executives in complex environments: Fostering administrative best practice. *Journal of Nursing Administration, 33*(11), 596–602.

Riverview Health Centre. (2006). Introducing the project team. *Interactions: Newsletter for Interprofessional Education for Geriatric Care Program. 1*(1), 4.

Shortell, S. M., Marsteller, J. A., Lin, M., Pearson, M. L., Wu, S.-Y., Mendel, P., et al. (2004). The role of perceived team effectiveness in improving chronic illness care. *Medical Care, 42*(11), 1040–1048.

Smith, D., Meyer, S., & Wylie, D. (2006). Leadership for teamwork and collaboration. In J. M. Hibberd & D. L. Smith (Eds.), *Nursing leadership and management in Canada* (3rd ed., pp. 519–547). Toronto, ON: Elsevier Mosby.

Stepans, M., Thompson, C., & Buchanan, M. (2002). The role of the nurse on a transdisciplinary early intervention assessment team. *Public Health Nursing, 19*, 238–245.

Sullivan, E., & Decker, P. (2005). *Effective leadership & management in nursing* (6th ed.). Upper Saddle River, NJ: Pearson Prentice Hall.

Temkin-Greener, H., Gross, D., Kunitz, S., & Mukamel, D. (2004). *Medical Care, 42*(5), 472–481.

Villeneuve, M., & MacDonald, J. (2006). *Toward 2020: Visions for nursing*. Ottawa, ON: Canadian Nurses Association.

Wagner, E. (2004). Effective teamwork and quality of care. *Medical Care, 42*(11), 1037–1039.

Wesorisk, B. (2002). 21st century leadership challenge: Creating and sustaining healthy healing cultures and integrated services at the point of care. *Nursing Administration Quarterly, 26*(5), 18–32.

Yoder-Wise, P. S. (2007). *Leading and managing in nursing* (4th ed.). St. Louis: Mosby Elsevier.

Zeiss, A. M. (2002). Measuring team performance in health care settings. In G. D. Heinemann & A. M. Zeiss (Eds.), *Team performance in health care* (p. 19). New York: Kluwer Academic/Plenum Publishers.

REASSESSING LEADERSHIP COMPETENCIES

CHAPTER 10

Complexity Interactions for the Nurse Leader: Critical Thinking, Decision Making, and Appreciative Inquiry

When I'm part of an organization entrusted by the community to provide service, I'm conscious that trust requires me to be a leader in finding ways to respond to community needs and be a just steward of resources in the organization.

—Sister Elizabeth M. Davis, RSM

Elizabeth Davis has made presentations to senior health executives around the world and has spoken extensively on transforming the health care system. She is a member of the Congregation of the Sisters of Mercy of Newfoundland and Labrador and is currently a doctoral student at the University of Toronto. She holds a BA and a BEd from Memorial University of Newfoundland, an MA (Theology) from the University of Notre Dame, and an MHSc (Administration) from the University of Toronto. Among her recent awards are the Humanitarian of the Year Award (Newfoundland and Labrador Chapter of the Canadian Red Cross), the 2001 Performance Citation Award (Catholic Health Association of Canada), the 2001 Award for Excellence in Distinguished Service (Canadian Health Care Association), and an honorary Doctor of Laws from Memorial University of Newfoundland (May 2002). Sister Elizabeth speaks regularly on leadership in today's changing world and on maintaining a values base in times of uncertainty.

Overview

The profession of nursing is in a dynamic state of complex change, redefining its practice and accepting accountability for competent care and safe client outcomes. As such, nurse leadership roles and responsibilities continue to evolve in response to the complexities of the health care system. For nurse leaders, the challenge of an increased emphasis on critical thinking is an integral component for making innovative, ethical, and independent decisions related to resolving clients' issues, stressful work environments, and health care mandates. Nursing, as a caring profession, requires critical thinking to enhance the quality of decision making. Nurse leaders strive to promote evidence-based decision making, which is an interactive process involving conscientious and judicious consideration of the available evidence to identify the best approaches to providing quality care. By applying the process of appreciative inquiry, nurse leaders have the potential to stimulate growth and change in the health care organization by focusing on individual and organizational strengths.

Objectives

By critically reflecting upon and processing knowledge throughout this chapter, you will be able to respond effectively to the following objectives:

1. Examine the concept of critical thinking as it applies to nurse leaders.
2. Critique the quality of critical thinking skills and dispositions needed in nursing practice.
3. Prepare a chart of the central components of critical thinking.
4. Illustrate your understanding of the different types of reflection.
5. Develop a scenario whereby a nurse leader might apply several dimensions of the revised Bloom's framework.
6. Appraise the nurse leader's role in facilitating a team to develop critical thinking skills.
7. Determine the importance of evidence-based decision making within the complexity of the health care system.
8. Compare and contrast the steps and procedures involved in problem solving and decision making within nursing practice.
9. Design a case study by which the nurse leader can demonstrate using the eight steps of the decision-making process.
10. Delineate the factors that affect a nurse leader's decision-making process.
11. Evaluate the importance of group thinking in an interdisciplinary team.
12. Analyse the importance of ethical decision making in today's complex health care system.
13. Apply the appreciative inquiry "4-D" cycle in your workplace.

Critical Thinking

Critical thinking is widely regarded in nursing as a concept and a process of central importance, both in nursing education and in nursing practice (Cody, 2002). As nurse leaders deal with complexity, increased demands, and greater accountability in the health care system, they must be able to think critically to provide the leadership that creates positive change (Valiga, 2009). It is important for the leader to form a fundamental understanding of the various definitions, components, and dimensions of critical thinking, which then can be used as an impetus for transforming the critical thinking process into the leadership action needed to enhance nursing practice (Porter-O'Grady et al., 2005). Nurses must be able to question, think and comprehend, apply, analyse, synthesize, and evaluate client and family health situations. In fact, critical thinking is the key in nursing practice (Profetto-McGrath, Smith, & Bulmer, 2003). Simpson and Courtney (2002) state that, in a variety of settings, nurses need to be able to recognize complex phenomena within relationships that have the potential for leading to creative personalized solutions. As depicted in Figure 10.1, critical thinking is a fundamental component of nursing practice. Building capacity for critical thinking to transform the practice environment is highly important for nurse leaders.

Definition

The concept of critical thinking was analysed extensively by Turner (2005). She used the evolutionary view of concept analysis because it focuses primarily on identifying and classifying the concept in its existing view. To identify the changes that have occurred in the concept of critical thinking over time, the years 1981 to 2002 were selected for study. This 20-year block of time was then divided into two time periods, 1981 to 1991 and 1992 to 2002, known as the first and second stratum. Three nursing databases were used for the analysis, and articles were obtained from Swedish, Canadian, and British journals for inclusion in the study.

Table 10.1 outlines the most frequently cited definitions of critical thinking found in the literature from 1981 to 2002. The most frequently cited definition originates from the American Philosophical Association Delphi Research Project. In examining scholarly articles and research studies, the majority of the more recent literature references the American Philosophical Association Delphi study definition of the early 1990s (Redding, 2001; Banning, 2006; Worrell & Profetto-McGrath, 2007; Valiga, 2009).

reflective **THINKING** What is your definition of critical thinking?

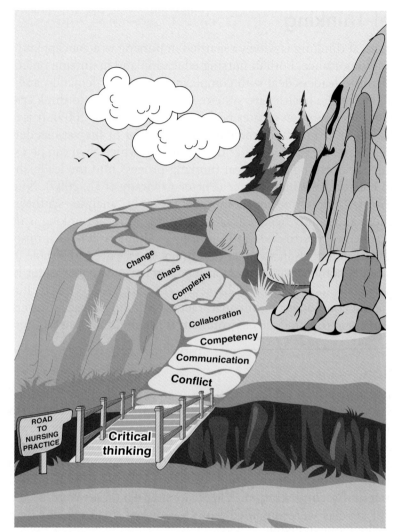

FIGURE 10.1 Road to nursing practice.

Turner (2005) concludes that in nursing, critical thinking is purposeful, self-regulatory judgment characterized by reasoning, interpretation, analysis, inference, and evaluation. Critical thinking requires consideration of the contextual evidence (facts pertaining to a particular situation or client) that results in safe, competent practice and improved decision making, clinical judgments, and problem solving. However, it is important to note that many complex and diverse definitions of critical thinking have been generated in various disciplines. Strong agreement exists among the experts that a critical thinker should possess certain skills, as well as dispositions, toward the process of critical thinking (Paul, 1984; Facione, Facione, & Sanchez, 1994; Norris, 1995).

TABLE 10.1	MOST FREQUENTLY CITED DEFINITIONS OF CRITICAL THINKING
Source of Definition	**Definition**
American Philosophical Association Delphi Report, Facione, P., 13 occurrences	• Purposeful, self-regulatory judgment that results in interpretation, analysis, evaluation, and inference, as well as explanation of the evidential, conceptual, methodological, criteriological, or contextual considerations upon which that judgment is based. • A nonlinear, recursive process in which a person forms a judgment about what to believe or what to do in a given context. • The process of purposeful self-regulatory judgment; an interactive, reflective, reasoning process. • The development and evaluation of arguments. Facione, P. (1990a). *Critical thinking: A statement of expert consensus for purposes of educational assessment and instruction. The Delphi Report: Research findings and recommendations.* Washington, DC: American Philosophical Association. Facione, P. (1990b). *Executive summary of critical thinking: A statement of expert consensus for purposes of educational assessment and instruction, the Delphi Report.* Millbrae, CA: California Academic Press.
Paul, R. W., 8 occurrences	• Thinking about your thinking while you are thinking in order to make your thinking better, more clear, more accurate, and more defensible. • A tool that is used to think about a subject, situation, or project accurately and clearly, as well as deeply and broadly. • The intellectually disciplined process of actively and skillfully conceptualizing, applying, analyzing, synthesizing, and/or evaluating information gathered or generated by observation, experience, reflection, reasoning, or communication as a guide to belief and action. Paul, R. W. (1992). *Critical thinking: How to prepare students for a rapidly changing world.* Santa Rosa, CA: Center for Critical Thinking. Paul, R. W. (1993). *Critical thinking: What every person needs to survive in a rapidly changing world.* Santa Rosa, CA: Foundation for Critical Thinking.
Watson and Glaser, 7 occurrences	• An attitude to being disposed to consider problems in a thoughtful manner within the range of one's experience. • A composite of attitudes, knowledge, and skills that include attitudes of inquiry that involve the ability to recognize the existence of problems and an acceptance of the general needs for evidence in support of what is asserted to be true; knowledge of the nature of valid inferences, abstractions, and generalizations in which the weight or accuracy of different kinds of evidence are logically determined; and skills in employing and applying the above attitudes and knowledge.

(table continues on page 258)

TABLE 10.1	MOST FREQUENTLY CITED DEFINITIONS OF CRITICAL THINKING (continued)
Source of Definition	**Definition**
	• The combination of abilities required to define a problem, select pertinent information for the solution, recognize stated and unstated assumptions, formulate and select relevant and promising hypotheses, draw conclusions, and judge the validity of inferences. Watson, G., & Glaser, E. M. (1964). *Critical thinking appraisal manual.* New York: Brace & World. Watson, G., & Glaser, E. M. (1980). *Critical thinking appraisal manual.* New York: Harcourt, Brace & Jovanovich.
Beyer, 4 occurrences	• A higher order thinking activity that transcends problem solving to involve reasoned judgment and evaluation. • Judging the authenticity, worth, or accuracy of something. Beyer, B. (1995). *Critical thinking.* Bloomington, IN: Phi Delta Kappa Educational Foundation.
Kataoka-Yahiro and Saylor, 4 occurrences	• A domain-specific process of cognitive activity that determines actions. • A process that is reflective and reasonable thinking. Kataoka-Yahiro, M., & Saylor, C. (1994). A critical thinking model for nursing judgment. *Journal of Nursing Education, 33*, 351–360.
Ennis and Millman, 4 occurrences	• Reasonable reflective thinking that is focused on deciding what to believe or do. It consists of three major components: mental operations, certain kinds of knowledge, and certain attitudes. It occurs only when all three of these components are engaged. • A unique cognitive thought process. Ennis, R. J., & Millman, J. (1985). *Cornell tests of critical thinking.* Pacific Grove, CA: Midwest Publications.

From Turner, P. (2005). Critical thinking in nursing education and practice as defined in the literature. *Nursing Education Perspectives, 26*(5), 272–277. Adapted and reproduced with the permission of National League for Nursing.

Skills and Dispositions

In addition to possessing a set of essential skills, such as those of analysis, inference, and evaluation, critical thinkers must also display a set of necessary and related dispositions to complement the skills, such as those outlined in Table 10.2. Nurses must be able to explore ideas and examine arguments while remaining open-minded and tolerant of divergent ideas. At the same time, they need to be able to entertain alternatives (Profetto-McGrath, 2005).

TABLE 10.2	KEY DISPOSITIONS AND CHARACTERISTICS OF THE CRITICAL THINKER
Disposition of the Critical Thinker	**Characteristics of the Critical Thinker**
Open-minded	▪ Has an appreciation of alternate perspectives ▪ Willing to respect the right of others to hold different opinions ▪ Seeks to understand other cultural traditions to gain perspectives on self and for others
Inquisitive	▪ Curious and enthusiastic in wanting to acquire knowledge ▪ Wants to know how things work, even when the applications of them are not immediately apparent
Truth seeking	▪ Courageous about asking questions to obtain the best knowledge ▪ Strives to find truth even if such knowledge might fail to support one's perceptions, beliefs, and interests
Analytical	▪ Uses verifiable information ▪ Demands the application of reason and evidence ▪ Inclined to anticipate consequences
Systematic	▪ Values organization ▪ Follows a focused and diligent approach to problems at all levels of complexity
Self-confident	▪ Trusts one's own reasoning and skills ▪ Inclined to use these skills rather than other strategies to respond to problems ▪ Makes decisions based on scientific evidence ▪ Responds to the values and interests of individuals and society

Adapted from Banning, M. (2006). Nursing research: Perspectives on critical thinking. *British Journal of Nursing, 15*(8), 458.

Profetto-McGrath, Hesketh, Lang, and Estabrooks (2003) studied the relationship between research utilization and the critical thinking dispositions of 141 nurses across four tertiary Canadian hospitals. The results indicated that open-mindedness was significantly correlated with overall, instrumental, and conceptual research utilization. In fact, open-mindedness is one of the most important dispositions for research utilization. This disposition implies that a nurse is comfortable at encountering conflicting views and can listen to new ideas before making decisions about the validity of new information. In this study, overall research utilization referred to the use of any kind of research findings, in any manner and in any aspect, of the nurses' work. Instrumental research utilization is the noticeable implementation of research findings in nursing practice. Meanwhile, conceptual research utilization was described as research findings used to change one's thought processes or assumptions about how certain client care, or other health care situations, should be approached.

> *reflective* **THINKING** Think about the dispositions and related characteristics identified in Table 10.2. What other dispositions do you deem important for a nurse leader who works on a pediatric clinical unit, for example?

Central Components

Riddell (2007) reminds us that the literature contains many different definitions of critical thinking. However, an oversimplification of the concept arises if one endeavours to reduce it solely to a definition. Given the complexity of the critical thinking process, it is important to describe critical thinking in terms of central components and features by which the concept may be recognized. Commonalities among the varying descriptions of critical thinking include the following:

- *Contextual awareness*: Understanding the context within which assumptions, and the actions arising from these, are developed
- *Inquiry, interpretation and analysis, reasoning, and judgment*: Progressing in the thought cycle with the intent of attaining inferences and further observations
- *Identification and appraisal of assumptions*: Scanning emerging patterns and perceived cues for the purpose of generating a hypothesis
- *Reflection*: Broadening the perspective, moving into uncharted waters, challenging assumptions, and reformulating issues (Brookfield, 1987; Mezirow, 1991; Cody, 2002).

Critical thinking can be considered the application of reasoning and reflection in a variety of health issues and discourses, along with the ability to identify evidence to support one's beliefs, evaluate its significance, and change one's thinking accordingly (Cody, 2002).

> *reflective* **THINKING** In what ways can you test assumptions about a client and family to determine whether they are correct?

Reflection

The need to reflect is another key element in developing the ability to think critically (Riddell, 2007). According to Mezirow (1991), critical thinking can be facilitated by skilled critical questioning to stimulate three types of reflection. These three reflections include:

1. *Content reflection*, which is the "what" of the problem.
2. *Process reflection*, which is the "how" of the problem.
3. *Premise reflection*, which is the "why" of the problem.

Both content and process reflections can change beliefs by reinforcing, negating, elaborating, conforming, or transforming them (Mezirow, 1991). On the other hand, premise reflection can give rise to a fully developed belief system that is more open, inclusive, discriminating, and integrative of experience. Riddell (2007) states "it is important to realize that content and process reflections change *belief schemes*; premise reflection can change *belief systems*" (p. 123). Ideally, the process of critical questioning will always facilitate the process of critical reflection, both for individuals and groups. Those who will use critical questioning effectively will be able to apply the skills of critical thinking and analysis to specific client-centred collaborative practice situations (Kearney, 2008). The intended outcome, however, is that all interdisciplinary teams are composed of individuals who have learned to develop their own habits of critical reflection, thus qualifying as real critical thinkers. The importance of reflection in nursing practice is indicated in the significant findings of two nursing research studies. Findings of Hartrick (2000) and Peden-McAlpine, Thomlinson, Forneris, and Meyer (2005) indicate that reflection, combined

---

Reflections on Leadership Practice

For several days you have been thinking about reflection. You have read that one powerful experience is to ask yourself the question, "Why am I caring for clients and families in this manner today?" Take time to reflect on your thoughts and reactions with clients. What have you learned by doing this exercise?

A second powerful experience is to ask a nurse colleague who is close to you to reflect back to you your own apparent attitudes, rationalizations, and habitual ways of behaving and asking while caring for clients and their families. Take time to reflect on the observations of your colleague. Have you become more aware of any particular assumptions and beliefs underlying your actions? Are you becoming more aware that your actions are affected by context as well as by personal histories? Realizing how your behaviour is seen by others is a crucial step to unravelling the complexities and assumptions that ultimately determine what you do in your practice.

with narrative and dialogue, has assisted in the transformation of nursing practice by bridging the gap between the theoretical ideals of nursing care and the realities of daily care-giving practices. Nurses who use reflection well can organize their thinking around context to develop effective critical thinking skills in practice.

The process of reflection occurs in many interrelated instances. The process is extremely important for nurses as they challenge old discrepancies and sift out new meanings. Reflection enables nurses to explore their assumptive world and question premises they have begun to take for granted.

Dimensions

The dimensions of critical thinking comprise both cognitive skills and affective dispositions (Simpson & Courtney, 2002). As a means of qualitatively expressing various kinds of cognitive skills, the Taxonomy of Educational Objectives was developed by Benjamin Bloom (1956). The taxonomy is a means of discussing higher order thinking. Page and Mukherjee (2007) state that the understanding of *critical thinking* is used interchangeably with what is meant by *reflective thinking* and by *higher order thinking*.

Original Bloom's Framework

The original Bloom's taxonomy provided a valuable framework for classifying cognitive learning in six major categories, ordered in increasing complexity, as follows:

1. *Knowledge*: Recall of factual information
2. *Comprehension*: Understanding of those facts
3. *Application*: Applying those facts, ideas, and principles in a particular context
4. *Analysis*: Separating parts into distinct elements to recognize connections, examine the meaningful parts, and discard the unneeded parts
5. *Synthesis*: Reassembling parts into a more meaningful whole; for example, developing a plan or proposing a strategy
6. *Evaluation*: Making a judgment on the basis of explicit and relatively complex criteria; for example, comparing proposals (Krathwohl, 2002; Page & Mukherjee, 2007)

Bloom's taxonomy has withstood the test of time for more than 50 years, and it remains useful for discussing higher order thinking (Krathwohl, 2002). For example, the cognitive activities of analysis, synthesis, and evaluation are generally considered to be higher order thinking. Nurses, who are involved in active learning, practice these skills in specific experiences with clients and families in either the clinical or community setting.

> **reflective THINKING** Select an article from the reference list at the end of this chapter. Use the process of analysis, synthesis, and evaluation while reading this article. What benefits have you derived from doing this exercise?

Revised Bloom's Framework

Recently, Bloom's taxonomy was updated to reflect changes in the pursuit of learning in the 21st century (Anderson et al., 2002). The framework provides a means of classifying cognitive learning through six levels of cognitive processes and four dimensions of knowledge (Krathwohl, 2002). Although the first three categories were included in the original taxonomy, metacognitive knowledge was added in the revised taxonomy. Metacognitive knowledge includes knowledge about cognition as well as awareness of, and knowledge about, one's own cognition (Pintrich, 2002). In combination, the dimensions of cognitive processes and knowledge form a two-dimensional framework. This framework is illustrated in Table 10.3.

Su, Osisek, and Starnes (2005) developed instructional designs for teaching and assessing implicit thought processes involved in clinical reasoning for a group of student nurses. They state that to achieve transfer of nursing knowledge, students must acquire knowledge of thinking paradigms in relation to the context of the subject matter. For example, in applying procedural knowledge,

TABLE 10.3 | THE DIMENSIONS OF KNOWLEDGE AND COGNITIVE PROCESS

The Knowledge Dimension	The Cognitive Process Dimension					
	Remember	Understand	Apply	Analyze	Evaluate	Create
Factual Knowledge	List	Summarize	Classify	Order	Rank	Combine
Conceptual Knowledge	Describe	Interpret	Experiment	Explain	Assess	Plan
Procedural Knowledge	Tabulate	Predict	Calculate	Differentiate	Conclude	Compose
Metacognitive Knowledge	Appropriate Use	Execute	Construct	Achieve	Action	Actualize

© 2005 Extended Campus, Oregon State University. Designer/Developer: Dianna Fisher, Director, Project Development and Training. Adapted and reproduced with permission.

students used a sequence of thinking strategies to make decisions while performing a task.

Meanwhile, in monitoring metacognitive knowledge, students analysed the thinking strategies used for different tasks, the knowledge of the conditions in which these strategies were used, and the extent that these strategies were effective. This process facilitated the students' self-awareness of the cognitive processes being used. During this learning process, the students acknowledged their realization of the connectedness of their individual cognitive abilities and were pleased with taking responsibility for their own learning (Su, Osisek, & Starnes, 2005).

---

reflective **THINKING** Describe what you experience when you think about your own thinking. (This is metacognition in action.)

Contemporary leaders in critical thinking have laid down strong foundations of the critical thinking process that nurse leaders can apply during these dramatic times of changing nursing practice (Porter-O'Grady et al., 2005). The complex needs of clients and family, and the expanding roles of professionals in the delivery of health care, require nurses to be critical thinkers and self-directed learners (Worrell & Profetto-McGrath, 2007).

The nurse leader must be aware that critical thinking skills need to be taught, supported, and nurtured, not only in undergraduate nursing education, but also in all settings where nurses practice. For example, the establishment of journal clubs is one way of developing critical thinking skills (Seymour, Kinn, & Sutherland, 2003). In addition, reviewing nursing research articles in a journal club format provides valuable motivation for evidence-based practice changes (Luby, Riley, & Towne, 2006).

Another way to promote critical thinking is by using reflective journals (Profetto-McGrath, 2005). These journals, created either from daily writings or from notes that focus on critical incidents, provide a means to personalize and reflect on relevant professional experiences. A review of the nursing literature indicates that for many nurses, the reflection process has been highly beneficial for their practice and the advancement of nursing knowledge (Craft, 2005).

---

reflective **THINKING** Keep a reflective journal for the next few days and write about a few significant clinical experiences you have had. In what ways has this experience helped you to realize new ways of looking at nursing? What new nursing knowledge have you created for yourself?

To accomplish these valuable professional developments, the nurse leader must provide a supportive environment whereby the staff nurses can explore, raise questions, challenge, and address rituals and the routine in ways that address sustainability and the need for adjustment or change (Hausman & Ignatavicius, 2002). Critical thinking is a strong indicator for high levels of excellence, and it is essential to expand evidence-based practice in the health care system (Profetto-McGrath, 2005).

Decision Making

Care providers represent wide ranges of educational preparation, competencies, and scopes of practices. The scope of practice of a professional group includes a range of services that the individuals in that group are authorized to provide, as determined by their education and by legislation in their profession. Decisions regarding which health care providers are qualified to provide service must be based on care competencies, needs of the client and family, and the context of practice (College of Registered Nurses of Manitoba, 2002).

Role of Nurse Leader

The effective nurse leader is aware that the process of decision making is a fundamental element in nursing practice. The decision-making process should consider the unique and shared competencies of each group of nurses. Further, the decisions should promote optimal use of the nurses' competencies in the interest of client and family care (Marquis & Huston, 2009). In this era of increasing complexity and cost-effective delivery of health care in organizational settings, decision making is a critical thinking process, by which the best actions are needed to ensure that the quality of care provided meets desired goals (Kozier et al., 2004). An important element of quality care in all aspects of nursing care, evidence-based decision making is essential to optimize outcomes for clients, improve nursing practice, and ensure accountability and transparency in decision making (Canadian Nurses Association, 2002).

reflective **THINKING**   Besides evidence, what other factors influence decision making in nursing practice?

Decision Making and Problem Solving

Decision making is a complex and challenging process engaging in the deliberation and choice of a particular course of action selected from generated alternatives. The importance of good decision-making skills, as a valuable competency for the leader, cannot be overemphasized. The leader's capacity to make decisions, and to assess the potential consequences of the chosen alternative, is particularly important (Pangman, 2004).

Problem solving, on the other hand, is an active process that assists the nurse leader to analyse the situation and choose a course of action (Tappen, Weiss, & Whitehead, 2004). Problem solving begins with a problem and ends with a solution. It includes a decision-making step of selecting the most appropriate strategy for the immediate problem. The well-known traditional problem-solving process consists of a series of seven steps, as follows:

1. Identify the problem.
2. Collect data.
3. Explore alternatives.
4. Evaluate the alternatives.
5. Select the most appropriate strategy.
6. Implement the strategy.
7. Evaluate the results (Marquis & Huston, 2009).

This process serves as a guide to work at any task or with any type of problem. However, the selection of the most appropriate solution takes into account the handling of the issue at hand, not necessarily eliminating the problem. One common limitation of problem solving is the failure to develop an initial objective. The setting of decision goals allows the decision maker to remain focused instead of becoming side-tracked (Marquis & Huston, 2009). Problem solving requires considerable time and energy to identify and alleviate the problem.

reflective **THINKING**   Identify a key stressor in your life. Use the seven-step approach to problem solving to analyse this difficult situation and choose a course of action.

Decision-Making Processes

Decision making can be thought of as a process with identified and structured steps. It can be defined as behaviour demonstrated in making a selection from among alternatives for dealing with an issue, and then implementing a course of action from among alternatives (Clancy, 2006). Although problem solving and decision making both use information and require critical thinking, they differ in several ways. Decision making is purposeful and goal directed, and it requires much consideration of context. It often involves discussion by the individuals who will be affected by the choice (Roussel & Swansburg, 2006).

Before the outset of the decision-making process, the issue or problem is clearly identified, and goals and objectives are set. Data are collected and criteria to be used to objectively evaluate the desirability of the alternatives are identified. Decision making requires generating and analysing alternatives, often by using some type of strengths, weaknesses, opportunities, and threats (SWOT) analysis (Marquis & Huston, 2009). A quantitative decision-making tool, such as a grid, is used to analyse objectively the alternatives by using the criteria determined earlier. The alternative that provides the greatest probability of an acceptable and desirable outcome, using available resources, is most likely to be selected (Roussel & Swansburg, 2006).

The next step in the decision-making process is to act on, or implement, the selected alternative. The knowledge and competency of the nurse leader transforms the selected alternative into action by completing the necessary plans to prepare for the implementation of the solution. The two final steps are to monitor the implementation and evaluate the outcomes. Table 10.4 outlines the eight steps of the decision-making process, with suggested guidelines to facilitate each step in the process. The effective nurse leader follows these eight steps in a logical sequence.

---

reflective **THINKING**   Evaluate your past decision-making process with the eight steps you are learning. Describe your findings.

These steps are similar to the rational model of decision making, with the exception of the development of the goal and objectives and identifying the criteria (Johns & Saks, 2008). If the goals and objectives are not developed, and if criteria are not determined, the decision may not be the most beneficial one for the issue at hand.

Decision-Making Tools

A variety of tools exist to help the nurse leader provide order and direction in obtaining the final decision (Clancy, 2006). One such tool is the decision-making grid (Marquis & Huston, 2009). By using this grid, in step five of the decision-making process, the nurse leader can visualize and use the same criteria to analyse each alternative. A comparison of alternatives is more feasible. An example of a decision grid is outlined in Figure 10.2. The alternatives are listed in the left-hand column, and the criteria appear in a row across the top of the grid. The nurse leader fills in the resulting cells with suitable comments to determine the decision. For example, the criteria could be client safety, cost

TABLE 10.4 | INDIVIDUAL DECISION MAKING

Decision-Making Steps	Details of Each Step

Identify: the issue/problem OR the *need* for a decision	• What is happening? Have a questioning attitude.
	• What is needed?
	  ▪ What are the presenting symptoms?
	  ▪ Who or what is involved? When? Where? How?

Set goal/objective	Develop goals and objectives.
	  ▪ What do you want to accomplish?
	  ▪ What, really, is desired? Write down main points.

Collect data	• What and who are the sources available?
	  ▪ What are the causes of the problem?
	  ▪ Who are the people involved, if any?
	  ▪ What do we know about the issue?
	  ▪ What articles or research findings are available on the issue/problem?

Identify criteria to be used to make the decision	• What is important in solving the issue/problem?
	  ▪ What values or interests need to be considered?
	  ▪ What personal preferences are relevant?
	  ▪ Which criteria demand greater weight than others?
	  ▪ What is the order of priority of the criteria?

Search for possible alternatives	• What educational/personal experience do you have regarding the issue/problem?
	  ▪ What have you tried before?
	  ▪ What worked? What did not work?
	  ▪ What alternatives are you able to create?
	  ▪ What other alternatives are available for exploration?

Compare alternatives with the criteria	• Are the tool(s) being used to analyse the alternatives, based on the criteria, valid and realistic?
	  ▪ How are you rating each alternative, based on the criteria?
	  ▪ Are you taking sufficient (or too much) time to carefully consider each alternative, based on the criteria?
	• How is this process affecting you professionally and personally?

Select the most appropriate alternative	• Does the alternative selected carry the most weight?
	  ▪ How will that alternative affect your goal and objectives?
	  ▪ Is that alternative the most obvious one?
	  ▪ Is there another alternative that will work better?

Decision-Making Steps	Details of Each Step
	• If this alternative was used before, what are the implications? • If this alternative was NOT used before, what are the implications? • What existing policy statement(s) need to be considered?

Implement the most appropriate alternative	• What preparatory steps are needed before explaining the decision to staff members concerned?
	  • What steps are needed to implement the decision?
	  • What resources are required before implementation?
	  • What final plans are required before implementation?

Evaluate the alternative and follow-up	• What are your evaluative criteria?
	  • What checklists, ratings, and rankings will you use to evaluate your decision?
	  • How is the alternative perceived by others?
	• What follow-up measure or indicator (such as an open-end questionnaire), to determine the acceptability of the decision, will be used?
	  • What arrangements have been made to record and display the results of feedback on the decision implemented?

From Pangman, V. C. (2004). Leadership in groups and teams. In L. West (Ed.), *Trends and issues in health care* (3rd ed., pp. 243–259). Toronto, ON: McGraw-Hill Ryerson Limited. Adapted and reproduced with the permission of McGraw-Hill Ryerson Canada, 2008.

factors, and staff morale. The alternatives might be to work 12-hour shifts, to implement a staff mix, or to rotate shift work more frequently. Other tools that can be used include decision-making trees, payoff tables, and critical paths. These tools reflect graphic illustrations or other protocols for making decisions (Clancy, 2006).

	CRITERIA				
Alternative	Client Safety	Cost	Staff morale	Time	Decision
#1.					
#2.					
#3.					
#4.					

FIGURE 10.2 Example of a decision-making grid.

Leadership Issue

*Y*ou are a nurse manager on a surgical unit. You are concerned about a new registered nurse who has been working on your unit for approximately 4 months. Essentially, you believe that he is following the Standards of Care. You are aware, however, that he continues to rely extensively on the other registered nurses, even for minor decisions regarding client care. He has not attended any staff development programs. Although you are relieved that he does not intervene in giving care completely on his own without consultation, you would like to see him become more independent and be attentive to his professional growth. Using the eight steps of the decision-making process, deliberate and decide how you will share your concerns with him. Develop a decision-making grid. List the criteria that will assist you in examining each of the alternatives. Discuss your decision.

Factors Affecting Decision Making

Decision making differs from problem solving, and it is influenced by many variables, including emotions, intuition, and knowledge (Rew, 2007). The knowledge a nurse brings to the issue at hand plays a critical role in determining how the problem will be interpreted, which clinical information data will be attended to, and in what priority (Bakalis & Watson, 2005). Values, life experiences, and individual thinking preferences also affect decision making and bring variability to the process. Certain personality factors, such as self-esteem and self-confidence, affect the extent to which one is willing to take risks in making decisions. Although the objective of having diverse nurse leaders is desirable, a balance must be maintained between independent decision making and the limitations of choice demanded by the organization. Yoder-Wise (2007) states that the qualities of a successful decision maker include self-awareness, energy, courage, the willingness to take risks, and the ability to be creative, flexible, and sensitive. Good decision makers often learn to think "outside the box" in a complex system. These decisions are often interconnected, and they evolve to bring about an emergence set, or order, without the need for centralized control (Clancy, 2006).

reflective **THINKING**   What factors have you experienced that affect your decision-making process?

Group Decision Making

Higher-quality decisions are more likely to result if the groups concerned are involved in the decision-making process. In fact, when health team members are allowed to introduce their thoughts and ideas into the process, they tend to function more productively, and generally, the quality of the decision is superior (Yoder-Wise, 2007). Collaboration is highly important for decision making, especially in an interdisciplinary team. Bailey (2006) states that it is essential that nurses be involved in the collaborative decision-making process, especially when the goal is to make the best ethically based decisions about an individual client's care.

One advantage of using groups is that the group can create a greater number of ideas and then can evaluate them more effectively. In addition, if groups understand the importance of making a decision, they tend to be more willing to see it through (Johns & Saks, 2008). Some of the disadvantages of group-made decisions include time constraints, intragroup conflict, and a control issue, either by several or even one member. Another disadvantage is that of groupthink, whereby the pressures for conformity prevent the group from critically appraising unusual, minority, or unpopular points of view (Langton & Robbins, 2007).

In deciding to use the group process, one needs to consider group size and composition. The nurse leader should provide a positive nonthreatening environment in which the group members are encouraged to participate actively. Providing positive feedback and keeping the group focused on the task are two important strategies to follow in creating a milieu conducive to productive decision making (Yoder-Wise, 2007).

Ethical Decision Making

Ethical decisions are both important and necessary at those times when value-based questions arise in selecting health care options or in determining the best respectful care in the course of health care interactions—especially on occasions of uncertainty (McPherson et al., 2004). They occur when issues such as the type or extent of medical or nursing care are involved. Ethical decisions are called for in maintaining client privacy and confidentiality, disclosing information to clients, dealing with interdisciplinary team or family conflicts, and accessing health and social resources (Rodney et al., 2002).

When health care professionals are faced with an ethical dilemma, the code of ethics of one's profession is consulted, and a decision is made based on that code. Consultation can be made with health care colleagues or with ethical experts. However, in the process of making the decision, the code of ethics remains the central and deciding factor in the decision. The nurse leader is responsible for determining who is affected, collaborating with the interdisciplinary team, selecting a course of action, pursuing that action, and taking full responsibility for the action (Harder, 2005).

For the nurse leader, the process of making decisions is one of the most important components in the nursing profession because it relates most often to the resolution of health care issues in nursing practice and to the achievement of organizational goals. Nurses at all levels need to be prepared to engage in decision making in matters that affect all aspects of the profession and nursing practice. Nurses are often encouraged to increase their analytical competencies, while engaged in decision making, instead of relying on intuition (Lamond & Thompson, 2000). Improved knowledge of, and skill in, making decisions enable nurse leaders to contribute more significantly to the viability of the organization. Decision making in nursing is teamwork that calls for cooperation, collaboration, and communication within a complex environment.

Appreciative Inquiry

Appreciative inquiry is a facilitative approach to organizational planning and change that often asks the question "What is working well in the environment and how do we build on it?" It is a strength-based methodology based on the major assumption that change can be leveraged by identifying what works and designing mechanisms to do more of what works (Havens, Wood, & Leeman, 2006). In the health care environment, appreciative inquiry allows nurse leaders to continuously scan the organization and to conduct inquiries to discover the greatest strengths and capacities in health team members and then build on them by offering opportunities to achieve the organizational goals and dreams. Appreciative inquiry stimulates organizational growth and transformational change. Through appreciative inquiry, an organizational culture develops that promotes success and creativity (Ricciardi, 2004).

Appreciative inquiry consists of a *four "D" cycle*, as outlined in Figure 10.3. The cycles occur in sequence:

1. *Discovery:* During *discovery*, the participants of the appreciative inquiry team focus on becoming both appreciative and open to what is happening. At this

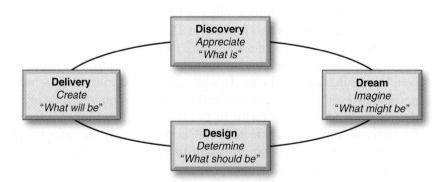

FIGURE 10.3 The four-D cycle of appreciative inquiry. (From Keefe, M. R. & Pesut, D. [2004]. Appreciative inquiry and leadership transitions. *Journal of Professional Nursing 20* [2], 103–109. Copied and reproduced with the permission of Elsevier © 2008.)

time, they engage in conversations designed to assess the present stage of the organization from a positive frame of reference.

2. *Dream:* During the *dream* phase, the dialogues of the participants focus on articulating dreams and desires. Many visioning activities are introduced to facilitate this phase. The participants think ahead and propose a compelling, positive vision. As the dream is enacted, the team summarizes the most convincing ideas. These ideas are then discussed with other stakeholders and become the basis for action plans.

3. *Design:* In the *design* phase, the appreciative inquiry teams examine processes and structures and determine what needs to be in place for the dream to become a reality. Some of the design elements include changes to committee structures, procedures and policies, meeting formats, communication links, and scheduling processes.

4. *Delivery:* The final phase, *delivery*, involves creating a vision, a set of goals, and outcomes. Participants focus on sustaining the team's approach to improvement. They make a habit of observing what is changing for the better, and they interact with others stating those observations (Havens, Wood, & Leeman, 2006; Keefe & Pesut, 2004).

Appreciative inquiry is an approach to leadership that nurse leaders can use within the health care organization. This approach to leadership involves appreciation, awareness, and creativity. It is the realization that a difference exists between issues and problems to be solved, and it includes aspirations to be realized to promote positive organizational change (Keefe & Pesut, 2004). For example, appreciative inquiry is a means to elicit enthusiasm and support for evidence-based practice in nursing and to sustain this change in the long term (Marchionni & Richer, 2007). The use of appreciative inquiry enables nurses to reflect on the positive experiences of evidence-based practice. This approach reinforces the notion that the team can achieve the goals they desire through dialogue and collaboration on values relevant to the implementation of evidence-based practice.

reflective **THINKING** As a nurse leader, what will you do to begin to use the approach of appreciative inquiry on your unit?

With a transformational style, the nurse leader can build a vision and take actions collectively with other health team members to make dreams a reality. Transformational leaders define a vision and communicate organizational values to achieve cohesion among health team members. Further research is needed to explore how appreciative inquiry facilitates change in the complex nature of the health care context.

WEBSITES

▪ Appreciative Inquiry

http://www.lib.uwo.ca/programs/generalbusiness/appinq.html

The "appreciative inquiry" construct was developed almost 20 years ago at Case Western Reserve University's Weatherhead School of Management. It is basically a positive approach to change that is constructed on an organization's strengths and strongest characteristics rather than on an attempt to correct perceived weaknesses or inadequacies. This site, developed by the University of Western Ontario, provides information and links to help you learn more about the approach.

▪ Critical Thinking: Student Resources

http://www.distance.uvic.ca/courses/critical

The goal of critical thinking is to evaluate in a reasoned and unbiased way what you read, hear, or observe in order to judge its validity or worth. Your reasoning should be guided by standards or habits of mind that include seeking clarity, accuracy, precision, relevance, depth, breadth, logic, and fairness in everything you encounter.

▪ Canadian Nurses Association Competencies

http://www.cna-aiic.ca/

The Canadian Nurses Association (CNA) provides a list of competencies for the registered nurse. Professional practice in nursing involves the demonstration of teamwork, leadership attributes such as decision making, basic management skills, advocacy, and political awareness. The links from CNA Home are as follows: Nursing in Canada>>Canadian Registered Nurse Examination>>Competencies.

REFERENCES

Anderson, L.W., Krathwohl, D. R., Airasian, P. W., Cruickshank, K. A., Mayer, R. E., Pintrich, P. R., Raths, J., & Wittrock, M. C. (2001). *A taxonomy for learning, teaching, and assessing: A revision of Bloom's Taxonomy of Educational Objectives.* New York: Longman.

Bailey, S. (2006). Decision making in acute care: A practical framework supporting the 'best interests' principle. *Nursing Ethics, 13*(3), 284–291.

Bakalis, N. A., & Watson, R. (2005). Nurses' decision-making in clinical practice. *Nursing Standard, 19*(23), 330–390.

Banning, M. (2006). Nursing research: Perspectives on critical thinking. *British Journal of Nursing, 15*(8), 458–461.

Beyer, B. (1995). *Critical Thinking.* Bloomington, IN: Phi Delta Kappa Educational Foundation.

Bloom, B. S., Engelhart, M. C., Furst, E. J., Hill, W. H., & Krathwohl, D. R. (1956). *Taxonomy of educational objectives: The classification of educational goals. Handbook 1: cognitive domain.* New York: David McKay.

Brookfield, S. (1987). *Developing critical thinkers: Challenging adults to explore alternative ways of thinking and acting.* San Francisco: Jossey-Bass.

Canadian Nurses Association. (2002). *Position statement: Evidence-based decision-making and nursing practice.* Ottawa, ON: Author. PS-63.

Clancy, T. R. (2006). Decision-making skills. In Huber, D. L. (Ed.), *Leadership and nursing care management* (3rd ed., pp. 149–178.). Philadelphia: Elsevier.

Cody, W. (2002). Critical thinking and nurse science: Judgment or vision? *Nursing Science Quarterly, 15*(3), 184–189.

College of Registered Nurses of Manitoba (CRNM). (2002). *Guidelines for decision-making regarding the appropriate nursing care provider.* Winnipeg, MB: CRNM.

Craft, M. (2005). Reflective writing and nursing education. *Journal of Nursing Education, 44*(2), 53–57.

Ennis, R. J., & Millman, J. (1985). *Cornell tests of critical thinking.* Pacific Grove, CA: Midwest Publisher.

Facione, N. C., Facione, P. A., & Sanchez, C. A. (1994). Critical thinking disposition as a measure of competent critical judgment: The development of the California Critical Thinking Disposition Inventory. *Journal of Nursing Education, 33*(8), 345–350.

Facione, P. (1990a). *Critical thinking: A statement of expert consensus for purposes of educational assessment and instruction. The Delphi Report: Research findings and recommendations.* Washington, DC: American Philosophical Association.

Facione, P. A. (1990b). *Executive summary of critical thinking: A statement of expert consensus for purposes of educational assessment and instruction, the "Delphi Report."* Millbrae, CA: California Academic Press.

Harder, J. (2005). Ethical decision making in health care. *Occupational Health Nurses Journal, 24*(3), 6–7, 24–25.

Hartrick, G. (2000). Developing health-promoting practice with families: One pedagogical experience. *Journal of Advanced Nursing, 31*(1), 27–34.

Hausman, K. A., & Ignatavicius, D. D. (2002). *Clinical companion for medical-surgical nursing: Critical thinking for collaborative care* (4th ed.). Philadelphia: Saunders.

Havens, D. S., Wood, S. O., & Leeman, J. (2006). Improving nursing practice and patient care. *Journal of Nursing Administration, 36*(10), 463–470.

Johns, G., & Saks, A. M. (2007). *Organizational behaviour: Understanding and managing life at work* (7th ed.). Toronto, ON: Pearson Education Canada.

Kataoka-Yahiro, M., & Saylor, C. (1994). A critical thinking model for nursing judgment. *Journal of Nursing Education, 33*, 351–360.

Kearney, A. J. (2008). Facilitating interprofessional education and practice. *Canadian Nurse, 104*(3), 22–26.

Keefe, M. R., & Pesut, D. (2004). Appreciative inquiry and leadership transitions. *Journal of Professional Nursing, 20*(2), 103–109.

Kozier, B., Erb, G., Berman, A. J., Burke, K., Raffin-Bouchal, D. S., & Hirst, S. P. (2004). *Fundamentals of nursing: The nature of nursing practice in Canada* (Canadian ed.). Toronto, ON: Pearson Education Canada.

Krathwohl, D. R. (2002). A revision of Bloom's Taxonomy: An overview. *Theory into Practice, 41*(4), 212–218.

Lamond, D., & Thompson, C. (2000). Intuition and analysis in decision making and choice. *Journal of Nursing Scholarship, 23*(4), 411–414.

Langton, N., & Robbins, S. P. (2007). *Fundamentals of organizational behaviour* (3rd Canadian ed.). Toronto, ON: Pearson Education Canada.

Luby, M., Riley, J., & Towne, G. (2006). Nursing research journal clubs: Bridging the gap between practice and research. *MEDSURG Nursing, 15*(2), 100–102.

Marchionni, C., & Richer, M.-C. (2007). Using appreciative inquiry to promote evidence-based practice in nursing: The glass is more than half full. *Nursing Leadership (203)*, 86–97.

Marquis, B. L., & Huston, C. J. (2009). *Leadership roles and management functions in nursing: Theory and application* (6th ed.). Philadelphia: Wolters Kluwer Health/Lippincott Williams & Wilkins.

McPherson, G., Rodney, P., McDonald, M., Storch, J., Pauly, B., & Burgess, M. (2004). Working within the landscape: Applications in health care ethics. In J. L. Storch, P. Rodney, & R. Starzomski (Eds.), *Toward a moral horizon: Nursing ethics for leadership and practice* (pp. 98–125.). Toronto, ON: Pearson Education Canada.

Mezirow, J. (1991). *Transformative dimensions of adult learning.* San Francisco: Jossey-Bass.

Norris, S. (1995). Format effects on critical thinking test performance. *The Alberta Journal of Educational Research,41*(4), 378–406.

Page, D., & Mukherjee, A. (2007). Promoting critical thinking skills by using negotiation exercises. *Journal of Education for Business, 82*(5), 251–257.

Pangman, V. C. (2004). Leadership in groups and teams. In L. West (Ed.), *Trends and issues in health care* (3rd ed., pp. 243–259.). Toronto, ON: McGraw-Hill Ryerson Limited.

Paul, R. (1984). Critical thinking: Fundamental to education for a free society. *Educational Leadership, 42*(1), 4–14.

Paul, R. W. (1992). *Critical thinking: How to prepare students for a rapidly changing world.* Santa Rosa, CA: Center for Critical Thinking.

Paul, R. W. (1993). *Critical thinking: What every person needs to survive in a rapidly changing world.* Santa Rosa, CA: Foundation for Critical Thinking.

Peden-McAlpine, C., Tomlinson, P., Forneris, S. G., & Meyer, S. (2005). Evaluation of a reflective practice intervention to enhance family care. *Journal of Advanced Nursing, 49*(5), 494–501.

Pintrich, P. R. (2002). The role of metacognitive knowledge in learning, teaching and assessing. *Theory into Practice, 41*(4), 219–227.

Porter-O'Grady, T., Igein, G., Alexander, D., Blaylock, J., McComb, D., & Williams, S. (2005). Critical thinking for nursing leadership. *Nurse Leader, 3*(4), 28–31.

Profetto-McGrath, J. (2005). Critical thinking and evidence-based practice. *Journal of Professional Nursing, 21*(6), 364–371.

Profetto-McGrath, J., Hesketh, K. L., Lang, S., & Estabrooks, C. A. (2003). A study of critical thinking and research utilization among nurses. *Western Journal of Nursing Research, 25*(3), 322–337.

Profetto-McGrath, J., Smith, K. B., & Bulmer, K. (2003). What's in a question? No matter how we phrase our questions, whether in daily practice or in a research capacity, critical thinking is key. *The Canadian Nurse, 99*(10), 29.

Redding, D. (2001). The development of critical thinking among students in baccalaureate nursing education. *Holistic Nursing Practice, 15*(4), 57–64.

Rew, L. (2007). Acknowledging institution in clinical decision making. *Journal of Holistic Nursing, 18*(2), 94–108.

Ricciardi, R. (2004). Appreciative inquiry: Promoting individual and organizational change. *Journal of Pediatric Health Care, 18*(6), 16A.

Riddell, T. (2007). Critical assumptions: Thinking critically about critical thinking. *Journal of Nursing Education, 46*(3), 121–126.

Rodney, P., Varcoe, C., Storch, J. L., McPherson, G., Mahoney, K., Brown, H., Pauly, B., Hartrick, D., & Starzomski, R. (2002). Navigating toward a moral horizon: A multi-site qualitative study of ethical practice in nursing. *Canadian Journal of Nursing Research, 34*(2), 75–102.

Roussel, L., & Swansburg, R. C. (2006). Decision-making and problem solving: Communication practices and skills. In L. Roussel, R. C. Swansburg, & R. J. Swansburg (Eds.), *Management and leadership for nurse administrators* (4th ed., pp. 81–112.). Toronto, ON: Jones and Bartlett.

Seymour, B., Kinn, S., & Sutherland, N. (2003). Valuing both critical and creative thinking in clinical practice: Narrowing the research-practice gap? *Journal of Advanced Nursing, 42*(3), 288–296.

Simpson, E., & Courtney, M. (2002). Critical thinking in nursing education: Literature review. *International Journal of Nursing Practice, 8*(2), 89–98.

Su, W. M., Osisek, P. J., & Starnes, B. (2005). Using the revised Bloom's Taxonomy in the clinical laboratory: Thinking skills involved in diagnostic reasoning. *Nurse Educator, 30*(3), 117–122.

Tappen, R. M., Weiss, S. A., & Whitehead, D. K. (2004). *Essentials of nursing leadership and management* (3rd ed.). Philadelphia: F. A. Davis.

Turner, P. (2005). Critical thinking in nursing education and practice as defined in the literature. *Nursing Education Perspectives, 26*(5), 272–277.

Valiga, T. (2009). Promoting and assessing critical thinking. In S. DeYoung (Ed.), *Teaching strategies for nurse educators* (2nd ed). Upper Saddle River, NJ: Pearson Education.

Watson, G., & Glaser, E. M. (1964). *Critical thinking appraisal manual.* New York: Harcourt, Brace & World.

Watson, G., & Glaser, E. M. (1980). *Critical thinking appraisal manual.* New York: Harcourt, Brace, & Jovanovich.

Worrell, J. A., & Profetto-McGrath, J. (2007). Critical thinking as an outcome of context-based learning among post RN students: A literature review. *Nurse Education Today, 27*(5), 420–426.

Yoder-Wise, P. S. (2007). *Leading and managing in nursing* (4th ed.). St Louis, MO: Mosby.

CHAPTER 11

CONFLICT RESOLUTION AND NEGOTIATION: CHALLENGING MOMENTS FOR THE NURSE LEADER

Make change—be strategic; use power and politics to influence; be a winner; be true to yourself and your values; develop and nurture key relationships; be accessible; stretch yourself; communicate.

—Judith Shamian, PhD

Presentation at Registered Nurses Association of Ontario
Creating Healthy Work Environments
Summer Institute, Haliburton, ON, August 2007

Dr. Judith Shamian is the president and CEO of Victoria Order of Nurses (VON) Canada, having been appointed in June 2004. From 1999 to 2004, Dr. Shamian was the Executive Director, Office of Nursing Policy, Health Policy and Communications Branch with Health Canada. Before 1999, she served for 10 years as vice president at Mount Sinai Hospital in Toronto. In that position, she developed and led the World Health Organization Collaborating Center at Mount Sinai, the first such centre based in a hospital setting. Dr. Shamian is a professor in the Faculty of Nursing, University of Toronto, where she maintains an active research portfolio as a principal investigator, co-investigator, and decision maker. Dr. Shamian's career in Canada began with her education in nursing at Shaare Zedek Hospital in Jerusalem. She attended Concordia University in Montreal, New York University, and earned her PhD from Case Western Reserve University, Cleveland, OH, in 1988.

Overview

Conflict is a basic aspect of all human interaction, and it is fundamental to the human experience. Health care organizations are particularly vulnerable to conflict because the nature and context of health care professionals' work can be difficult and stressful on a daily basis. In addition, uncertainties caused by changes in roles and role relationships with new health care workers, varying perceptions of health team members, and complexities within organizations add to the perplexing work environment. These elements often lead to conflict in the workplace.

The literature and findings from research studies indicate that nurses encounter conflict in varying degrees, and this often interferes with providing quality care for the client and family. Conflict also reduces productivity in health care settings. When nurse leaders encounter conflict situations, they need to be able to accept conflict as a normative challenge and use effective conflict management approaches and other alternatives to transform conflict into an opportunity for growth. The process of negotiation is an effective interactive approach that emphasizes the need to maintain ongoing relationships and to share power and control. Nurse leaders use negotiation as one conflict intervention that enhances the spirit of the health care team while benefiting the client and the organization as a whole.

Objectives

By critically reflecting upon and processing knowledge throughout this chapter, you will be able to respond effectively to the following objectives:

1. State the meaning of conflict as you understand it.
2. Compare and contrast the perspectives of conflict.
3. Analyze the different types of conflict.
4. Prepare a chart to differentiate the components, effects, and desired outcomes of conflict.
5. Debate the effects of diversity on conflict.
6. Examine the various models of conflict.
7. Recognize situations in which several conflict management strategies can be used.
8. Critique the concept of conflict transformation.
9. Compare and contrast the various styles of negotiation.
10. Apply the negotiation process to a conflict situation in a health care setting.

The Dynamics of Conflict

Conflict among nurses has been identified as a significant issue within health care settings globally (Almost, 2006). A recent Canadian study showed that the frequency of conflict with nursing coworkers is on the rise (Hesketh et al., 2003). As a result of conflict, the work climate becomes disruptive, reduced collaboration occurs within the health care team, and client care suffers. The degree of conflict that occurs in any setting is an important factor to consider when analyzing its effects (Grohar-Murray & DiCroce, 2003). Nurse leaders in particular need to review the dynamics of conflict and be attentive to factors affecting the well-being of nurses within the health care team. Managing conflict is one of the greatest challenges a nurse leader faces in any setting.

> reflective **THINKING** From your own experience, describe a conflict situation in which you were involved with a coworker. What elements contributed to the conflict?

Definition

There is no single definition of conflict. Thomas (1992) explains that the term *conflict* has two broad usages in the behavioural sciences. The first usage denotes an incompatible response tendency within an individual—a form of dilemma. The second usage refers to a phenomenon that involves two or more individuals. Thomas (1992) defines conflict as "the process that begins when one party perceives that the other has negatively affected, or is about to negatively affect, something he or she cares about" (p. 653). One of the benefits of this definition is that it is simple and sufficiently broad to cover a variety of conflict issues and events.

Generally, conflict stems from discordance that arises in values, beliefs, thoughts, feelings, or behaviours of two or more parties. Warner's (2001) research findings indicate that during conflict situations, nurses identified similar attributes regarding the onset of conflict. A few other attributes mentioned were differences in priorities, practices, and perceptions among individuals.

Perspectives of Conflict

The *traditional view* of conflict maintained that it was disruptive and dysfunctional and needed to be avoided. The early understanding of conflict assumed that all conflict was harmful and bad (Cox, 2006). However, despite this early prevailing attitude, researchers began to examine the positive dynamics of conflict and the consequences of them.

The *human relations view* of conflict argues that conflict is a natural phenomenon and is inevitable in any group or organization. Because it is natural and inevitable, conflict should be accepted (Cox, 2006). In fact, conflict can even contribute to the effectiveness of group performance.

The current *interactionist view* of conflict depicts it as exerting both positive and negative effects and consequences. Conflict is now recognized as being a multidimensional construct (Almost, 2006). The presence of conflict can have an organization-wide impact by calling to mind problem areas that, when recognized, can lead to improved decision making, resulting in fundamental changes within organizations (Callanan & Perri, 2006). Recognizing the functional aspects of conflict has shifted the emphasis to the management of conflict (Rahim, 2002). By relying on interdependence and professional collaboration, all parties involved grow and benefit, including the organization and the population being served (Hendel, Fish, & Berger, 2007). It is important for nurse leaders to have a clear understanding and working knowledge of the approaches to conflict. It is important as well to be aware of the various alternatives to managing conflict.

> *reflective* **THINKING** What is your personal point of view regarding conflict? How does a nurse leader deal with a personality conflict from a traditional view compared with an interactionist view?

Types of Conflict

Three types of conflict exist: intrapersonal, interpersonal, and intergroup. In each, a tension is produced within an individual or party because needs, goals, or objectives have not been met (Hibberd, Valentine, & Clark, 2006). Figure 11.1 depicts the tension in nurses in all three types of conflict.

Intrapersonal Conflict

Intrapersonal conflict refers to discord or stress that develops within an individual and which usually arises because of a choice the individual must make between two alternatives (Ellis & Hartley, 2008). An example of intrapersonal conflict in nursing occurs when the nurse is caring for many clients and must decide whether to be with a family member whose loved one is dying or deal with another significant priority elsewhere on the unit.

Interpersonal Conflict

Interpersonal conflict is a dynamic process that occurs between or among individuals as they experience negative emotional reactions to differences in ideas, values, perceptions, or goals (Barki & Hartwick, 2001). Ethical issues, such as stem cell research, gene therapy, and do-not-resuscitate orders, often result in conflict between those who are responsible for the delivery of care (Ellis & Hartley, 2006).

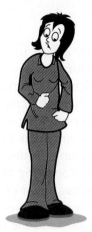

Intrapersonal

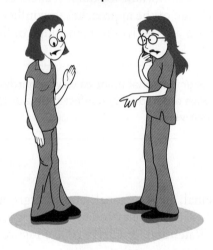

Interpersonal

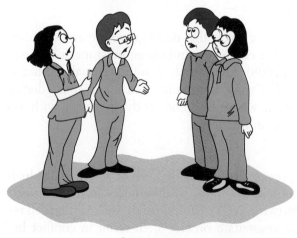

Intergroup

FIGURE 11.1 Three types of conflict.

For example, two nurses might have conflicting views about when to ambulate clients or on the importance of having advance directives for seriously ill clients.

Intergroup Conflict

Intergroup conflict occurs between or among two or more groups; it often involves client care issues, style of management, policies, and procedures (Ellis & Hartley, 2006). For example, nurses and physicians sometimes disagree about policies regarding prepping procedures in the operating room. Sometimes conflict arises between departments or units as groups. That is, competition can occur among various departments that are each vying for available resources. The nurse leader should be aware of the different types of conflict that can occur within a health care setting.

Cox (2000) tested a structural equation that examined the relationship among individual and contextual variables and intragroup conflict, job satisfaction, team performance effectiveness, and anticipated turnover. The findings of the study indicated that less intragroup conflicts exist on units where perceptions are high on unit morale and interpersonal relations. The nurse leader should strive to create a work environment that supports a team-oriented culture. In fact, every effort should be made to manage conflict in order to create a win–win situation.

> *reflective* **THINKING** Think of an intrapersonal conflict you recently experienced. What was the basis of the felt stress? How was it resolved?

Components, Effects, and Outcomes of Conflict

To further one's understanding of the dynamics of human conflict, it is necessary to examine briefly the components, effects, and the desired outcomes of conflict.

Components

Three components of conflict include relationships, tasks, and processes. Table 11.1 differentiates among the three components and provides relevant nursing examples and tips for nurse leaders.

Effects

The effects of conflict can be viewed as either functional or dysfunctional, depending on how each individual perceives, manages, and resolves the conflict (Vivar, 2006). Conflict is functional when it improves the quality of decisions, stimulates creativity, and fosters an environment of self-evaluation and change (Cox, 2006). In essence, conflict is productive when it actually improves the

TABLE 11.1	COMPONENTS OF CONFLICT		
	Relationship	**Task**	**Process**
Description	Interpersonal tensions arise among persons that are related to their personal characteristics and relatedness per se—not to the task at hand.	Disagreements occur about the nature of the work to be performed.	Disagreements flare about how the work should be organized and accomplished.
Example	Personality clashes	Differences about the specific goals being worked toward or about certain technical matters of the task	Disagreements about responsibility, resource allocation, and the authority of the work
Tips for the Nurse Leader	Accommodate and adjust for differences in perception among individuals.	Provide clearly worded information packages and policy statements related to the task at hand.	Be aware of different possible interpretations of meaning and personal biases that members of the group might have.

Adapted from Johns, G., & Saks, A. M. (2008). *Organizational behaviour*. Toronto, ON: Pearson Education Canada; Porter-O'Grady, T. (2003). When push comes to shove: Managers as mediators. *Nursing Management, 34*(10), 34–40.

performance of members and supports the goals of the organization. Meanwhile, conflict is dysfunctional when it promotes infighting among members, slows the process of communication, or reduces the cohesiveness of the group (Cox, 2006). That is, dysfunctional conflict hinders organizational performance (Kreitner, Kinicki, & Cole, 2007).

Outcomes

According to Kreitner, Kinicki, and Cole (2007), three desired outcomes of conflict are as follows:

1. *Agreement:* Fair and equitable agreements between and among members of an organization are the best.
2. *Stronger relationships:* Good agreements facilitate the conflicting members to build bridges of trust and good will for future use. Moreover, conflicting members who trust each other are more likely to keep their end of the bargain.
3. *Learning:* Functional conflict can promote greater self-awareness and critical thinking in dealing with complex situations in health care organizations.

In nursing, desired outcomes include effective and safe client care as well as client and family satisfaction, improved collaboration and relationships, personal and professional growth, and the efficient use of resources. Trust plays an important role in the outcome of a conflict because trust affects the manner in which one perceives the actions of others. These valuable perceptions are arrived at through one's interpretations of existing actions and previous events (Dirks & Ferrins, 2001). On the other hand, negative outcomes include burnout, increased turnover, the lack of professional growth, and less than efficient use of resources (Cox, 2006).

Nurse leaders are challenged to strive for desired outcomes after conflictual situations between and among health team members in times of uncertainty and unpredictability in health care. Nurse leaders need to clearly communicate goals to members of the health care team. The nurse leader also needs to provide accurate and timely feedback as well as praise and suitable rewards for jobs well done.

> *reflective* **THINKING**   Recall a conflict that occurred on your unit.
> Describe the component of the conflict, the effect, and the outcome.

Role of Diversity

The concept of diversity is well known in organizations. At times, differences are perceived in the extent of power and status that individuals attain or are assigned. Such situations frequently result in the potential for conflict.

Cross-Cultural Conflict

When two or more different cultures are represented in a health care organization, differing assumptions often arise among members about how to think and act in various situations. The most important cultural factor in shaping attitudes regarding conflict is an orientation toward either individualism or collectivism. In individualistic cultures, such as the case in Canada, the needs, rights, and goals of each individual are considered to be highly important, and the people have the right to stand up and speak out for themselves. Meanwhile, in collectivistic cultures—more common in Asia and Latin America—the concerns of the group are considered to be more important than the needs of the individual. The assertive behaviour that is appropriate in North America would seem insensitive and rude in collectivistic cultures (Adler, Ross, Proctor III, & Towne, 2009). Individuals from collective cultures are more likely than those from individualistic cultures to manage disagreements through avoidance or problem solving (McShane, 2006). Although the awareness of cultural differences in styles of managing conflict is beneficial, it is important not to make sweeping generalizations that define styles of everyone in a particular culture (Folger, Poole, & Stutman, 2005).

Nurse leaders need to be aware that certain elements contribute to the ability of an organization to become more culturally competent. These elements include the following:

- Gain knowledge about culture and culture dynamics.
- Value diversity by accepting and respecting differences.
- Become aware of the "dynamics" inherent when cultures interact (Barker, 2006).

Such awareness will undoubtedly assist nurse leaders to cope successfully and effectively with conflict situations.

Intergenerational Conflict

Nurse leaders must be aware that differences frequently arise among the four generations currently in practice in nursing: the Traditionalists, Baby Boomers, Generation X, and Generation Y (Barker, 2006). The coexistence of these particular generations in nursing is leading to episodes of tension and intergenerational conflict (Swearingen & Liberman, 2004). Key generational differences that arise focus on values, work ethics, expectations, and life experiences. Each generation reacts and responds differently to similar events. For example, Generation X members are more team based than their Baby Boomer counterparts, who expect their individual achievements and contributions to be recognized and rewarded (Weston, 2001).

To understand the individual's beliefs, values, and attitudes about the workplace requires considerable time, effort, and insight on the part of the nurse leader. The ability to plan with input from others and to react calmly, to reframe potentially negative to potentially positive responses, and to provide a new course of action are of utmost value (Hansten, 2003). Nurse leaders who work with people from Generation X and Generation Y take time to teach and coach in an informal sense. Typically, members of younger generations rely more on technology, rather than people or books, to meet their learning needs.

The nurse leader will need to mediate intergenerational conflicts when individuals from different generations interact. Recognizing and responding to generational expectations can dramatically help the nurse leader to improve communications and the effectiveness of work teams (Weston, 2001). However, it is important that the nurse leader identify and recognize her or his own unique biases and realize how these biases influence interactions with others.

reflective **THINKING**   In what way can you as a nurse leader assess the extent to which you have biases regarding individuals in different generations? What can you do about these biases?

Models of Conflict

Scholars have described the dynamics of conflict across a temporal sequence of stages or phases (Filley, 1975; Thomas, 1992; Robbins, 2003). The resulting models provide considerable understanding into the nature of the conflict phenomenon (Cox, 2006).

Thomas Model

The model developed by Thomas (1992) is often cited in nursing textbooks (Almost, 2006). Figure 11.2 outlines the five stages: awareness, thoughts and emotions, intentions, behaviours, and outcomes. Brief explanations of each stage follow:

- *Awareness:* Perceiving or experiencing a change in a situation that one cares about. A difference of opinion occurs, which leads to a variety of thoughts and emotions.
- *Thoughts and emotions:* The awareness is experienced primarily in terms of thoughts or cognitions that the individual uses to make sense of the conflict and the emotions, or affect, which interact with the thoughts. These two elements are especially important in understanding the conflict process. Thoughts and emotions define the individual's subjective interpretation of the reality that is at the core of the conflict.
- *Intentions:* The next event in the conflict episode is the decision to act in a certain way. Intentions intervene between the individual's thoughts and feelings and the overt behaviour. For example, attributes such as cooperation, collaboration, self-defence, and competition are not themselves behaviours, but are intentions, or purposes, that serve to explain patterns of observed behaviour.
- *Behaviour:* After the formation of intentions, the next event in the conflict episode is overt behaviour. Behaviours refer to observable actions performed by individuals. They may be in a form of avoiding, competing, or collaborating.
- *Outcomes:* The final element in this model involves the outcome(s) of the conflict episode. When behaviours relevant to the conflict cease, some set of outcomes are presumed to have occurred. In fact, the most obvious is the decision—or the lack of decision—reached regarding the conflict issue (Thomas, 1976). The outcomes of a given situation determine whether a subsequent episode on the same issue will recur in the future. Productivity or efficiency will either increase, stay the same, or decrease (Hibberd, Valentine, & Clark, 2006; Donohue, 2007).

Almost (2006) examined the concept of conflict in nursing work environments using the evolutionary approach to concept analysis. Articles written over the last 25 years were examined from relevant databases to identify major themes, areas of agreement and disagreement across disciplines, changes in the concept over time, and emerging trends. Figure 11.3 outlines the theoretical model of antecedents and consequences that the researcher developed.

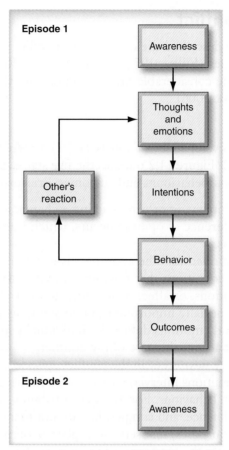

FIGURE 11.2 Process model of conflict episodes. (From Thomas, K. W. [1992]. Conflict and negotiation processes in organizations. In M. D. Dunnette & L. M. Hough [Eds.], *Handbook of industrial and organizational psychology* [vol. 3, 2nd ed.]. Palo Alto: CA. Consulting Psychologists Press [p. 658]. Reproduced with permission of Consulting Psychologists Press, Inc.)

Antecedents and Consequences of Conflict Model

According to Almost's model, the *antecedents of conflict* are individual characteristics, such as differing opinions and values, that create the potential for conflict. Other antecedents include interpersonal factors, such as perceptions of injustice or disrespect; one's communication style, either verbal, or nonverbal; or just the absence of communication (Warner, 2001). Organizational factors, such as organizational changes and time pressures due to short staffing, intense workload, or overtime, are also attributes towards conflict. The *consequences of conflict* tend to centre on individual effects, interpersonal relationships, and organizational interactions (Almost, 2006). In regard to the effects of conflict on people, Cox (2003) found that higher levels of intragroup conflict resulted in lower levels of job satisfaction in nurses. In one Canadian study, several nurses admitted that

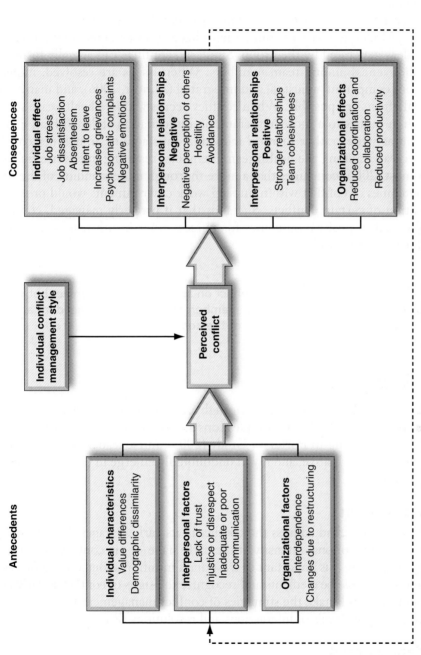

FIGURE 11.3 Antecedents and consequences of conflict. (From Almost, J. [2006]. Conflict within nursing environments: Concept analysis. *Journal of Advanced Nursing,* 53[4], 444–453. Courtesy of Wiley-Blackwell Publishing, Ltd., Oxford, UK.)

they had reduced their hours of work because of conflict with nursing coworkers (Warner, 2001).

Regarding interpersonal relationships, conflict can have positive consequences. Moderate levels of conflict have been shown to contribute to the quality of ideas generated by the group. Similarly, conflicts can actually foster internal cohesiveness among team members. When issues are resolved, individuals feel more competent, adjusted, and integrated (Almost, 2006), and many organizational effects are possible. When conflict occurs within a health care setting, a shift often occurs to a more autocratic or authoritarian style, with an increased focus on activities rather than on individual satisfaction. Sometimes collaboration decreases among the health team members, resulting in lower efficiency.

Almost (2006) concludes that a more thorough understanding of the sources and outcomes of conflict within nursing work environments would promote the prevention of certain conflicts. She adds that if properly managed, conflict can actually lead to positive outcomes for nurses, other health team members, and health care organizations.

> **reflective THINKING** Reflect on an interpersonal conflict between yourself and another health team member. List all of the antecedent attributes. What was the consequence of the conflict?

Conflict Resolution

To resolve conflict effectively, a thorough assessment of the situation is of prime importance. Table 11.2 outlines questions and points to consider for assessment purposes. According to Porter-O'Grady (2003), nurse leaders should remember that conflict is normative, and it will undoubtedly emerge in the course of human relationships.

Conflict Assessment

It is best to assess and address the conflict in its earliest stages. For example, the relatively low emotional intensity at the early stage of the conflict makes it more readily resolvable. It is important to trust one's intuition about a potential conflict. It is good to assess the elements and recognize the signs of conflict as early as possible and then undertake the strategies of conflict management to move individuals toward higher levels of interactions and resolutions (Porter-O'Grady, 2004a).

Conflict Management

Conflict management refers to the modes used by both individuals and groups to cope with conflict (Hendel, Fish, & Berger, 2007). Conflict management can achieve a successful resolution that can lead to higher trust, greater effectiveness,

TABLE 11.2	CONFLICT ASSESSMENT
Questions	**Points to Consider**

What is the issue?	• The stated/observed issue(s), as indicated by the individuals concerned
	• Antecedents
	 • Perceptions of the individuals concerned
	 • Cultural, generational, or experiential differences
	 • Values
	  • Of the individuals concerned
	  • Organizational

Who is involved?	• One or two individuals? • Several individuals? • Nursing? • Interdisciplinary? • Clients only? • Clients and staff? • Others?
Where is/was the conflict taking place?	• On the unit? • In the board room? • Other? • What relevant factors, if any, does the location of the conflict bring to the management of it?

Which is the best conflict management style to activate?	• Time factor
	 • How long has the conflict been going on?
	 • When was it first observed?
	 • When must it be resolved?
	• Emotional and logical matters that need to be addressed
	• Expertise to manage conflict
	 • Yours
	 • The individuals involved
	 • Others who might be affected
	 • Colleagues whose input and/or assistance you might seek. Before you proceed to seek outside help:
	  • Who will you ask? In what way(s) might they be of assistance to you?
	  • For what duration do you expect to require their assistance? Should you share such expectations with them at the outset?
	  • When the time comes, how will you advise them that you no longer require their assistance?
	  • What is your decision regarding outside help?
	• Outcome
	 • Immediate requirements
	 • Possible long-term requirements

and more transparency (Jacinta, 2006). Five common approaches, or strategies, to conflict resolution have been identified in the literature (Johns & Saks, 2008; Vivar, 2006; Jacob, 2006). The five conflict management strategies, with definitions for each strategy, uses, and outcomes, are presented in Table 11.3.

In a study of conflict management strategies in nursing, Valentine (2001) compared the use of five conflict management strategies used by staff nurses, nurse managers, and deans of schools of nursing. The findings indicated that staff nurses ranked the five strategies in the following order of preference: *avoiding, accommodating, compromising, collaborating,* and *competing.* It is assumed that avoidance was used most frequently because of the sense of powerlessness generally associated with the staff nurse role. *Avoidance* was selected by half of the nurse managers as the strategy of choice for the same reason.

The deans selected *compromising* as their first choice. The *collaboration* strategy was not a popular choice, even though it maintains positive relationships and is most rewarding (Valentine, 2001). For nurse leaders, collaboration is the preferred method for conflict resolution to meet the current problems facing the health care system (Blais, Hayes, Kozier, & Erb, 2006). However, because collaboration takes time, energy, and the willingness and skills to work with one another, it may not be the most popular option for many nurses (Barker, 2006).

It would be interesting to replicate Valentine's (2001) study and examine the results in light of the four generations of nurses working in a variety of settings. Perhaps staff nurses would consist mainly of Generations X or Y. Meanwhile, one might expect nurse managers to consist of Baby Boomers, as would deans of faculties of nursing.

> *reflective* **THINKING**   Formulate the research question for a study to examine conflict management strategies in nursing.

Understanding and effectively applying conflict management strategies is a fundamental of good leadership. Further, the leader must make a broad commitment to develop conflict management programs that operate as part of the workplace structure (Porter-O'Grady, 2004b). A significant finding by Meyer (2004) indicated that when the amount and intensity of a conflict in the workplace escalates, the results are inefficiencies and poor performance. It is essential that nurse leaders create safe and positive environments for all team members in the workplace.

Conflict Transformation

Chinn (2008) states that conflict transformation involves ways of knowing and doing that are central to "peace and power" processes. For example, conflict transformation draws especially on the *power of diversity*, encouraging creativity

TABLE 11.3 | CONFLICT MANAGEMENT STRATEGIES

Strategy	Description	Use
Avoiding	It features low assertiveness, passive withdrawal, or active suppression of the issue.	When trivial issues are encountered To allow parties to calm down and regain perspective *Strength:* It buys time. *Limitation:* It is a temporary fix.
Accommodating	It allows cooperation with others while not asserting one's own interests. It serves to minimize differences among individuals.	To maintain harmony with others and smooth out issues *Strength:* It encourages cooperation. *Limitation:* It is a temporary fix.
Competing	This strategy maximizes assertiveness and power, and it minimizes cooperative responses, while fostering low concern for others.	In minor issues, when a deadline is near, or when quick decisions are needed. It enforces upon others the facts of discipline and rules. *Strength:* It is quick. *Limitation:* The style is somewhat forceful.
Compromising	This is the "give-and-take" approach where all concerned are encouraged to present their views. It combines intermediate levels of assertiveness and cooperation.	It can achieve temporary settlements to complex issues. It can serve as a back-up plan for times when collaboration or competition fail. *Strengths:* It is a democratic process. It has no losers. *Limitation:* Resulting dissatisfactions sometimes tend to stifle creative decision making briefly.
Collaboration	This strategy features the group meeting, where members are encouraged to present views, listen, suggest alternatives, be supportive, and contribute.	It maximizes both assertiveness and cooperation. It merges insights from different perspectives to find an integrative solution. *Strengths:* It has longer-lasting impact. It deals with the underlying problem. *Limitations:* It is a time-consuming process.

Adapted from Kreitner, R., Kinicki, A., & Cole, N. (2007). *Fundamentals of organizational behaviour: Key concepts, skills and best practices* (2nd Canadian ed.). Toronto, ON: McGraw-Hill Ryerson; Valentine, P. (2001). A gender perspective on conflict management strategies of nurses. *Journal of Nursing Scholarship, 33*(1), 69–74; Johns, G., & Saks, A. (2008). *Organizational behaviour: Understanding and managing life at work* (7th ed.). Toronto, ON: Pearson Education Canada.

Reflections on Leadership Practice

*R*eview the theoretical model of antecedents and consequences that the researcher (Almost, 2006) developed. Notice that in Figure 11.3, she has highlighted in bold individual conflict management style as well as perceived conflict. Take time to reflect on the following case study:

You are a female nurse assigned to caring for a 15-year-old male quadriplegic client. He is beginning to direct sexual comments and suggestive facial gestures towards you while you are providing his basic care. Yesterday, it was so annoying that you became frustrated and did not complete his basic care. You are reluctant to say anything to the client directly because the doctor in charge of his medical care is the client's uncle. In addition, the client has told you that he will report you to his uncle for not completing his basic care, especially if you make a formal report of his behaviour to the nurse unit manager. It is anticipated that this client will remain on your unit for at least several weeks. What will you do to handle the conflict?

What were the antecedents in this situation? How is the situation perceived by the client, and by you? What conflict management style would you initially advocate? For what reasons? What style, if any, would you use later? Explain your rationale.

and valuing alternative views; *power of solidarity*, integrating variety within the group; and *power of responsibility*, owning one's actions and encouraging criticism and self-criticism for each individual and the group. Enacting these powers is not an easy task, nor is it always possible. When a group of individuals is unable to integrate diversity, the group becomes engaged in divisive conflict. Table 11.4 cites examples of individuals who nurture diversity, as opposed to those who engage in divisiveness. It is beneficial for the nurse leader always to be aware of how the health team members overcome instances of divisiveness and move toward valuing diversity (Chinn, 2008).

Conflict transformation begins before there is conflict in the group. Groups can develop three important mechanisms during times of relative calm that build a strong foundation for transforming conflict. The three modes of action are as follows:

1. *Nurturing an enduring sense of rotating leadership within a group*: A group that rotates its leadership can turn to others who have vision, clarity, and energy to address a conflict constructively.
2. *Practicing critical reflection*: This practice enables the shift out of interactive styles of blaming, hostility, and damaging verbal assaults to embracing constructive growth and change.
3. *Practicing ways to value diversity*: By forming habits to value diversity, a foundation is laid to remain open to alternative options, even when emotions and tensions rise (Chinn, 2008).

TABLE 11.4 DIVERSITY AND DIVISIVENESS COMPARED		
Situation at hand	**Diversity**	**Divisiveness**
I am convinced that my point of view is the only reasonable one.	I still take the time to find out what other people think.	I keep repeating it to make sure that everyone hears it.
Things have become tense in a discussion, and sides are being taken.	I encourage discussion so that each point of view is presented fully.	I usually know which side I am on and grow impatient with drawn-out discussions.
In a meeting or online. . .	I make sure I express my point of view and limit my comments so that others may also speak to the issue.	I make sure I express my point of view at length so that others don't miss out on all the implications of my insights.
I am aware that something I have said or done has bothered others.	I stop to consider what has happened and try to put myself in their shoes.	I decide it is their problem and it is up to them to work it out.
When others are expressing their views. . .	I actively listen and hear them out before framing my response. Online, I read carefully and make sure I understand their points of view.	I usually already know what they are trying to say and jump in to say what I have to say to move the discussion along.
There is disagreement in the group.	I invite everyone to express their viewpoints so that we can all hear and consider these in reaching a decision.	I think the best way to deal with it is simply to agree to disagree and not get caught up in trivia.
I am unable to attend a scheduled meeting or unable to be online for a period of time	I make sure someone knows my concerns about relevant issues and is willing to take them to the group.	I reason that I can catch up later and let people know then what I think.

Reprinted with permission from Chinn, P. L. (2008). *Peace and power: Creative leadership for building community* (7th ed., p. 124). Sudbury, MA: Jones & Bartlett Publishers.

Conflict is everyone's responsibility. Through conflict and its resolution, every individual learns, gains new insights, and experiences new possibilities. The peace-and-power process for transforming conflict is growth producing. The process can, with practice, be learned, and it can become a common ground of understanding that grows among individuals (Chinn, 2008).

> reflective **THINKING** Think of a situation in which you have had a conflict recently with a friend. Role-play how you can transform this conflict.

Dynamics of Negotiation

Negotiation occurs during interactions and reactions of almost all individuals, whether they are in groups or in a large organization (Langton & Robbins, 2007). In the day-to-day activity within health care organizations, negotiation is an ongoing effective strategy that emphasizes the need to maintain good working relationships. In fact, negotiation employs communication skills, the power of persuasion or debate, the ability to articulate a point of view or a position, the capability to acknowledge the other individual's position, and a commitment to a course of action (Koerner & Huber, 2006; Hibberd, Valentine, & Clark, 2006). For nurse leaders in health care settings, effective negotiation skills are called upon more frequently than ever to resolve conflict so that teams can work together more productively.

> reflective **THINKING** What are some of the issues that nurse leaders are required to negotiate with health team members?

Styles of Negotiation

The literature describes three methods or approaches to negotiation:

- Distributive negotiation or bargaining
- Integrative negotiation or bargaining
- Principled bargaining.

The hard or soft negotiation is similar to distributive and integrative negotiation (Tomey, 2009). *Distributive negotiation or bargaining* results in a win–lose situation in which a fixed amount of assets is to be divided between parties. In theory, the parties will move more or less toward some compromise. At times, the parties might make threats or give ultimatums. This process builds animosities, and it deepens the divisions among individuals when they must work together later on an ongoing basis (Langton & Robbins, 2007).

In contrast to distributive bargaining, *integrative negotiation or bargaining* results in a win–win situation that assumes that collaborative problem solving can advance the interest of both parties. It requires a degree of creativity to enlarge the assets. In addition, differences between parties can be framed as opportunities (Johns & Saks, 2007). Integrative negotiation bonds negotiators and allows both parties to leave the bargaining process feeling that they have achieved a victory (Langton & Robbins, 2007).

A third negotiation style, known as *principled bargaining* (Fisher, Ury, & Patton, 2004), is based on a collaborative process, and it insists on fair standards. A strong advantage is that it decides issues on their merits and looks for mutual gains for both parties. It promotes trust and emphasizes the need to maintain ongoing relationships. Finally, it is generally the style of choice of nurse leaders (Hibberd, Valentine, & Clark, 2006). Four basic points to principled negotiation follow:

1. Separate the people from the problem.
2. Focus on interests instead of positions.
3. Generate a variety of options before deliberating and deciding what action to take.
4. Insist that the outcome be based on an objective (Finkleman, 2006; Koerner & Huber, 2006; Fisher, Ury, & Patton, 2004).

These characteristics comprise the focus of principled bargaining. Within a negotiation, it is imperative to be aware that people have issues, positions, and interests. Issues are items that are specifically placed on the table for discussion. Positions are the individual's stand on issues, either in an affirmative or negative way. Finally, interests are the underlying concerns that are affected by the negotiation resolutions (Langton & Robbins, 2007).

reflective **THINKING** What style of negotiating or bargaining appeals to you? Give a few reasons.

Negotiation Process

Browman, Snider, and Ellis (2003) state that the nurse leader can create conditions for an explicit negotiating environment. These conditions are as follows:

- Plan for the right parties to get together in an environment conducive for discussion.
- Enlighten the parties in regard to what the mutual (agreed upon) goals are.
- Establish ways to achieve these goals.
- Allow for the expression of different beliefs, values, and opinions.
- Subject the issue(s) to detailed analysis in a respectful, fair, and objective way.

■ Respect the differences that occur in the interpretations of the analysis created by the varying perceptions of the individuals.
■ Provide an appeal mechanism when both sides feel that compromise is difficult to attain.
■ Place a closure on issues such that, even though there is disagreement between parties, they can live with the differences.
■ Give voice to concerns.
■ Allow all issues to be aired equally.
■ Stay with the issues on the agenda as listed, even though difficult.

The process of negotiation usually proceeds through a series of steps that encircle the conditions.

Step 1: Analyzing

During the analysis the nurse leader analyses the context of the conflict situation. A negotiation checklist is outlined in Box 11.1 that the nurse leader can use as a guide to prepare for the upcoming negotiation.

Emphasis must be placed on the following four components:

1. *About You*: Identify the issue and overall goal to be achieved. Develop a detailed and accurate scoring system. Assign points to issues listed; the sum of maximum points across issues should be 100. List the range of possible settlements for each issue and assign points to the possible outcomes. Give the maximum number of points to the preferred settlement for that issue. Then rank and assign points to the possible settlements, ranging from the best to the worst (Simons & Tripp, 2003). Develop the best alternative to negotiated agreement (BATNA). The BATNA is a plan that determines the key negotiation powers. It consists of the target point that defines the highest outcome achievable and a resistant point that marks the lowest acceptable outcome (Langton & Robbins, 2007).
2. *About the Other Side*: Identify who is involved and what their needs and limits are. Attempt to estimate the priorities of the other party.
3. *The Situation*: Be aware of all possible contextual factors. Be flexible with regard to time. Doing so can be a definite strength. Be aware of cultural differences and perceptions.
4. *The Relationship Between Parties*: Determine the trust factor and style of problem solving.

Step 2: Planning

During the planning phase, each of the four components is again considered, and additional options and criteria are developed. Both parties consider a proposed course of action for negotiations. There can be mutual exploration, using objective standards, of how to meet the concerns of the other party (Tomey, 2009).

BOX 11.1 NEGOTIATION CHECKLIST

The negotiation checklist is a systematic way to ensure you are well prepared before your next negotiation.

Check off each item as it is accomplished.

A. About You
    1. What is your overall goal?
    2. What are the issues?
    3. How important is each issue to you?

    Develop a scoring system for evaluating offers:
      a) List all of the issues of importance from step 2.
      b) Rank order all of the issues.
      c) Assign points to all the issues (assign weighted values based on a total of 100 points).
      d) List the range of possible settlements for each issue. Your assessments of realistic, low, and high expectations should be grounded in health care norms and your best-case expectation.
      e) Assign points to the possible outcomes that you identified for each issue.
      f) Double-check the accuracy of your scoring system.
      g) Use the scoring system to evaluate any offer that is on the table.

    4. What is your "best alternative to negotiated agreement" (BATNA)?
    5. What is your resistance point (i.e., the worst agreement you are willing to accept before ending negotiations)? If your BATNA is vague, consider identifying the terms you can possibly accept and beyond which you must recess to gather more information.

B. About the Other Side
    1. How important is each issue to them (plus any new issues they added)?
    2. What is their best alternative to negotiated agreement?
    3. What is their resistance point?
    4. Based on questions B.1, B.2, and B.3, what is your target?

C. The Situation
    1. What deadline exists? Who is more impatient?
    2. What fairness norms or reference points apply?
    3. What topics or questions do you want to avoid? How will you respond if they ask anyway?

D. The Relationship Between the Parties
    1. Will negotiations be repetitive? If so, what are the future consequences of each strategy, tactic, or action you are considering?

(box continues on page 300)

> **BOX 11.1**   NEGOTIATION CHECKLIST (continued)
>
> **2.** Trust:
>   **a)** Can you trust the other party? What do you know about them?
>   **b)** Does the other party trust you?
> **3.** What do you know of the other party's styles and tactics?
> **4.** What are the limits to the other party's authority?
> **5.** Consult in advance with the other party about the agenda.

Reprinted with permission from Simons, T., & Tripp, T. M. (2003). The negotiation checklist. In R. J. Lewicki, D. M. Saunders, J. W. Minton, & B. Barry (Eds.), *Negotiation: Readings, exercises, and cases* (p. 51). New York: McGraw-Hill/Irwin.

Step 3: Negotiating

The strategies of negotiation are implemented. Some interactive skills enhance the process, whereas others impede it. Empathy, being genuine and caring, is an important facilitative skill. On the other hand, blaming, becoming angry, and crying will block the process. Try to understand emotions by making them explicit and legitimate. Use symbolic gestures of goodwill, such as shaking hands and sending a note of acknowledgement. Effective communication is critical to successful negotiations (Hibberd, Valentine, & Clark, 2006).

Step 4: Follow-Up

The final step involves the evaluation, which ensures that the problem has been successfully resolved. Summarize the agreement and then write a letter specifying your understanding of the agreement. There is a definite need to ensure that the plan of action successfully addressed the conflict and that no further intervention is required (Hibberd, Valentine, & Clark, 2006).

Leadership Issue

*Y*ou want your budget request for equipment and staffing needs to be approved by your administration. Administrators have emphasized that no additional funds are available and that your unit must use the resources available. This is the second year that your request has been rejected. Apply the steps of the negotiation process to resolve this conflict.

For a nurse leader, the most important step in learning to deal with conflict is recognizing that it is normal and manageable. Understanding that it is a natural outcome of interacting with others, and that various approaches exist, are critical to maintain relatedness among health team members. Improving working relationships is beneficial, not only for the nurse leader's well-being, but for that of the health care team as well. Communication, collaboration, and respect maintained among the team members are vital components in contributing to the safe quality care of clients and their families.

WEBSITES

▧ Canadian Federation of Nurses (CFN)

http://nursesunions.ca/

The CFN is the national voice for nurses. Representing 158,000 nurses, members, and associate members, they advance solutions to improve patient care, working conditions, and the public health care system.

▧ Ontario Nurses Association (ONA)

http://www.ona.org/

How are collective agreements negotiated? There are two scenarios for the start of collective bargaining. One focuses on a trade union that has just been certified and has given the employer written notice of its desire to bargain. The second focuses on an employer and a union who are already bound by a collective agreement. This site provides extensive links to many current issues and interests in nursing.

▧ Canadian Nurses Protective Society (CNPS)

http://www.cnps.ca/

The CNPS is a nonprofit society, owned and operated by nurses for nurses, that offers legal liability protection related to nursing practice to eligible registered nurses by providing information, education, and financial and legal assistance.

REFERENCES

Adler, R., Rolls, J., Proctor III, R., & Towne, N. (2009). *Looking out/looking in* (brief Canadian ed.). Toronto, ON: Nelson Education.

Almost, J. (2006). Conflict within nursing work environments: Concept analysis. *Journal of Advanced Nursing, 53*(4), 444–453.

Barker, A. (2006). Human resource management strategies. In A.M. Barker, D.T. Sullivan, & M.J. Emery (Eds.), *Leadership competencies for clinical managers: The renaissance of transformational leadership* (pp. 213–235). Sudbury, MA: Jones and Bartlett.

Barki, H., & Hartwick, J. (2001). Interpersonal conflict and its management in information system development. *MIS Quarterly, 25*, 195–228.

Blais, K., Hayes, J., Kozier, B., & Erb, G. (2006). *Professional nursing practice: concepts and perspectives* (5th ed.). Upper Saddle River, NJ: Pearson Education.

Browman, G., Snider, A., & Ellis, P. (2003). Negotiating for change. The healthcare manager as catalyst for evidence-based practice: changing the healthcare environment and sharing experience. *Healthcare Papers, 3*(3), 10–22.

Callanan, G. & Perri, D. (2006). Teaching conflict management using a scenario-based approach. *Journal of Education for Business, 81*(3), 131–139.

Chinn, P. (2008). *Peace and power: creative leadership for building community* (7th ed.). Mississauga, ON: Jones and Bartlett.

Cox, K. (2000). The effect of unit morale and interpersonal relations on conflict in the nursing unit. *Journal of Advanced Nursing, 35*(1), 17–25.

Cox, K. (2003). The effects of intrapersonal, intragroup, and intergroup conflict on team performance effectiveness and work satisfaction. *Nursing Administration Quarterly, 27*(2), 153–163.

Cox, K. (2006). Power and conflict. In D.L. Huber (Eds.), *Leadership and nursing care management* (3rd ed., pp. 501–542). Philadelphia: Elsevier.

Dirks, K. & Ferrin, D. (2001). The role of trust in organizational settings. *Organization Science, 12*(4), 450–467.

Donohue, M. (2007). Conflict: The cutting edge of change. In P.S. Yoder-Wise (Ed.), *Leading and managing in nursing* (4th ed., pp. 459–480). St. Louis, MO: Mosby.

Ellis, J., & Hartley, C. (2008). *Nursing in today's world: trends, issues & management* (9th ed.). Philadelphia: Wolters Kluwer Health/Lippincott Williams & Wilkins.

Filley, A. (1975). *Interpersonal conflict resolution.* Glenview, IL: Scott, Foresman and Company.

Finkelman, A. W. (2006). *Leadership and management in nursing,* Upper Saddle River, NJ: Pearson Prentice hall.

Fisher, R., Ury, R. Y., & Patton, W. Y. (2004). *Getting to yes: negotiating agreement without giving in.* Boston: Houghton Mifflin.

Folger, J., Poole, M., & Stutman, R. (2005). *Working through conflict: strategies for relationships, groups and organizations.* Boston: Pearson Education.

Grohar-Murray, M., & DiCroce, H. (2003). *Leadership and management in nursing.* Upper Saddle River, NJ: Pearson Education.

Hansten, R. (2003). Star search: finding the next generation of nurse leaders. *Nurse Leader, 1*(3), 46–49.

Hendel, T., Fish, M., & Berger, O. (2007). Nurse/physician conflict management mode choices: implications for improved collaborative practice. *Nursing Administration Quarterly, 31*(3), 244–253.

Hesketh, K., Duncan, S., Estabrooks, C., Reimer, M., Giovannetti, P., Hyndman, K. & Acorn, S. (2003). Workplace violence in Alberta and British Columbia hospitals. *Health Policy, 63,* 311–321.

Hibberd, J., Valentine, P., & Clark, L. (2006). Conflict resolution and negotiation. In J. M. Hibberd & D. L. Smith (Eds.), *Nursing leadership and management in Canada* (3rd ed., pp. 649–668). Toronto, ON: Elsevier Canada.

Jacinta, K. (2006). An overview of conflict. *Dimensions of Critical Care Nursing, 25*(1), 22–28.

Jacob, S. (2006). Human resource development: managing a culturally diverse work force. In L. Roussel, R. C. Swansburg, & R. J. Swansburg (Eds.), *Management and leadership for nurse administrators* (4th ed., pp. 181–214). Sudbury, MA: Jones and Bartlett.

Johns, G., & Saks, A. (2008). *Organizational behaviour: understanding and managing life at work* (7th ed.). Toronto, ON: Pearson Education Canada.

Koerner, J., & Huber, D. (2006). Communication, persuasion, and negotiation. In D. L. Huber (Eds.), *Leadership and nursing care management* (3rd ed., pp. 407–438). Philadelphia: Elsevier.

Kreitner, R., Kinicki, A., & Cole, N. (2007). *Fundamentals of organizational behaviour: key concepts, skills and best practices* (2nd Canadian ed.). Boston, MA: McGraw-Hill Ryerson.

Langton, N., & Robbins, S. (2007). *Fundamentals of organizational behaviour.* Toronto, ON: Pearson Education Canada.

McShane, S. (2006). *Canadian organizational behaviour* (6th ed.). Toronto, ON: McGraw-Hill Ryerson.

Meyer, S. (2004). Organizational response to conflict: future conflict and work outcomes. *Social Work Research, 28*(3), 183–190.

Porter-O'Grady, T. (2003). When push comes to shove: managers as mediators. *Nursing Management, 34*(10), 34–40.

Porter-O'Grady, T. (2004a). Embracing conflict: building a healthy community. *Health Care Management Review, 29*(3), 181–187.

Porter-O'Grady, T. (2004b). Constructing a conflict resolution program for health care. *Health Care Management Review, 29*(4), 278–283.

Rahim, M. (2002). Toward a theory of managing organizational conflict. *International Journal of Conflict Management, 13*, 206–235.

Robbins, S. (2003). *Organizational behavior* (10th ed.). Englewood Cliffs, NJ: Prentice-Hall.

Simons, T., & Tripp, T. (2003). The negotiation checklist. In R. J. Lewicki, D. M. Saunders, J. W. Minton, & B. Barry (Eds.), *Negotiation: readings, exercises and cases* (4th ed., pp. 50–53). New York,: McGraw-Hill.

Swearingen, S., & Liberman, A. (2004). Nursing generations: an expanded look at the emergence of conflict and its resolution. *The Health Care Manager, 23*(1), 54–64.

Thomas, K. (1976). Conflict and conflict management. In M. D. Dunnette (Ed.), *The handbook of industrial and organizational psychology* (pp. 889–935). Chicago, IL: Rand McNally.

Thomas, K. (1992). Conflict and negotiation processes in organizations. In M. D. Dunnette & L. M. Hough (Eds.), *Handbook of industrial and organizational psychology* (2nd ed., vol. 3, pp. 651–717). Palo Alto, CA: Consulting Psychologists Press.

Tomey, A. M. (2009). *Guide to nursing management and leadership* (8th ed.). St. Louis, MO: Mosby.

Valentine, P. (2001). A gender perspective on conflict management strategies of nurses. *Journal of Nursing Scholarship, 33*(1), 69–74.

Vivar, C. (2006). Putting conflict management into practice: a nursing case study. *Journal of Nursing Management, 14*(3), 201–206.

Warner, I. (2001). Nurses' perceptions of workplace conflict: Implications for retention and recruitment. *Journal of Advanced Nursing, 53*(4), 444–453.

Weston, M. (2001). Coaching generations in the workplace. *Nursing Administration Quarterly, 25*(2), 11–21.

12

TIME MANAGEMENT AND DELEGATION: MAXIMIZING THE PRODUCTIVITY AND PERFORMANCE OF THE NURSE LEADER

In the College's Standards for Nursing Practice (2003), an indicator for professional leadership standard (Standard 5) states: "The registered nurse demonstrates professional judgment and accountability when delegating or assigning tasks or functions to other members of the healthcare team."

College of Registered Nurses of Nova Scotia (CRNNS)
Delegation Guidelines for Registered Nurses
Copyright © 2004, CRNNS

The CRNNS, through provincial legislation, has the legal accountability to regulate nursing in the public interest. Through the same legislation, the *Registered Nurses Act* (2001), individual registered nurses have the authority and accountability to provide nursing services and to practice in accordance with standards established by the College (CRNNS, 2004, p. 3).

Overview

With today's organizational restructuring, technological innovation, and over-abundance of information, along with the introduction of new management principles in the health care environment, time management has become a significant challenge for nurse leaders and nurses alike. As increasing emphases are placed on speed and timeliness, stress is created within individuals and impacts all levels of productivity within the scope of nursing practice. Time management is a process that includes aspects of data analysis, planning, and prioritizing, as well as implementing such strategies as delegation to enhance performance.

Delegation is key to time management because it encompasses workload distribution. To delegate, the registered nurse (RN) must be accountable and responsible, taking into consideration the competence of the available staff and the client's needs. Delegated tasks must fall within the staff's scope of practice.

Objectives

By critically reflecting upon and processing knowledge throughout this chapter, you will be able to respond effectively to the following objectives:

1. Describe time management from your own perspective.
2. Analyze the different types of stress in the workplace.
3. Recognize a situation whereby several of the seven habits can be applied.
4. Critique the three prominent barriers of time management.
5. Debate the positive versus the negative outcomes related to time management.
6. Apply the time management process to your nursing practice.
7. Examine the definitions of delegation promoted by professional nursing bodies.
8. Analyze what is understood by the registered nurses' scope of practice.
9. Evaluate the process of delegation by the registered nurse to regulated health workers compared with unregulated health workers.
10. Apply the principles of delegation to a nursing situation in a health care setting.
11. Examine the benefits of delegation and barriers to delegation.

Time Management in Nursing Practice

Effective time management results in greater effectiveness and efficiency in the delivery of quality nursing care. According to Finkelman (2006), effectiveness means doing the right thing and efficiency means doing the right thing right. Time management is a process that takes into account analyzing work data and planning and implementing appropriate strategies to ensure that time is invested in activities leading toward the achievement of priority goals (Pettigrew, 2007). Quality performance and high productivity are critical to organizations and are essentially dependent on effective management of time. The use of one's time impacts individuals in different and complex ways. The ability of a nurse leader to manage health team members who have differing perceptions of time involves endless patience and extensive knowledge of the time management process.

> reflective **THINKING**   What is your meaning of time? How do you perceive your ability to manage time personally and professionally?

Stress in the Workplace

The current intent of health care organizations often includes trying to do more with less, in financial matters as well as staffing. Consequently, such conditions have led to high demands, resulting in extensive stress being placed on health team members (Pettigrew, 2007). Any change that affects the distribution of time that health care professionals spend on their health service activities can have a considerable effect on the quality of client and family care. Among common factors related to the use of time are workload, personal time management, work habits, and more.

Workload

The combined effects of restructuring and downsizing have exerted tremendous impacts on nurse leaders and staff nurses alike. Nurses face stress arising from heavy workloads involving physical and mental strain; daily life-and-death situations; the need for knowledge on how to be technologically wise with complex equipment; interpersonal conflict with staff, physicians, other departments, and families; and the awareness of the serious consequences of mistakes (Tomey, 2009). Figure 12.1 depicts such a stressed nurse. Nurses are reporting growing stress levels, high levels of job insecurity, and poor morale. With rising nursing shortages, the workload is increasing dramatically in most health care settings.

Greenglass, Burke, and Fiksenbaum (2001) examined the relationship between workload, burnout, and somatization in a sample of 1,363 nurses employed in Ontario hospitals undergoing organizational restructuring. They concluded

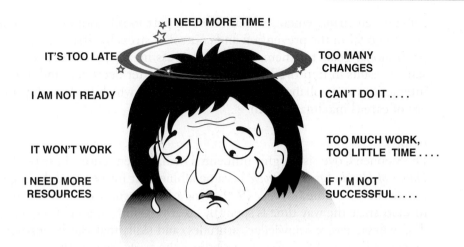

FIGURE 12.1   Stress in nursing practice.

that the nurses' perceptions of increased workload were positively related to emotional exhaustion. Human Resources and Social Development Canada (2005) state that work-related stress, work–life conflict, and work–life balance (WLB) constitute a growing concern for employees and employers in the workplace. Both administration and staff are well aware that the increasing costs of benefits, absenteeism, and productivity losses present a most serious issue in the workplace.

To begin taking the necessary steps to moderate stress to manageable levels, nurse leaders face the need to assess all levels and all types of stress that occur in health team members. As a start, the nurse leader can begin support groups, organize team-building activities, and initiate and coordinate stress management programs.

reflective **THINKING**   As a nurse leader in the workplace, what are some of the elements that contribute to your stress level?

Read the article "Time spent with family during a typical workday, 1986 to 2005" by Turcotte (2007), listed in the Reference section. How much time do you spend at work compared to time spent with your family?

Personal Time Management

A close relationship exists between stress and time management. That is, when competing demands create stress, the effective management of one's time becomes increasingly important (Cox & Huber, 2006). Time management is actually self-management, which refers in part to self-awareness. Nursing leaders can go far in the prevention and control of stress by first setting personal and professional goals for themselves. Less stress means less wear and tear on oneself. It results in improved critical thinking, better decisions, and more effective interactions and collaboration with others, all of which leads to improved delivery of care (Finkelman, 2006).

Habits

Dr. Stephen Covey is a highly influential management guru whose book *The Seven Habits of Highly Effective People* became a blueprint for personal development and for maximizing time (Covey, 1990). One of his premises is that individuals need to reorganize the way time is spent by creating habits of good time management. The habits involve knowledge, attitudes, and skills that can be learned through practice (Tomey, 2009). Box 12.1 outlines the *seven habits*, with a brief description of suggested personal time management practices for each habit.

It has been said that an individual's coping ability is the major variable in being able to modulate stress and control its outcome (Cox & Huber, 2006). In addition, nurse leaders can manage stress beginning with an understanding of their own value system. Such leaders can influence others to enhance their own coping strategies and learn how to provide essential support for one another. Nurse leaders can model the seven habits and inspire hope and vision for the future in health care for their health team members.

> reflective **THINKING**   Try practicing the last habit, "Sharpen the saw." What activities do you practice for self-renewal?

Barriers to Time Management

In developing new habits, the nurse leader may encounter barriers that affect the ability to manage time effectively. Being aware of such obstacles alerts the leader to possible pitfalls (Grohar-Murray & DiCroce, 2003). Figure 12.2 depicts a nurse leader who is frazzled and weary, primarily as a result of combating the three looming barriers. These three barriers—procrastination, perfectionism, and pessimism—affecting time management are discussed below, with suggested coping techniques. Other barriers are also discussed briefly.

Procrastination

Procrastination is the chronic delay in planning and carrying out strategies that are necessary to accomplish important tasks (Rider Ellis & Love Hartley, 2008). Being aware of the tendency to procrastinate is important in understanding time man-

BOX 12.1 TIPS FOR PERSONAL TIME MANAGEMENT

Be Proactive
This means that one needs to start by being proactive and accepting responsibility for his or her own actions and attitudes. As one exercises freedom to choose responses, the more proactive one becomes. As a result, opportunities are fed and problems are starved.

Begin With the End in Sight
We should have a clear understanding of the desired direction and destination. If things are created mentally before they are created physically, quality is designed and built in.

Put first things first. Personal management is organizing and managing based on personal priorities to get to where you want to go. Give less time to urgent things that are not important, such as nonproductive meetings called by an anxious supervisor. Spend more time on things that are important but not urgent, such as relationships, prevention, planning, preparation, taking opportunities, and recreation.

Think Win–Win
Effectiveness is often accomplished by the cooperative efforts of two or more people. A win–win attitude explores options until a mutually satisfactory solution is reached. This is an abundance mentality that builds on synergy, rather than a scarcity mentality that leads to win–lose strategies.

Seek First to Understand, Then to Be Understood
Good communications are essential to building win–win relationships. Our perceptions come from our experiences. Credibility problems usually involve differences. Empathetic listening is therapeutic. When people feel they are understood, they lower their defences. Once one understands the other person's point of view, it is easier to arrive at a win–win solution by problem solving.

Synergize
Synergy comes from teamwork or creative cooperation. Synergy results from bringing different perspectives together in a spirit of mutual respect to seek the best solution.

Sharpen the Saw
The longer one saws, the duller the saw gets, and the harder one works to get less and less accomplished. People need physical, spiritual, mental, social, and emotional self-renewal. One needs to give priority to a balanced program of self-renewal.

Adapted from Covey, S. R. (1990). *The 7 habits of highly effective people: Powerful lessons in personal change.* New York: Fireside/Simon & Schuster; Tomey, A. M. (2009). *Guide to nursing management and leadership* (8th ed., pp. 33–45). St. Louis, MO: Mosby.

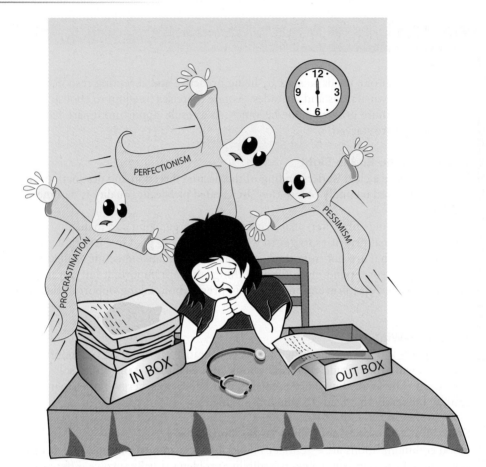

FIGURE 12.2 Barriers to time management.

agement. Techniques such as scheduling, maintaining "to do" lists, and adhering to them could break the habit of procrastination (Barker, 2006). However, the practice of these techniques on a daily basis is essential.

Perfectionism
Perfectionism is the tendency to become caught up in the details of work. The result is that work accomplished is never perceived to be good enough. The recognition of the need to be perfect is important not only for time management, but also for one's self-esteem (Barker, 2006). Overcoming perfectionism requires considerable effort, so patience and practice are essential (Pettigrew, 2007).

Pessimism
Pessimism is having a negative outlook on life, both personally and professionally. It colours one's work, and all effort seems to be dismal and disappointing.

Pessimism can be a companion of procrastination and perfectionism. Becoming aware of one's attitude is critical to initiating change. It is important to focus on the positive side of life. Humour and leisure activities often go far to facilitate a lighter aspect of life.

Other Barriers: Personal and System

Other barriers to time management include personal issues, such as physical and mental health problems that may interfere with time management. For example, nurses who are experiencing physical health problems are not able to move consistently with the speed required for direct care interventions (Rider Ellis & Love Hartley, 2008). Meanwhile, nurses who experience mental health problems, such as depression, may experience serious limitations in their ability to initiate and complete tasks (Adler et al., 2006). Nurses often need to consult with the human resources department to identify other work positions that mesh better with their current health status (Rider Ellis & Love Hartley, 2008).

System issues, such as information overload brought on by pile-up of e-mails, voice and text messages, and routine meetings, often interfere with one's time management. Being interrupted and disorganized and not delegating effectively can drain one's time and energy. But, all of these barriers can be overcome, even though the amount of time in a day remains the same (Finkelman, 2006).

> *reflective* **THINKING** What uncontrollable events, considered to be barriers to time management, can you identify?

Positive Outcomes Related to Time Management

Effective time management can result in important benefits for the nurse leader personally and professionally for the delivery of care within the organization. The essential benefits include:

- *Conserving personal energy* by minimizing the number of demands at work and taking breaks.
- *Having peace and clarity of mind* by prioritizing tasks and maintaining a safe environment that retains staff and results in quality client care.
- *Establishing trust with team members* by role modeling a calm attitude and keeping on top of work activities; doing this demonstrates satisfaction and team spirit (Barker, 2006; Finkelman, 2006).
- *Accomplishing what is important* by focusing attention on important tasks, being fluid, flexible, and in process. Doing this helps one gain momentum during work (Vaccaro, 2003).

Negative Outcomes Related to Time Management

A few of the negative consequences of poor time management are as follows:

- *Being frazzled and weary.* Fatigue and feeling overworked produces an undesirable impact of noncaring about oneself and others.
- *Displaying a negative attitude.* Being dismal and short tempered affects others, especially when they rely on the leader's input into projects.
- *Promoting distrust.* By not following through on promised decisions and actions, the nurse leader may find that team members have begun to distrust him or her (Barker, 2006).

---

reflective **THINKING**   What positive and negative outcomes of time management have you experienced in your clinical practice? As a nurse leader, what suggestions do you have to overcome the negative outcomes?

Evidence Related to Negative Outcomes of Time Management

A study was conducted to identify the types and extent of nursing care regularly missed as a result of time pressures on a medical-surgical unit (Kalisch, 2006). The findings indicated that routine omissions included basic care measures, such as ambulation, turning, delayed or missed feeding, and hygiene, as well as the more professional behaviours of client teaching, discharge planning, emotional support, intake and output documentation, and surveillance. The results of this study suggest a number of actions that nursing leaders can use to decrease the problems of missed nursing care.

One of the actions is to collect and analyze data related to missed nursing care on the units. Another action is to create a culture of quality and safety that ensures attention to the honest reporting of omissions of nursing care. Once the issue is recognized, then strategies can be implemented on the unit to address the problems. Moreover, nurses are often distracted by inadequate staffing, poor teamwork, and the acuity of clients. The recognition of these problems, followed by appropriate attention to their solutions within the organization, helps greatly to increase the amount of time spent in the delivery of quality care. The importance of delegation should be emphasized so that nurses can more appropriately manage the staff working with them (Kalisch, 2006).

A Canadian study explored the relationship between busyness in nursing and nurses' research utilization. The researchers defined busyness as "an individual perception of internalized pressure created by a situation where there is a shortage of time to accomplish valued work and often results in a reduced energy level" (Thompson et al., 2008, p. 542). They found that maintaining busyness was an expectation of both nurses and hospital administrators. In fact, a culture of busyness in nursing was created that supported the familiarity of nursing tasks over the unfamiliarity of research utilization. One example of the culture of busyness is the shift report, which takes up much of the nurse's time rather than scanning research findings from studies.

The researchers conclude that if nursing is committed to advancing evidence-based practice, then work environments must be modified so that less time is spent on "busyness" and time required to use research in practice is a recognized and valued component of nursing practice (Thompson et al., 2008).

> *reflective* **THINKING**   What is your concept of busyness? What are examples of busyness in your clinical experience?

Time Management Process for Nurse Leaders

Time is a manageable resource. Today, in health care organizations, it has become critical to manage time effectively because nursing leaders and team members are expected to be decisive and to focus on the "now" while considering long-term goals (Finkelman, 2006). Time management implementation is an ongoing process that requires flexibility, meaningful adjustments, and self-discipline as situations change (Pearce, 2007). Box 12.2 outlines the key elements in the time management process. Nurse leaders can begin to maximize their time by conducting an inventory of their activities. A tool to assist them is found in Table 12.1.

The findings from the following research studies provide insight into the strategies used to manage time in health care.

- *Bowers, Lauring, and Jacobson (2001)* conducted a study to determine how nurses manage time in long-term care. Time was an extremely salient work condition for the nurses interviewed. The results indicated that the nurses, under the conditions of having too little time and many interruptions, compensated by developing strategies either to keep up or catch up. These strategies included *minimizing the time spent doing required tasks, creating new time*, and *redefining work responsibilities*. The researchers concluded that increased staffing would allow nurses time to improve the quality of care in long-term care facilities.

BOX 12.2   TIME MANAGEMENT PROCESS

Conduct Time Inventory
- Develop self-awareness by using the tool found in Table 12.1.
- Record activities for a week (or other reasonable duration).
- Assess and evaluate time wasters.

Set Goals and Priorities
- Write down realistic goals (daily goals and also broader weekly, monthly ones).
  - Carry them with you (use a day planner or handheld computer).
  - Assess required tasks daily (to keep them fresh and to remain sensitive to opportunities that will help you reach your goals). Adjust time blocks as needed.
- Evaluate tasks by importance first and urgency second. See Barker et al. (2006, p. 84) for a suggestion of a quadrant system using high–low importance versus high–low urgency.
- Set priorities. Be mindful of the Pareto principle (known as the 80/20 principle) suggesting that 80% of satisfying outcomes are a result of just 20% of the time that you spend. Many other variations of this principle can be found.
- Ask questions:
  - Could the task be done differently to require less time?
  - Is this a weekly, monthly, quarterly, or annual task?
  - What is the best way to schedule it to meet deadlines?
  - Is it necessary to consult with anyone before work can begin?
  - What will happen if this task is not done?
  - Can I delegate parts or all of it to someone else?
  - Is this task worth the time required to do it?

Plan Strategies and Draw Up the Schedule
- Begin by planning the day:
  - Some will do so at the end of the day for the next day.
  - Some will plan out the whole week and others (say, in applying direct care) will need to focus on planning at the beginning of the day or shift.
- Determine a plan to stay focused and accomplish tasks:
  - Be prepared to alter or adjust the daily plan based on appointments, meetings, phone calls, rounds, report or documentation, necessary reading (literature or reports).
  - Develop a "to do list." But keep it focused. It is easy to keep adding to the list until it is unrealistic to accomplish all items in the allotted time.
  - Include time to deal with the unexpected.
  - Be aware of your prime internal time—best time to work alone.
  - Be aware of your best external time—best time to work with others.

BOX 12.2 TIME MANAGEMENT PROCESS (continued)

- Remember that no schedule is perfect:
  - There will always be interruptions, crises, staff changes, changes in direction of the project.
  - Tasks often take longer than expected.
  - Schedules need to be reevaluated to make them more reasonable.
- It is better to make many alterations to a schedule than to have no schedule.

Learn Time Management Techniques
- Being able to say "no" graciously is a skill.
- Use transition time:
  - Mail can be read while one is "on hold" or when returning phone calls.
  - Use speed-reading techniques. The more they are practiced the better one becomes at them.
- Set a "batch time"—blocks of time to work on particular tasks.
- Streamline paper work—organize into low- and high-priority piles.
- Control social time.
- Adhere to self-discipline. Over scheduling makes it difficult to cope with the unexpected.

Adapted from Finkelman, A. W. (2006). *Leadership and management in nursing.* Upper Saddle River, NJ: Pearson Education; Barker, A. M., Taylor Sullivan, D., & Emery, M. J. (2006). *Leadership competencies for clinical managers: The renaissance of transformational leadership.* Toronto, ON: Jones & Bartlett.

- *Waterworth (2003)* explored how nurses organize and manage their time. This researcher also found that time management is complex and that nurses use a range of time-management strategies and a repertoire of actions. Six time strategies were identified: *prioritizing, routinization, concealment, catch up, juggling,* and *extending temporal boundaries.* The researcher discusses two of such strategies. One is routines, which are habituated ways of responding to occurrences in everyday life, and the other is prioritizing, which is a prerequisite for effective work performance and is an expected strategy. Prioritizing almost always becomes an integral part of a nurse's routine. This study also indicates how the two management strategies—routinization and prioritization—are influenced by others (team and organization). Failure to address these two variables may lead to missed opportunities in focusing on issues in organizing nurses' work and coordinating care involving other health care providers.
- *Hendry and Walker (2004)* searched databases regarding priority setting in nursing. The publications found were used in a selective descriptive review.

TABLE 12.1 | ANALYSIS OF TOOL FOR TIME MANAGEMENT

Use the following scoring system for each answer below.
Place an X in the column that is appropriate for you.
1 = Never; 2 = Rarely; 3 = Occasionally; 4 = Usually; 5 = Always

	1	2	3	4	5
I feel calm and in control of my time.					
I spend the majority of my time in meaningful work that contributes to the positive work on my clinical unit.					
I spend the majority of my time doing activities that I find satisfying.					
I complete my paperwork and projects on time.					
I follow through on promises I make to my staff, boss, and others.					
I delegate tasks to others in my clinical unit.					
I assess tasks for their importance and their urgency.					
I am able to control interruptions.					
I set aside time each day for planning.					
I complete one task before undertaking a new one.					
I spend the right amount of time looking for information.					
I repeat only those actions that need to be repeated.					
I prepare myself for meetings, shift, and report.					
I take time to talk with my clients and family members.					
I return all my phone calls and e-mails.					
TOTALS: For each column, multiply the number of Xs in the column by the number at the top. Insert the scores in the spaces to the right.					

Your five-column scores can provide you with a quick personal analysis profile of your time management habits.
Adapted from Finkelman, A. W. (2006). *Leadership and management in nursing* (p. 407). Upper Saddle River, NJ: Pearson Education; Barker, A. M., Taylor Sullivan, D., & Emery, M. J. (2006). *Leadership competencies for clinical managers: The renaissance of transformational leadership* (p. 81). Toronto, ON: Jones & Bartlett.

They found that *priority setting* is a highly important skill in nursing, and that a priority setting deficit can have serious consequences for clients and their families. According to these investigators, priority setting can be defined as "the ordering of nursing problems, using notions of urgency and/or importance, in order to establish a preferential order for nursing actions" (p. 427). Although a number of factors have been identified that may impact on priority setting, such as the expertise of the nurse, the availability of resources, and nurse–client relationships, a scant number of empirical studies have been conducted in this area. The researchers recommend that further study of priority setting in a range of clinical practice settings is necessary.

Time management strategies are recognized as an important component of work performance and professional nursing practice (Waterworth, 2003). Further research is needed in this area to determine more precisely the strategies nurses can implement to achieve the desired levels of productivity and performance in their practice.

reflective **THINKING**   As a nurse leader, you decide to conduct a research study regarding priority setting. What research question would you develop for this study?

Reflections on Leadership Practice

*R*eview the key elements in the time management process Box 12.2. Take time to reflect on the following case study:

You are a recent BN graduate assigned to a medical unit. Yesterday, you completed the orientation and were assigned a mentor. Today is your first day on the unit. You are mildly nervous, but as you meet the nurse unit manager, who appears calm and caring, you are put at ease. He introduces you to the entire health team, and everyone seems warm and friendly. The mentor assures you that if you have any questions, she is nearby to assist you. As you enter the room to meet one of your two assigned clients, you observe that this client's facial colour is ashen and that he is clutching his chest. You become extremely anxious and, while providing care to this client, you neglect the other client completely. You also forget to inform the mentor of the situation. After the crisis has passed, the nurse unit manager calls you into his office and questions your time management skills.

- In reviewing your day, what should you have done before beginning your care?
- What realistic goal could you have developed before starting your care?
- Reflect on your behaviour and begin again to plan your nursing care. What would this plan of care entail?
- If you were a nurse leader, how would you handle the situation?

Benefits of Effective Time Management

Effective time management strategies benefit all team members in the organization. Nurse leaders who use their time well are highly organized. They are able to assist their staff to manage their time, resulting in improved productivity in their clinical practice. Nurse leaders who are in control of their own workload are likely to achieve a balance between organizational roles and their personal lives (Arnold & Pulich, 2004). The result is that they will be viewed positively and considered trustworthy by others in the organization.

Delegating Effectively

Delegation has become increasingly important for nurse leaders as the nursing profession experiences changes within the dynamic health care environment. The complex nature of the health care system, coupled with complicated client and family situations, require the RN to provide a full range of care requirements. That is, the RN is responsible and accountable for overall assessments, the determination of client status, care planning, strategies, and care evaluation (College of Registered Nurses of British Columbia, 2007). The issue of delegation, to health team members with different educational backgrounds, requires that nurses be vigilant in ensuring that client safety and well-being are maintained (Marthaler & Angkaw, 2008). Efficient delegation of care protects the client and family and provides effective outcomes (Canadian Nurses Association [CNA], 2003; Fisher, 2000).

reflective **THINKING** Have you had the experience of delegating a task to another health care worker? Describe your experience briefly.

Definition of Delegation by Professional Bodies

Several professional organizations have contributed to the definition of delegation:

- *College of Nurses of Ontario (2007)* defines delegation as a formal process by which a regulated health professional, who has the authority and competence to perform a procedure under one of the controlled acts, delegates the performance of that procedure to others under certain conditions.
- *Canadian Nurses Protective Society (2001)* defines delegation when either the employer or nurse transfers authority to a health care worker in a selected situation to do work traditionally performed by a nurse. For example, an unlicensed worker may measure vital signs, but the nurse analyses the data for comprehensive assessment, nursing diagnosis, and planning care.

All delegation involves at least two individuals, the delegator, who possesses the authority to delegate, and the delegatee, who receives direction for the task from the delegator. The relationship between the two health team members exists within the workplace environment. It is important to note that the delegation does not change the delegator's accountability or responsibility for task completion (Mutzebaugh, 2007).

reflective **THINKING**   What is your definition of delegation?

To be effective in accomplishing goals, the RN who is delegating must take on a leadership role. With successful delegation, the health care needs of the client and the family are addressed, and the nurse's professional goals are also addressed (Marthaler & Angkaw, 2008).

Scope of Practice

The practice of RNs and other professional health care providers is regulated by professional and licensing bodies who define and sanction the scope of their work. Regulated health care providers are responsible and accountable for competent practice. Unregulated health care workers are caregivers who provide care to individuals while being supervised by regulated care providers. Regulated care providers are responsible for the care given by unregulated health care workers

Regulated Care Providers

Regulated care providers (RNs, licensed practical nurses [LPNs], and registered psychiatric nurses [RPNs]) are accountable to the public through legislation. They are expected to adhere to their provincial/territorial standards of practice, code of ethics, and speciality practice standards (CNA, 2003). According to the Association of Registered Nurses of Newfoundland and Labrador (ARNNL) (2006), the scope of practice is defined as "the range of roles, functions, responsibilities, and activities which RNs are educated and authorized to perform" (p. 3). This broad scope of practice reflects all of the roles and activities undertaken by RNs to be present to the full range of human experiences and responses to health and illness. According to the Code of Ethics (CNA, 2002), nursing practice is directed toward the goal of assisting clients to achieve and maintain optimal health to maximize quality of life across the lifespan. The scope of practice of the individual nurse is influenced by the nurse's knowledge, practice setting, health care agency requirements, and the needs of the client. It is often described in job descriptions and/or illustrated in practice settings as competencies (ARNNL, 2006). Regulated health care providers are responsible for practicing within their own level of competence and are responsible for their own practice.

When an RN, LPN, or RPN decides to delegate components of nursing care to another regulated health care provider, he or she is accountable for the decision to delegate that particular component of care and for assessing and determining that the provider has the necessary knowledge and skills to perform the competency safely and competently (College of Registered Nurses of Manitoba, 2002).

Unregulated Health Care Workers

Unregulated health care providers do not have a regulatory body or a legally defined scope of practice. They do not have mandatory education or regulatory practice standards (Saskatchewan Registered Nurses' Association, 2004). The unregulated health care workers are caregivers who provide personal care or support for activities of daily living to individuals. To maintain client safety, the RN, LPN, or RPN who assigns tasks or procedures must ensure certain requirements are met before the assignment. One such condition is that the health care worker has the ability to perform the task safely. When nursing tasks or procedures are assigned to an unregulated health care worker, the worker must be under the supervision of an RN, LPN, or RPN. The degree of supervision required by the unregulated worker must be established by the RN, LPN, or RPN who is delegating the task or procedure and upon the complexity of the task or procedure being delegated. One of the responsibilities of all unregulated health care workers is to know what procedures they are qualified to perform as approved by their employers (College of Registered Nurses of Manitoba, 2002). They must ascertain that the nursing tasks performed have been approved by their employer as tasks or procedure that can be performed by unregulated health care workers.

reflective **THINKING**   What tasks could a nurse leader delegate to an unregulated health care provider? What factors do you need to consider when delegating tasks?

Principles of Delegation

The scope of practice of the RN implies that the nurse is the most comprehensive, versatile, and flexible of all nurse care providers. Consequently, RNs have the knowledge, skill, and judgment to make a broader range of decisions with greater ease than other health care providers (CNA, 2002). Delegation occurs in practice settings when decisions must be made to provide quality care while recognizing the reality of maximizing the utilization of every health care provider. In determining the most appropriate practitioner to provide services, RNs and/or health care agencies must consider client/patient needs, context of practice, and the competencies of the health care providers (CRNNS, 2004).

Delegation decisions must be made in the best interest of the client. When the competencies of an RN are needed, client safety should not be compromised through the substitution of less qualified health care providers (CRNNS, 2004). RNs must be familiar with the scope of practice and job description of the health care providers to whom they decide to delegate a nursing task (Timm, 2003).

The essential elements of delegation are reflected in the five principles and are found in Figure 12.3. For example, when considering delegating the right tasks to the right person, one should check the provincial or territorial nurse practice acts, the policies and procedures of the agency, and the description of jobs of all staff involved (Marthaler & Angkaw, 2008).

Evidence on the Effects of Delegation

Canadian researchers examined the views of case managers on delegation. After focus group sessions, they collected the comments and analyzed the content for key themes. Based on their findings, a model of delegation was developed for use within home care. The model was used to encourage the performance of appropriate delegation practices and to detect inappropriate ones through sensitivity to the ways that delegation decisions are developed (Hirst & Foley, 2001). The researchers conclude that within any health care service, including home care, policies and procedures should address delegation.

Timm (2003) analyzed the concept of delegation and explained how the delegation process can be used effectively by professional home care nurses. A comprehensive definition of delegation resulted from this concept analysis:

> "Delegation is a legal and management concept and a process that involves assessment, planning, intervention, and evaluation in which selected nursing tasks are transferred from one person in authority to another person, involving trust, empowerment, and the responsibility and authority to perform the tasks. In delegation, communication is succinct, guidelines are clearly delineated in advance and progress is constantly monitored in which the person in authority remains accountable for the final outcomes." (p. 264)

The researcher concluded that competent delegation skills are essential and that professional nurses often fail to fully understand delegation. The concept analysis described in this study provides a timely insight into proficient delegation practices (Timm, 2003).

Benefits of Delegation

Through effective delegation, many benefits result. One such benefit is that team members feel more involved and can undertake tasks that interest them (Curtis & Nicholl, 2004). That is, delegation serves the purpose of enhancing the health care provider's professional development, and it prepares them to assume greater

Registered Nurse

#1 Right Context	Ask	Is the decision to delegate based on client health care needs?	No	Do not delegate
Identify appropriate rationale for delegation		Is the decision to delegate based on evidence-based practice?		
		Is the decision to delegate based on sound nursing judgment?		

Yes

#2 Right Task	Ask	Is this task within the RN's scope of practice?	No	Do not delegate
Identify task required for delegation		Do the *Standards of Nursing Practice* and *Code of Ethics* support this delegation?		
		Is this task appropriate for delegation in this context of practice?		

Yes

#3 Right Person	Ask	Is the health care provider (delegatee) competent?	No	Do not delegate
Identify appropriate health care provider		Is client safety a low-risk issue?		
		Is the client's health status stable with predictable outcomes?		

Yes

#4 Right Communications	Ask	Has the decision to delegate the task been appropriately communicated?	No	Do not delegate
Identify appropriate communication		Is the decision supported by appropriate supervision?		
		Has the delegation been followed up with appropriate documentation?		

Yes

#5 Right Resources	Ask	Is this delegation supported with educational resources?	No	Do not delegate
Identify appropriate evaluation and follow-up		Is the delegation supported by policy and procedures?		
		Is the delegation supported by the RN Act and other relevant legislation?		

Yes

Delegate

FIGURE 12.3 Five principles of delegation. (Adapted from College of Registered Nurses of Nova Scotia [2004]. *Delegation Guidelines for Registered Nurses* [p. 9]. Halifax, NS: Author. Reproduced with permission.)

Reflections on Leadership Practice

*Y*ou are facing a heavy assignment today on the surgical unit. Several of your clients have been taken to surgery, and a few have already returned to the unit. While examining your assignment sheet, you realize that you have not removed the sutures from one of your clients who is due for suture removal. You have data to enter and a few other tasks before you. You decide to delegate this task.

Describe the five principles of delegation that you must follow. Write down these steps and the data that are needed.

---

responsibilities in the future. For a nurse leader, delegation should be evaluated in terms of its effectiveness with respect to a health care worker's job performance and satisfaction (Tourigny & Pulich, 2006). Regarding the benefits to the organization, delegation can be assessed through improved client care and services.

Barriers to Delegation

Delegation involves risk. Detrimental outcomes may occur when the nurse leader is unaware of the competencies, or the scope of practice, of health team members. That is, delegating a task that results in it being completed unsafely translates into harming the client and seriously undermining the goal of the organization (Marthaler & Huber, 2006). At times, possibly to enhance self-image, a nurse leader will invest time in self-enhancement activities rather than delegating to others (Tourigny & Pulich, 2006). Frequently, nurse leaders have chosen not to delegate because they believe that they are ultimately responsible for client outcomes. Consequently, nurse leaders may perceive delegation as a means of avoiding responsibilities.

> *reflective* **THINKING** What are other benefits of delegation to the health care provider, client and family, and health care organization?

Delegation is a highly effective means through which nurse leaders can take advantage of the varying skill levels of available staff. When delegation is conducted effectively, it can reduce burnout, improve job satisfaction, enhance time management, clarify accountability, and facilitate access to care. Delegation can contribute to a reduction in health care costs. Well-trained unregulated health care workers can be very cost-effective and important members of the interdisciplinary team as the delivery of care continues to evolve (Quallich, 2005).

With a clear understanding and application of delegation principles to their daily practice, nurse leaders can experience an increase in job satisfaction and loyalty, high performance, and improved productivity (Timms, 2003).

WEBSITES

▓ Statistics Canada – Social Trends

http://www.statcan.ca/english/ads/11-008-XIE/cumulative.htm
Statistics Canada produces *Canadian Social Trends*, which contains articles written by professionals on various issues, such as time use and many others. The "Search" feature is excellent.

▓ Three Frameworks for Delegation by Registered Nurses

http://www.crnm.mb.ca/ Follow the links: Publications, Standards of Practice, Fact Sheets, *Decision making—A framework for delegation.*
http://www.crnbc.ca/downloads/429.pdf
http://www.srna.org/nurse_resources/2004_RN_assignment_delegation.pdf

REFERENCES

Adler, D. A., McLaughlin, T. J., Rogers, W. H., Chang, H., Lapitsky, L., & Lerner, D. (2006). Job performance deficits due to depression. *American Journal of Psychiatry, 163*(9), 1569–1576.

Arnold, E., & Pulich, M. (2004). Improving productivity through more effective time management. *The Health Care Manager, 23*(1), 65–70.

Association of Registered Nurses of Newfoundland and Labrador. (2006). *Scope of nursing practice: Definition, decision-making & delegation.* St. John's, NL: Author.

Barker, A. M. (2006). Managing personal resources: Time and stress management. In A. M. Barker, D. Taylor Sullivan, & M. J. Emery (Eds.), *Leadership competencies for clinical managers: The renaissance of transformational leadership* (pp. 77–92). Toronto, ON: Jones & Bartlett.

Bowers, B. J., Lauring, C., & Jacobson, N. (2001). How nurses manage time and work in long-term care. *Journal of Advanced Nursing, 33*(4), 484–491.

Canadian Nurses Association. (2002). *Code of ethics for registered nurses.* Ottawa, ON: Author.

Canadian Nurses Association. (2003). *Position statement: Staffing decisions for the delivery of safe nursing care.* Ottawa: ON: Author. PS-67.

Canadian Nurses Protective Society. (2001). Delegation to other health care workers. *Nursing in Focus, 2*(2), 23–24.

College of Nurses of Ontario. (2007). *Practice Guideline: Authorizing mechanisms.* Toronto, ON: Author. Publication no. 41075.

College of Registered Nurses of British Columbia. (2007). *Assigning and delegating to unregulated care providers.* Vancouver, BC: Author. Publication no. 98.

College of Registered Nurses of Manitoba. (Rev. 2002). *Fact sheet: Decision making: A framework for delegation.* Winnipeg, MB: Author.

College of Registered Nurses of Nova Scotia. (2004). *Delegation guidelines for registered nurses.* Halifax, NS: Author.

Covey, S. R. (1990). *The seven habits of highly effective people: Restoring the character ethic.* New York: Fireside.

Cox, K. S., & Huber, D. L. (2006). Managing time and stress. In D. Huber (Ed.), *Leadership and nursing care management.* (3rd ed., pp. 83–94). Philadelphia: Elsevier.

Curtis, E., & Nicholl, H. (2004). Delegation: A key function of nursing. *Nursing Management, 11*(4), 26–31.

Finkelman, A. W. (2006). *Leadership and management in nursing.* Upper Saddle River, NJ: Pearson Education.

Fisher, M. (2000). Do you have delegation savvy? *Nursing 2000, 30*(12), 58–59.

Greenglass, E. R., Burke, R. J., & Fiksenbaum, L. (2001). Workload and burnout in nurses. *Journal of Community & Applied Social Psychology, 11*(3), 211–215.

Grohar-Murray, M. E., & DiCroce, H. R. (2003). *Leadership and management in nursing.* Upper Saddle River, NJ: Pearson Education.

Hendry, C., & Walker, A. (2004). Priority setting in clinical nursing practice: Literature review. *Journal of Advanced Nursing, 47*(4), 427–436.

Hirst, S. P., & Foley, L. (2001). Delegation: The views of case managers. *Home Health Care Management & Practice, 13*(4), 301–307.

Human Resources and Social Development Canada. (2005). *Addressing work-life balance in Canada – introduction.* Retrieved May 2008 from http://www.hrsdc.gc.ca/en/lp/spila/wlb/awlbc/02introduction.shtml

Kalisch, B. J. (2006). Missed nursing care: A qualitative study. *Journal of Nursing Care Quality, 21*(4), 306–313.

Marthaler, M., & Angkaw, J. P. (2008). Delegation of nursing care. In P. Kelly, & H. Crawford (Eds.), *Nursing leadership and management* (1st Canadian ed., pp. 237–248). Toronto, ON: Nelson Education.

Marthaler, M., & Huber, D. (2006). Delegation. In D. Huber (Ed.), *Leadership and nursing care management* (3rd ed., pp. 543–560). Philadelphia: Elsevier.

Mutzebaugh, C. A. (2007). Delegation: An art of professional practice. In R. A. Patronis Jones (Ed.), *Nursing leadership and management: Theories, processes and practice* (pp. 345–356). Philadelphia: F. A. Davis.

Pearce, C. (2007). Ten steps to managing time. *Nursing Management, 14*(1), 23.

Pettigrew, A. C. (2007). Self-management: Stress and time. In P. S. Yoder-Wise (Ed.), *Leading and managing in nursing* (4th ed., pp. 531–554). St. Louis, MO: Mosby.

Quallich, S. A. (2005). A bond of trust: Delegation. *Urologic Nursing, 25*(2), 120–123.

Rider Ellis, J., & Love Hartley, C. (2008). *Nursing in today's world: Trends, issues, & management* (9th ed.). Philadelphia: Wolters Kluwer Health / Lippincott Williams & Wilkins.

Saskatchewan Registered Nurses' Association. (2004). *Practice of nursing: RN assignment and delegation.* Regina, SA: Author.

Thompson, D. S., O'Leary, K., Jensen, E., Scott-Findlay, S., O'Brien-Pallas, L., & Estabrooks, C. A. (2008). The relationship between busyness and research utilization: It is about time. *Journal of Clinical Nursing, 17*(4), 539–548.

Timm, S. E. (2003). Effectively delegating nursing. *Home Healthcare Nurse, 21*(4), 260–265.

Tomey, A. M. (2009). *Guide to nursing management and leadership* (8th ed.). St. Louis, MO: Mosby.

Tourigny, L., & Pulich, M. (2006). Delegating decision making in health care organizations. *The Health Care Manager, 25*(2), 101–113.

Turcotte, M. (2007). Time spent with family during a typical workday, 1986 to 2005. *Canadian Social Trends, 83*(Summer), 2–11.

Vaccaro, P. J. (2003). Forget about time management. *Family Practice Management, 10*(5), 82.

Waterworth, S. (2003). Time management strategies in nursing practice. *Journal of Advanced Nursing, 43*(5), 432–440.

REFRAMING LEADERSHIP

13

ROLE TRANSITION INTO CAREER DEVELOPMENT

Leaders are those individuals in formal and informal leadership roles who are recognized by their peers and colleagues as experts in their practice, who consider patient care and nursing excellence as their priorities, who can be trusted and with whom it is easy to have a conversation about one's dreams and vision for one's career.

—Gail J. Donner, RN, PhD and
Mary M. Wheeler, RN, MEd, PCC

From Donner G. J., & Wheeler, M. M. (2004).
New strategies for developing leadership.
Nursing Leadership, 17(2), 27, 28.

Gail Donner is Professor and Dean Emeritus in the Lawrence S. Bloomberg Faculty of Nursing at the University of Toronto and a partner in donnerwheeler Career Planning Consultants. Her research and consulting interests include career development, health policy, and nursing administration. In addition to presenting papers, seminars, and workshops on a variety of health care topics, Dr. Donner has been active on a number of boards and committees and is currently a member of the Board of Trustees of the Hospital for Sick Children in Toronto; Chair of the Board of the Change Foundation in Toronto; and book editor of the *Canadian Journal of Nursing Leadership*. For her contributions to nursing and the community, she has received the Order of Ontario, an honorary Doctor of Science from Ryerson University in Toronto, the Registered Nurses Association of Ontario Award of Merit, and the Ontario Medical Association Centennial Award.

Mary M. Wheeler is a certified coach with more than 15 years of consulting expertise in career, organization, and human resource development. She has published extensively in the area of career development, coaching, and mentoring. In addition to her work with donnerwheeler Career Planning Consultants, she has co-led Career Cycles Getaways for the Ontario Medical Association Physician Health Program and acts as an executive coach and as an associate of Development-by-Design. Mary is an active member in the International Coach Federation, the Association of Career Professionals International, and the Career Planning and Adult Development Network, for which she is a book reviewer. She is also a book proposal reviewer for Sigma Theta Tau International. She is currently a member of the Nursing Advisory Committee, Ryerson University, and a member of the International Council of Nurses Bank of Experts (in the field of Human Resources/Planning and Development and/or Nursing Remuneration-Working Conditions).

Overview

The process of change unfolds gradually during the span of a nurse's professional career. The change begins with the transition from student nurse to nurse and then from nurse to nurse leader. These changes are usually accompanied by considerable uncertainty about the challenges of the workplace. During the transition, expectations tend to be high that the nurse will rapidly begin to function as a professional practising nurse or as a competent nurse leader. Managing change effectively is a learned skill, and it is a necessary component of career planning. The acquisition of the skills needed to navigate through the various phases of the career cycle is a critical journey that calls for perseverance and patience. Senior nurse leaders have a prime responsibility to assess the needs and behaviours of aspiring new nurses and nurse leaders. Second, they need to develop strategies that will assist new nurses to cope and grow personally and professionally. These efforts are essential not only for the transition of nurses into the work environment, but also to promote the retention of nurses in today's complex health care environment.

Objectives

By critically reflecting upon and processing knowledge throughout this chapter, you will be able to respond effectively to the following objectives:

1. Explain the importance of a successful role transition.
2. Conduct a debate about the differences between the transition of a student nurse to a nurse and nurse to a nurse leader.
3. Compare the similarities and differences of the nurse leader's role in the transition processes with that of the novice nurse and the new nurse leader.
4. Design a chart to list the evidence provided in the chapter to assist nurse leaders in facilitating transition processes for nurses.
5. Justify the importance of a conceptual framework for career planning and development.
6. Compose and write your own resume.
7. Create a role-play situation for an applicant being interviewed by a potential employer.
8. Describe the importance of the advanced nurse practitioner and certified nurse in today's health care system.

Role Transitions

According to Meleis, Sawyer, Im, Messias, and Schumacher (2000), transitions are a result of, and result in, changes in health, life, relationships, and environments. Transitions are multidimensional, complex, and universal. Role transitions are best comprehended as challenging opportunities when moving from one phase in a career to another. Regardless of the complexity of the transition, the cumulative effect is the inevitability of change and predictable discomfort that an individual experiences. The strategies used to navigate transitional change are critical. Several of the strategies include accepting the reality of change, recognizing that pain accompanies growth, remembering previous successes, maintaining a balance in life, and identifying areas of relative constancy (Haynes, 2004).

Delaney (2003) states, "Within the nursing profession, the transition from student to nurse is a common rite of passage experienced by all graduate nurses" (p. 437). The orientation phase of the new nurse's first work experience marks the beginning of a journey and is perhaps the most critical part of the transition. The experience and immediate emotional reactions of this phase carry an impact on both immediate and long-term outcomes in the process of becoming an expert nurse. From the time nurses enter the workforce, career preferences and attitudes toward nursing practice continue to develop within them at varying rates (Hayes et al., 2006).

> *reflective* **THINKING** In what ways are you preparing yourself for the transition phase from student nurse to a graduate, and later to a registered nurse?

From Student Nurse to Nurse

New graduate nurses bring to their work an extensive repertoire of knowledge and beginning competencies that are sufficient for a successful role transition from nursing student to professional nurse (Haynes, 2004). However, Ellerton and Gregor (2003) found that the extensive documentation during the first 3 months of employment as a graduate nurse represent the most stressful time in the nurse's career. Casey, Fink, Krugman, and Propst (2004) examined the stress and challenges experienced by cohorts of graduate nurses working in six hospitals during specific time periods: at baseline, 3 months, 6 months, 12 months, and an additional continued follow-up of specific groups for a longer employment period. They found that the most difficult role-adjustment time period for graduate nurses was between 6 and 12 months after hire. The findings were consistent across the six hospitals, indicating that the transition process takes time and requires both mentoring and support.

> reflective **THINKING**   How can the novice nurse evaluate her or his professional growth during the first year of the nursing career?

Other nursing researchers, Schoessler and Waldo (2006), conducted an interpretative study whereby the participating graduate nurses met regularly during the first 18 months of nursing practice to share their experiences and discuss their concerns. The primary author facilitated and audio-recorded the conversations. During the nurses' discussions with the investigator, four themes and marker events emerged, as outlined in Table 13.1. These descriptions of the nurses' experiences indicate that the transition of the first 18 months in practice is incredibly challenging.

As a result of the study, the researchers proposed a framework entitled *Novice to Competent Nurse: A Process Model* for understanding the developmental experience of the graduate nurse. The researchers concluded that it is highly important for nurse leaders to understand the nurse's experience, as the nurses live it, and then to focus on organizational supports and theoretical frameworks to ease the transition and promote professional development.

> reflective **THINKING**   Review the article by Schoessler and Waldo (2006), "The First 18 Months in Practice: A Developmental Transition Model for the Newly Graduated Nurse," found in the reference section. Take time to reflect on the model proposed. Try to discover ways this framework would promote and/or ease the process during transition in one's nursing career.

Implications for Nurse Leaders

Nurse leaders need to be aware of the lived experiences and the turmoil that novice nurses encounter as they progress through their transition. Supportive collaboration is needed among nurse leaders in education and service to promote a successful transition (Hayes et al., 2006).

Nurse Educators

Almost all student nurses eventually become nurse educators in one form or another. Frequently, nurse educators in academia encounter situations where their learners either have been, or are exposed to, the effects of transition. To ease the transition, a valuable strategy is to increase the number of clients in the student's clinical assignments. Doing so helps students to overcome the anxiety associated with real-world nursing (Delaney, 2003).

Related strategies to facilitate meaningful experiences for student nurses include, for example, having them participate frequently in interdisciplinary teams,

TABLE 13.1	TRANSITION THEMES AND MARKER EVENTS		
Theme	Ending (0–3 Months)	Neutral Zone (4–9 Months)	New Beginning (10–18) Months
Patient/ family	• Learning tasks/procedures • Client conditions as challenges	Fear of clients asking questions that the new nurse cannot answer	• Family emerges as a new demand • Comfort with procedural care • Inability to remember all clients by name
Organization	Struggling with shift organization	Shift organization improves as some tasks become more routine	• Organization has improved • Others have noticed the improvement
Team	• Dependent on the team • Importance of preceptor role • The team is talking about me • Physician interactions approached with trepidation	• Integrating with the team • Physician communication seen as problematic • Issues of efficiency vs. quality of care situated in staffing and budget	• Unit is "my home" now • Concerns with staffing patterns remain • Physicians' relationships remain problematic; however, there is value in building collaborative relationships
Marker events	• First patient death • First error • Development of new skills	"Other staff are asking me questions (and I know some answers)!"	• Beginning to be a preceptor to newer nurses • Comparing self to current new graduates • Becoming able to complete the shift on time • Assuming charge nurse responsibilities

From Schoessler, M., & Waldo, M. (2006). The first 18 months in practice: A developmental transition model for the newly graduated nurse. *Journal for Nurses in Staff Development 22*(2), 47–52. Adapted and reproduced with the permission from Lippincott Williams & Wilkins. Copyright © 2008.

manage information electronically, and practice relational skills, such as active listening and empathizing (Delaney, 2003; Ferguson & Day, 2007). To accommodate the various learning patterns of students, nurse educators must be creative in their approaches. Examples include using critical inquiry and providing simulated learning experiences in directing their learning (Arhin & Cormier, 2007). Encouraging words from nurse educators to students about their potential as future nurse leaders can be powerful influences in their career choices (Sherman & Bishop, 2007).

The College of Registered Nurses of Manitoba (CRNM) stresses the importance of expected graduated/entry-level competencies to serve as a guide to curriculum development in entry-level nursing programs. These competencies are designed to inform the public and the potential employer of the practice expectations of entry-level registered nurses (RNs) (CRNM, 2007a). In Canada, Black and her project participants worked from 2004 to 2006 to develop and refine entry-level RN competencies (Black et al., 2008). It was the first time that 10 Canadian jurisdictional nursing regulatory bodies collaborated on a project to enhance consistencies of competencies for RNs. Besides enhancing consistency, the project's purpose was to support reciprocity of registration and mobility of the workforce within Canada.

Clinical competence is perhaps the most important characteristic, because it requires much of the knowledge, skills, and judgment inherent in the practice of nursing (Evans & Donnelly, 2006). The CRNM has developed a fact sheet entitled *Profile of the Newly Graduated/Entry-Level Registered Nurse*. This document provides an overview of the practice expected of the newly graduated RN. CRNM supports the expectation that new graduates gain confidence, skill, and knowledge in a workplace that values and supports their contribution to the health care team (CRNM, 2007b).

reflective **THINKING** One of the entry-level competencies for RNs in Manitoba is *professional responsibility and accountability*. Take time to search for entry-level competencies for RNs in your province.

Different factors, such as ineffective placements, stilted interactions, and poor learning environments, can contribute to a difficult student-to-nurse transition and unmet career expectations as new nurses enter the workplace. According to Donner and Wheeler (2001), nurse educators should be attentive to students' interests and goals and assist them to achieve the appropriate skills so they can prepare themselves for constant change in their roles and responsibilities.

Senior Leaders

According to Ferguson and Day (2007), nurse leaders in the clinical setting are in an ideal position to create and sustain supportive practice environments that facilitate new nurse integration and professional practice in various practice settings.

Many benefits accrue to both the organization and the new nurse, especially when the nurse leader assists novice nurses to achieve a level of performance whereby they can make decisions confidently while focusing on effective client outcomes (Ferguson & Day, 2007). In fact, transformational leaders can use a combination of behaviours that provide new nurses with special opportunities for focused professional development (Raup, 2008). When new nurses enter practice, nurse leaders must be particularly aware that the new nurses need access to good quality evidence to support their practice. This support can be provided by current reference texts and journals and by promoting access to internet resources and the library (Ferguson & Day, 2007). Belonging to interdisciplinary journal clubs can be especially encouraging and can spark exchanges of knowledge and ideas about effective client and family care.

reflective **THINKING** What are a few other advantages of belonging to an interdisciplinary journal club for a new nurse?

The complexity and scope of professional nursing practice require that new nurses be engaged in a positive mentoring practice to facilitate career progression (Thomka, 2001). Good mentoring relationships in nursing can provide the guidance, support, and encouragement that new nurses require as they assimilate the knowledge, skill, judgment, and confidence needed to practice nursing successfully (Thomka, 2001; Evans & Donnelly, 2006). Nurses must view their ongoing development as a necessary component of their professional lives.

Research Studies How Nursing Leadership Affects Nursing Practice or Effect of Nursing Leaders on Nursing Practice

Manojlovich (2005) conducted a study to understand the effect of nursing leadership on the relationship of structural empowerment (opportunity, information, support, and resources) and nursing self-efficacy (belief in one's self-worth) to professional nursing behaviours. She found that nurses are able to practice more professionally when they perceive strong and effective leadership. That is, when nurse leaders provide more access to structural empowerment, they in turn influence the nurses' self-efficacy, which leads to more professional practice behaviours. Manojlovich (2005) states that the implication of this finding for nurse leaders is that leadership development is important. The knowledge and competencies acquired can enhance leadership skills and provide strong advantages for novice or senior nurses on the unit.

reflective **THINKING** What do you think are a few leadership competencies that can enhance the professional development of the novice nurse?

> **BOX 13.1** MAIN COMPONENTS FOR EASING ORIENTATION
>
> 1. Offer a reassuring and warm welcome when a new nurse begins employment. Consider all new members with humanity.
> 2. Provide complete and precise training from the beginning.
> 3. Train supervisors and provide them with tools to measure the continuing progress of professional competence.
> 4. Provide constant support for new nurses.
> 5. Evaluate frequently the effectiveness and appropriateness of the orientation program. Make alterations as warranted. Use feedback information from earlier participants.

Adapted from Lavoie-Tremblay, M., Viens, C., Forcier, M., Labrosse, N., Lafrance, M., Laliberté, D., et al. (2002). How to facilitate the orientation of new nurses into the workplace. *Journal for Nurses in Staff Development, 18*(2), 80–85.

The orientation of novice nurses into the workplace is a challenge. A team of researchers from Laval University and the Centre Hospitalier Universitaire de Quebec used a descriptive and participative research method to understand how to facilitate the orientation of new nurses (Lavoie-Tremblay et al., 2002). Box 13.1 outlines the findings—five main components that must be considered by nurse leaders to create a successful work orientation for the new RN.

The nurse leader plays a vital role in designing and carrying out overall orientation programs that encourage creative thinking and foster integration into the health care organization and nursing profession (Santucci, 2004). A new graduate's transition from student to professional nurse requires constant support and professional development, especially during the first year of practice. Leaders must continue to model professional development, encourage career planning, and support the nurses' personal career choices (Tomey, 2009).

From Nurse to Nurse Leader

The transition from the role of staff nurse caring for a number of clients to that of novice nurse leader responsible for the health team members on a unit is an exciting and challenging career opportunity (Twedell & Jackson Grey, 2007). However, this opportunity to undertake greater responsibility can be accompanied by a high degree of anxiety and much uncertainty. Figure 13.1 depicts a staff nurse wondering whether she really is ready for this role.

Becoming a new leader requires a fairly extensive background of professional leadership development. Such development helps nurses make the transition from focusing on their own personal performance to collaborating and coordinating efforts of members on a health care team (Redman, 2006). Frontline leaders are pivotal because they link the organizational vision, goals, and strategic

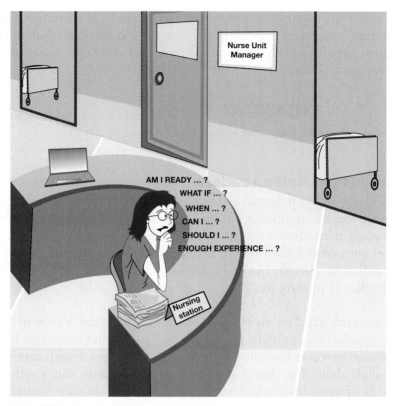

FIGURE 13.1 Role transition.

plan with clinical practice at the unit level for the delivery of effective quality client care (Sherman, Bishop, Eggenberger, & Karden, 2007).

Although developing a new identity as a leader is important, the nurse must also focus on learning leadership competencies—either from experiences or from educational means. Arnold and Nelson (2008) state that almost overnight, the frontline leader becomes an administrative representative and change agent, and as such, is expected to articulate and implement policy and assure accountability for those policy outcomes. In addition, the nurse leader must manage budgets, resolve conflicts, facilitate and promote the learning of complex technology, coach nurses to improve their performance, and foster collaboration among health team members. Together, these tasks are intended to encourage mutual respect for one another's competencies and foster reciprocal concern for providing quality client care (Arnold & Nelson, 2008; Upenieks, 2003). However, most new nurse leaders receive little support in the form of guidance, direction, feedback, and support from administration (Kirby & DeCampli, 2008; Heller et al., 2004). In fact, Tourangeau (2003), a Canadian scholar and researcher, states that despite the fact that some nurses are involved in educational programs, most nurses have learned to be leaders on the job through trial and error. That is, nurses are frequently thrust into managerial positions without being sufficiently prepared for the transition into these roles.

> *reflective* **THINKING**   How do you think administrative support can be gained for the nurse leader role?

Implications for Nurse Leaders

Both the career potential and the significance of the nurse leader role need to receive special attention from nurse leaders in academia and from senior service leaders in health care organizations. If new leaders are to flourish, the expert leaders must rethink their role in the organization and determine ways in which they can best support the novice leader so, together, they can advance the professional practice of nursing in all health care settings (Cardin & McNeese-Smith, 2005).

Research Studies on How Leaders Perceive the Value of Their Role

Upenieks (2003) conducted a study to gain further understanding of how nurse leaders perceive the value of their roles in today's health care setting and their beliefs about how power and gender interface with role worth. She found that 83% of nurse leaders believe that to be effective in their positions, nurse leaders need informal and formal power, access to information and resources, and opportunities to grow with new challenges. Other factors that had notable influence toward increasing the effectiveness of the nurse leader role included:

- Supportive organizational cultures where nurses are recognized and valued based on their professional expertise.
- Organizational commitment to the professional qualities of nurses.
- Distinctive leadership attributes demonstrated by nursing administration, including a passion for nursing, visibility, responsiveness, and business astuteness.
- Collaborative and respectful teamwork among nurses and their collegial health care workers.
- Compensation whereby nurses are awarded adequate and necessary resources—to attend leadership conferences, for example.

Upenieks (2003) states emphatically that the findings suggest that organizational efforts that focus on access to information, resources, support, and opportunity carry the definite potential to enhance leadership. In organizations, senior nurse leaders are well positioned to play key roles in implementing these supportive structures. Nurse leaders who are successful in their roles are visionary, knowledgeable, and responsive. They are given power at the administrative level to do what they passionately feel is necessary to create a positive environment for the novice nurse leader.

> *reflective* **THINKING** In your health care setting, what signs indicate that the new nurse leader is succeeding in the organization?

Research Studies on Needs of New Unit Managers

A study was conducted to investigate leadership needs and experiences of nurse unit managers with all levels of experience and all types of clinical environments across the health care system (Sullivan, Bretschneider, & McCausland, 2003). In describing the developmental needs of new nurse managers, the researchers found that most participants focused on the description of basic and introductory managerial skills. Box 13.2 outlines the developmental and educational needs of new nurse managers.

BOX 13.2 TWENTY DEVELOPMENTAL AND EDUCATIONAL NEEDS OF NEW NURSE MANAGERS

- Role transitioning
- Goal setting and evaluation
- Interactional skills
- Organizational and prioritization skills
- Institutional policies and procedures
- Introduction to key personnel and support department staff
- Role expectations and description
- Managing a balance of life and work responsibilities
- Time management
- Performance management, including staff counselling and evaluation
- Computer skills
- Financial management, budgetary, and payroll skills
- Human resources issues
- Staffing and scheduling skills
- Conflict resolution skills
- Regulatory agency compliance issues
- Skills for leading staff meetings
- Structured orientation program
- Formal mentoring program
- Intradepartmental and interdepartmental delegation

Adapted from Sullivan, J., Bretschneider, J., & McCausland, M. P. (2003). Designing a leadership development program for nurse managers: An evidence-driven approach. *Journal of Nursing Administration*, *33*(10), 544,548.

Sullivan, Bretschneider, and McCausland (2003) state ". . . all participants unanimously agreed that a formal structured orientation program with a systematic mentoring process would greatly benefit future new managers" (p. 547). This finding supports the recommendation of other nursing scholars and researchers that leadership training for nurse mangers should be formalized (Noyes, 2002; Tourangeau, 2003; Scoble & Russell, 2003). Each noted independently certain commonalities for competency development in these programs. Examples include leadership practices, behaviours and skills, the business of health care with financing and budgeting, and the use of self in personal effectiveness and communication skills, critical thinking and decision making, delegation, and effective staffing strategies (Sherman et al., 2007; Heller et al., 2004). Recently, Porter O'Grady and Malloch (2007) argued that nurse leaders must have emotional competence to work effectively in today's health care field. An individual with high emotional intelligence undoubtedly has the potential to learn how to be emotionally competent. The behaviours that demonstrate leadership's emotional competence include self-awareness, passionate optimism, and compassion and impulse control.

Targeting potential nurse leaders early in their career and making effective learning opportunities available to them are important components of leadership development (Redman, 2006). In addition, coaching and mentoring by senior nurse leaders are essential throughout the leadership development program (McCall, 2004). However, for different learning needs, it is critical that nurses engage in participatory roles in their learning experiences (Griscti & Jacono, 2006).

reflective **THINKING**   What type of effective learning opportunities should be made for the novice nurse leader to facilitate his or her transition to the leadership role?

Research Studies on Competencies

Sherman, Bishop, Eggenberger, and Karden (2007) investigated 120 nurse managers regarding their views about the contemporary nurse manager role. This study also sought to gain perspective on the crucial leadership competencies needed to build a nursing leadership competency model. The findings resulted in six competency categories to form a nursing leadership model, which is found in Figure 13.2. Brief explanations of the six categories follow:

1. *Personal mastery*: begins with an awareness of one's self, which is the true hallmark of leadership.
2. *Interpersonal effectiveness*: includes the ability to communicate with a variety of individuals and, most of all, be visible and present to health team members.

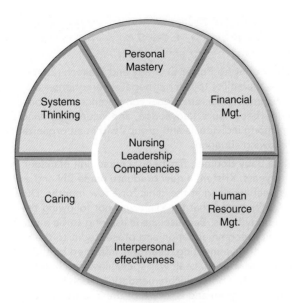

FIGURE 13.2 Nursing leadership competency model. (From Sherman, R. O., Bishop, M., Eggenberger, T., & Karden, R. [2007]. Development of a Leadership Competency Model. *The Journal of Nursing Administration, 37*[2], 85, 88.)

3. *Human resource management*: recognizes that retention begins with sound selections and an orientation process carefully designed to assist health team members to manage conflict.

4. *Financial management*: involves taking time and opportunities to become knowledgeable regarding budgets and different staffing patterns

5. *Caring for staff, clients, and self*: requires the ability to maintain a connectedness to health team members, which begins with self-care.

6. *Systems thinking*: includes developing an understanding of how the unit the leader leads fits into the whole organization and acknowledges the need to respect the viewpoints of other disciplines.

Developing a formalized career program in which potential and aspiring nurse leaders can assume nurse manager positions demonstrates a healthy professional commitment. Such a commitment ensures continuity when vacancies occur, and it makes good business sense. Supporting, nurturing, and strengthening the leadership skills of the nurse leader will effectively improve the professional and client outcomes. Excellent nurse leadership is vital to manage successfully the changing complex health care environment (Sherman et al., 2007).

> ## Reflections on Leadership Practice
>
> According to Porter O'Grady and Malloch (2007), impulse control or self-regulation—the ability to temper negative emotions—is an important pillar of emotional competence. Emotional competence is composed of a collection of perceptions, behaviours, knowledge, and values that enable a leader to manage meaning among individuals and groups within an organization. Take time to reflect on the following situation.
>
> Leah, a Baby Boomer, has been a nurse unit manager in a community clinic for a number of years. Kristen, a new graduate nurse BN and a Generation X-er hired by Leah, has been working at the clinic for a few months. During her third month on the job, Kristen noted that the clinic was not following the protocol for handling blood and body fluids. Because she is aspiring to be a nurse leader one day, she wrote a policy recommendation and presented it to the clinic's executive director. At an administrative meeting, Leah was informed by the director of the new policy that Kristen had written. Leah was speechless and upset because she knew nothing of Kristen's written policy recommendation. Leah has just taken the leadership development program and is aware of the importance of emotional competence.
>
> If you were Leah, how would you approach Kristen about the matter?
>
> What errors did Kristen make as a member of a health care team?
>
> What should Leah do and say to Kristen to teach her about the importance of being a respectful and contributing member of a health care team?

Change and Challenges: Career Guide for the Nurse

The nursing profession has encountered a multitude of complex changes in recent years. Many of these changes resulted from events such as the restructuring of the health care system, burgeoning technology and health information, increasing mobility of nurses within and between countries, escalating multi-generational workforce, increasing cultural diversity in the workplace, and changing population demographics (Anthony, 2006; Tomey, 2009). The compound effects of these changes have had a profound impact on contemporary nursing. They include new health care roles, innovative work environments, new practice models, increased number of interdisciplinary teams, collaborative exchange, and well-educated, career-oriented nurses (Donner & Wheeler, 2001; D'Amour, Ferrada-Videla, San Martin Rodriguez, & Beaulieu, 2005; Gottlieb & Feeley, 2006).

Nurses have come to realize that nursing is a career and a profession and not just a job. If this is the case, nurses must continue to take charge of their careers and develop solid career goals by keeping abreast of the national, global, economic, and political forces while, at the same time, remaining attuned to the ever-changing health care organization (Top Rhine & Davies, 2007). Life-long learning, including career planning and development, is the responsibility of each nurse, as well as of the profession as a whole (Finkelman, 2006). Approaching their career in a planned, organized, and thoughtful manner will lead nurses to greater professional success. Further, career commitment within the profession of nursing is highly important, primarily in terms of recruitment, career satisfaction, and retention of nurses in health care organizations (Anthony, 2006).

> *reflective* **THINKING**   Develop a career goal for a Canadian nurse leader who wishes to travel to, and work in, several countries, such as South Africa, England, and Australia.

Career Planning and Development

Today in Canada, and in most other countries, the nursing profession comprises highly knowledgeable and well-educated professionals. The basic preparation for a nursing career is itself invaluable, because many new opportunities in both practice and administration have evolved (Rodts & Lamb, 2008).

A Dynamic Process

Donner (2004) states, "Career planning can play a crucial role at every stage of one's career" (p. 5). It allows the nurse to thrive on the opportunities now available in the health care field and to respond and grow with ongoing changes. Nurses' careers can be outlined as moving through five stages; the key elements of each stage are described briefly in Table 13.2.

Career planning is not stagnant. Instead, it is a dynamic process that continually changes and adapts to the individual's world (Donner, 2004). The main objective of career planning is for nurses to take charge of their career and their future. Career planning perpetuates the development of those attitudes and skills deemed essential for nurses to be active participants in their career and to collaborate with other nurses in everyday work-related decisions involving nursing practice (McGillis Hall, Waddell, Donner, & Wheeler, 2004). This essential process is closely associated with career satisfaction, and it can influence factors such as staff retention, client and family satisfaction, and quality of care (Perry, 2008). The results of studies indicate that nurse career satisfaction is directly linked to determining quality client outcomes (Eaton, 2000; Kramer & Schmalenberg, 2004).

TABLE 13.2	STAGES AND KEY POINTS OF A NURSE'S CAREER
Stage	**Key Points**
1. Learning	• Introduction to the nursing profession • Concerned with learning "how to. . . ."
2. Entry phase	• Selection of first work place • Examination of employment options for best fit (person-position) • Seek mentor
3. Commitment phase	• Evaluation of clinical areas (likes vs. dislikes) • Examination of career goals • Commitment to a career
4. Consolidation phase	• Dedication to career and commitment to continuous learning • Makes contributions to health care and to society
5. Withdrawal stage	• Preparation for retirement or career change

Adapted from Donner, G. J. (2004). Taking control of your nursing career: The future is now. In G. J. Donner & M. M. Wheeler (Eds.), _Taking control of your nursing career_ (2nd ed., pp. 3–11). Toronto, ON: Elsevier Canada.

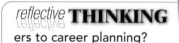 **reflective THINKING**   What do you consider are some of the barriers to career planning?

Conceptual Framework

Gail Donner and Mary Wheeler, internationally renowned, Canadian nursing scholars and consultants in career development, created the Donner-Wheeler Career-Planning and Developmental Model, as shown in Figure 13.3. Career development is a dynamic, continuously evolving, nonlinear process that requires ongoing contemplation and planning on the part of the nurse (Donner, 2004). The model relates to serial phases of self-assessment that integrate the knowledge of self with environmental opportunities. Essentially, it urges the nurse to assess his or her qualities and limitations in order to be prepared for the ever-changing workplace environment (Donner & Wheeler, 2001).

Following is a brief description of the five discrete phases of the model:

1. _Scanning_ is the process of viewing the environment and taking time to comprehend the current realities within the health care delivery system. It calls for examining the work environment, present and future trends in the local,

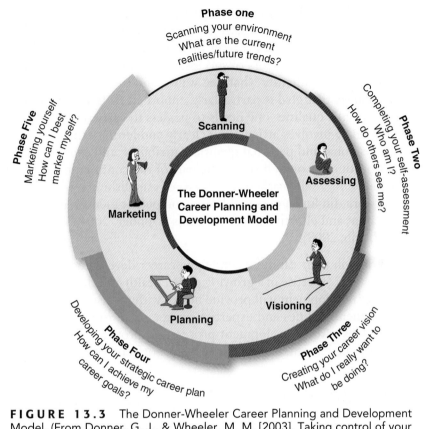

FIGURE 13.3 The Donner-Wheeler Career Planning and Development Model. (From Donner, G. J., & Wheeler, M. M. [2003]. Taking control of your nursing career [2nd ed., p. 6]. Ottawa, ON: Mosby; and http://www.donner-wheeler.com/model. Copyright Donner & Wheeler. All rights reserved. Reprinted with permission.)

national, and global levels within and outside of health care, and the nursing profession. Scanning is an activity that should become part of professional development because it will lay the foundation for a strong career-planning process.

2. *Assessing* means examining new and unexplored career opportunities and identifying knowledge, values, qualities, and limitations in combination with the environmental scan to develop a career vision. A reality check encourages the nurse to seek feedback regarding his or strengths and limitations, and it enables one to grow by reflecting upon the perspectives of others. Personal self-assessment is a critical component in developing a career plan.

3. *Visioning* requires projecting into the potential future, considering other career possibilities, and focusing on what seems possible and realistic, both

in the short and long term. One's career vision is the essential link between one's self-identity and what one has the potential to become.

4. *Planning* in the strategic career plan should include goals, resources, timelines, and indicators of success. The ability to set short-term and long-term goals, to identify what one wants, and to determine the steps necessary to achieve that goal is particularly important. It is also fruitful to determine the specific qualities one needs to possess to carry out the career plan.

5. *Marketing* involves articulating clearly and letting others know one's professional and personal qualities, attributes, and expertise. Promoting and advocating for oneself should be part of the continuum that demonstrates consistency. Self-marketing consists of establishing a wide professional network, finding a personable and competent mentor, and developing pleasant and effective relational skills (Donner, 2004; Waddell, 2008; Rodts & Lamb, 2008).

Through their carefully conducted career development plans, nurses can articulate their expertise in a growing global health care delivery system. Each phase in career development will provide nurses with precise steps to develop a clear vision of their qualities and expertise as they strive to fit into a unique marketing niche. This career development process can provide nurses with greater autonomy, personal worth, respect, and career satisfaction (Top Rhine & Davis, 2007).

Leadership Issue

*Y*ou have been a nurse leader on a medical unit for several years. For some time, you have felt called to consider a career change. An area that interests you is palliative care in the community. Using the five stages of the career planning and development model, develop each stage to the best of your ability to provide a guide to help you achieve your career goal and pursue your career vision.

Career Strategies

One important career strategy is to carefully develop and prepare a resume and a professional e-mail communication to an agency or organization for use with a job application. An additional strategy includes preparing for an interview and choosing appropriate professional references.

Electronic Resume

A resume is a brief summary of one's highlights, professional experience, and education, as outlined in Box 13.3. According to Waddell (2008), a resume should be honest, easy to read, and appealing. Most employers want to see a re-

BOX 13.3 SAMPLE RÉSUMÉ

LANA HEART
123 Chamber Way
Winnipeg, Manitoba
R3T 567

Highlights:
- Registered Nurse (RN) with professional experience in medical nursing
- Strong medical-evaluation and health promotion planning skills through clinical practice experience
- Knowledgeable about nursing care, client teaching, and discharge planning
- Reliable, ethical health care provider with the ability to remain calm in crisis situations, facilitate interdisciplinary groups, collaborate on interdisciplinary teams
- Consistently builds positive relationships with clients, family members, physicians, and other health care professionals

Professional Experience:

11/2007–5/2008   **Registered Nurse**   Lakeside Community Health Centre
Brandon, MB

- RN at a hospital with 500 beds
- Served in the medical unit and played a key role on an interdisciplinary team of health care professionals
- Actively participated in the development and implementation of individual health-care plans for clients with a broad range of medical concerns
- Ensured that physicians' orders were effectively and efficiently carried out

Key Accomplishments:
*Selected as only one of 10 student nurses to the medical unit
*Refined unit procedures in the area of diabetes management
*Responded to numerous family situations and earned the respect of families and healthcare team members

9/2006–10/2007   **Student Nurse/**   Sunnyway Health Centre
Clinical Rotations   Winnipeg, MB

- Provided nursing care, treatment, and clinical electronic documentation for cardiac palliative and medical surgical patients under the mentorship of an RN
- Was responsible for medication administration, dressing changes, IVs, and all other aspects of nursing care
- Facilitated admissions, discharges and transfers; prepared chart notes and other documentation

(box continues on page 348)

BOX 13.3 SAMPLE RÉSUMÉ (continued)

Key Accomplishments:
*Managed an average of 6 clients daily (100 percent of student caseload)
*Excelled in client health teaching and advanced health promotion practices with clients and families
*Earned a reputation for excellence in care as indicated by an excellence award in clinical practice

Education:

10/2007   **Bachelor of Nursing**   University of Manitoba Faculty of Nursing

- Relevant coursework includes: Human Growth & Development, Leadership in Nursing Practice, and Restoration & Maintenance
- Completed a Senior Practicum of 150 hours on a medical unit
- Worked extensively with clients to promote their participation in health promotion activities, identify problems and solutions in order to enhance their coping skills

Key Accomplishments:
*Dean's Honour List
*Highest grade in Skills Lab among fourth year nursing students

Affiliations:

12/2007–Present	**Member**	College of Registered Nurses of Manitoba
9/2003–8/2007	**Volunteer**	Golden Road Long Term Care Facility Brandon, MB

Additional Information:
Demonstrated patient advocate and team player

References:
Available upon request

Source: Courtesy Cosette Taylor-Mendes, MEd, Communications Instructor, Faculty of Nursing, University of Manitoba
Contact: Cosette_taylor-mendes@umanitoba.ca

sume rather than a curriculum vitae (CV) because the resume focuses on selected information (Finkelman, 2006). Many employers prefer to receive resumes by e-mail. Resumes can be formatted as a Microsoft Word file and printed on high-quality, letter-size typing paper using a laser printer. A resume should never be handwritten. Before sending the resume, one should check the grammar, spelling, language (or usage), and punctuation.

> reflective **THINKING** Reflect on your own professional life. Use the resume outline in Box 13.3 and create your own resume.

Professional E-mail

A professional e-mail communication should be developed (see Box 13.4) and sent with the attached resume. The e-mail should focus on the reason for the resume. It should be brief and catch the potential employer's attention (Finkelman, 2006). The e-mail should include an expression of appreciation, thanking the reader for taking the time to review the material.

Interview

An interview provides the employer with an opportunity to determine the extent to which the applicant meets the requirements for the position being sought. Moreover, the interview allows the applicant to ask questions and to obtain additional information about the position and the agency (Tomey, 2009). Often the first interview is conducted by telephone, especially if the employer is in a different province, or city, or if the applicant is in a remote community. If the applicant appears to be well qualified, then a face-to-face interview is arranged. In either case, the interviewer's aim is to learn about the applicant's dependability, responsibility, and way of interacting and working with others. First impressions are always important. The interviewer will quickly assess the applicant's attitude, manners, and appearance (Tomey, 2009).

> reflective **THINKING** Consider which criteria you would use in making hiring decisions for a nurse on a paediatric unit.

References

Professional/employment references play a key part in marketing one's professional qualities to potential employers (Waddell, 2008). The applicant's choice of referees should be specific to the position for which she or he is applying. Referees must be contacted and asked if they are willing to provide a positive reference; then the applicant can provide the referees with an updated resume and a description of the career position (Waddell, 2008). If possible, referees should be informed about when they might be contacted by the employer. If the referee is required to complete a form, provide him or her with sufficient time to do so. Be sure to provide the referee with a stamped and addressed envelope.

BOX 13.4 TIPS ON HOW TO WRITE A PROFESSIONAL E-MAIL

The way you write to your friends and the way you write to your potential employer should be different. Some of the key differences are summarized below:

When writing to friends and family, it is common to use:	When writing to professors or other professionals, it is *better* to use:
Emoticons ☺, :0 Informal language Incomplete sentences Misspelling Poor grammar Spelling the word the way it sounds, not how the word is spelled. For example, "bizness" for "business" Nicknames A funny or profane e-mail address domain or subject heading Lots of exclamation marks Ellipsis. . . (the little dots) between ideas instead of complete sentences Words in all CAPITAL LETTERS Reductions such as "RU" instead of "are you" or other text message language	Formal language Complete sentences Accurate spelling Correct grammar The reason for your e-mail stated concisely at the start of your message Formal titles, such as Dr. Ateah Punctuation A separate professional e-mail address without a funny or profane name or phrase Days of the week *and* dates Use an appropriate subject entry **Tip:** Edit your language and your content for any mistakes before you press send **Avoid:** Emoticons, writing in all capital letters, exclamation marks **Also:** If your intention was to attach a document, do remember to attach it.

Example:
From: superstah@gmail.org
To: jane@healthyheartcarefacility
Re: important!!!!!
Hello,
I want to apply for the position posted in the *Winnipeg Press* on the cardiac unit. See attached resume.
Thanks,
Kate

Change to:
From: kate@umanitoba.ca
To: jane@healthyheartcarefacility
Re: Posting 489 Cardiac Unit
Good Afternoon Ms. Morris,
I am writing in application for Posting 489 on the Cardiac Unit at your facility. The attached resume demonstrates the ways in which I could contribute to your organization. I look forward to hearing from you.
Thank you for your time and consideration,
Katie Blanc

Career Choices

According to the Canadian Nurses Association (CNA) (2008), trends in the delivery of health care are providing nurses with exciting opportunities to expand their current roles and create new ones. As nurses move along the continuum of their careers, they can choose from a variety of diverse and equally valuable practice opportunities, of which advanced practice nursing is one. Advanced practice nurses use their education and experience to take a professional nursing practice to new levels as they progress from a range of supportive responsibilities to a leading role in client and family care. Current advanced nursing practice roles in Canada are the clinical nurse specialist and the nurse practitioner (CNA, 2003a; CNA, 2003b).

The application of certification programs has gathered momentum each year to reflect the rate at which nurses commit to a national standard of professional competence to demonstrate a comprehensive understanding of their speciality and a commitment to continuing competence (CNA, 2007). The certification credential is an important indicator to clients, employers, the public, and professional licensing bodies that the nurse is qualified, competent, and current in the nursing speciality of her of his choice.

As advancing technology and increasing knowledge and demand combine to change the ways in which health care is delivered, nurses may often pause to reconsider their careers and to advance their knowledge and nursing practice, either in an advanced practice role or through certification in a speciality. Both advanced practice and certification provide nurses with the opportunity to build their expertise in the growing complexity of care.

---

reflective **THINKING** Reflect on your understanding of nursing practice as it relates to societal change and changes in the health care environment. What actions might you take to develop and promote your own nursing practice?

Nurse leaders play a pivotal role in contributing to quality client care and career satisfaction, along with nurse recruitment and retention in the health care system. They contribute extensively in developing the criteria for selection, and they structure their interviews for new nurse applicants accordingly. Once nurses are hired, they must be continually nurtured by nurse leaders to develop their competencies in challenging practice environments (Tomey, 2009). With the guidance of the nurse leader, professional development can be enhanced through well-chosen mentors, both for the beginning and the experienced nurse. Support during the transition process is critical in the development of the nurse's career path.

WEBSITES

■ The Health Action Lobby (HEAL)

http://www.physiotherapy.ca/heal/english/index.htm

HEAL is a coalition of national health and consumer associations and organizations dedicated to protecting and strengthening Canada's health care system. It represents more than half a million providers and consumers of health care. HEAL was formed in 1991 out of concern over the erosion of the federal government's role in supporting a national health care system.

■ DonnerWheeler Publications

http://www.donnerwheeler.com/Programs_and_Services/Publications

Gail Donner and Mary Wheeler have been acknowledged for their career planning and development model, their evidence-based practice, and their publications. Details are available at their Website.

REFERENCES

Anthony, M. K. (2006). Professional practice and career development. In D. L. Huber (Ed.), *Leadership and nursing care management* (3rd ed., pp. 61–81). Philadelphia: Elsevier.

Arhin, A., & Cormier, E. (2007). Using deconstruction to educate generation Y nursing students. *Journal of Nursing Education, 46*(12), 562–567.

Arnold, L., & Nelson, G. (2008). Developing the new frontline manager. *Nurse Leader, 2*(6), 50–53.

Black, J., Allen, D., Redfern, L., Muzio, L., Rushowick, B., Balaski, B., et al. (2008). Competencies in the context of entry-level registered nurse practice: A collaborative project in Canada. *International Nursing Review, 55*(2), 171–178.

Cardin, S., & McNeese-Smith, D. (2005). A model for bridging the gap: From theory to practice to reality. *Nursing Administration Quarterly, 29*(2), 154–161.

Casey, K., Fink, R., Krugman, M., & Propst, J. (2004). The graduate nurse experience. *Journal of Nursing Administration, 34*(6), 303–311.

Canadian Nurses Association. (2003a). *Position statement: The nurse practitioner.* Ottawa, ON: Author. PS – 68.

Canadian Nurses Association. (2003b). *Position statement: Clinical nurse specialist.* Ottawa, ON: Author. PS – 65.

Canadian Nurses Association. (2007). *Position statement: Advanced nursing practice.* Ottawa, ON: Author. PS – 92.

Canadian Nurses Association. (2008). *Obtaining CNA certification.* Ottawa, ON: Author. Retrieved June 2008 from http://www.cna-aiic.ca/

College of Registered Nurses of Manitoba. (2007a). Entry level competencies for registered nurses in Manitoba. Winnipeg, MB: Author. Retrieved June 2008 from http://www.crnm.mb.ca/downloads/entrylevelcompetencies_web.pdf

College of Registered Nurses of Manitoba. (2007b). Fact sheet: Profile of the newly graduated entry-level registered nurse. Winnipeg, MB: Author. Retrieved June 2008 from http://www.crnm.mb.ca/downloads/newgrad_web.pdf

D'Amour, D., Ferrada-Videla, M., San Martin Rodriguez, L., & Beaulieu, M.-D. (2005). The conceptual basis for interprofessional collaboration: Core concepts and theoretical frameworks. *Journal of Interprofessional Care,* S-1, 116–131.

Delaney, C. (2003). Walking a fine line: Graduate nurses' transition experiences during orientation. *Journal of Nursing Education, 42*(10), 437–443.

Donner, G. J. (2004). Taking control of your nursing career: The future is now. In G. J. Donner & M. M. Wheeler (Eds.), *Taking control of your nursing career* (2nd ed., pp. 3–11). Toronto, ON: Elsevier Canada.

Donner, G. J., & Wheeler, M. M. (2001). Career planning and development for nurses: The time has come. *International Nursing Review, 48*(2), 79–85.

Donner, G. J., & Wheeler, M. M. (2004). New strategies for developing leadership. *Nursing Leadership, 17*(2), 27–32.

Eaton, S. (2000). Beyond unloving care: Linking human resource management and patient care quality in nursing homes. *International Journal of Human Resource Management, 11*(3), 591–616.

Ellerton, M.-L., & Gregor, F. (2003). A study of transition: The new nurse graduate at 3 months. *The Journal of Continuing Education in Nursing, 34*(3), 103–107.

Evans, R. J., & Donnelly, G. W. (2006). A model to describe the relationship between knowledge, skill, and judgment in nursing practice. *Nursing Forum, 41*(4), 150–157.

Ferguson, L. M., & Day, R. A. (2007). Challenges for new nurses in evidence-based practice. *Journal of Nursing Management, 15*(1), 107–113.

Finkelman, A. W. (2006). *Leadership and management in nursing.* Upper Saddle River, NJ: Pearson Education.

Gottlieb, L. N., & Feeley, N., with Dalton, C. (2006). *The collaborative partnership approach to care: A delicate balance.* Toronto, ON: Elsevier Canada.

Griscti, O., & Jacono, J. (2006). Effectiveness of continuing education programmes in nursing: Literature review. *Journal of Advanced Nursing, 55*(4), 449–456.

Hayes, L. J., Orchard, C. A., McGillis-Hall, L., Nincic, V., O'Brien-Pallas, L., & Andrews, G. (2006). Career intentions of nursing students and new nurse graduates: A review of the literature. *International Journal of Nursing Education Scholarship, 3*(1), Article 26.

Haynes, L. C. (2004). Transition into practice. In L. C. Haynes, H. K. Butcher, & T. A. Boese (Eds.), *Nursing in contemporary society: Issues, trends, and transition to practice.* (pp. 401–416). Upper Saddle River, NJ: Pearson Education.

Heller, B. R., Drenkard, K., Esposito-Herr, M. B., Romano, C., Tom, S., & Valentine, N. (2004). Educating nurses for leadership roles. *The Journal of Continuing Education in Nursing, 35*(5), 203–233.

Kirby, K. K., & DeCampli, P. (2008). Nurse manager development beyond the classroom. *Nurse Leader, 6*(2), 44–47.

Kramer, M., & Schmalenberg, C. (2004). Development and evaluation of essentials of magnetism tool. *Journal of Nursing Administration, 34*(7–8), 365–378.

Lavoie-Tremblay, M., Viens, C., Forcier, M., Labrosse, N., Lafrance, M., Laliberté, D., et al. (2002). How to facilitate the orientation of new nurses into the workplace. *Journal for Nurses in Staff Development, 18*(2), 80–85.

Manojlovich, M. (2005). The effect of nursing leadership on hospital nurses' professional practice behaviors. *Journal of Nursing Administration, 35*(7/8), 366–374.

McCall, M. W. (2004). Leadership development through experience. *Academy of Management Executive, 18*(3), 127–130.

McGillis Hall, L., Waddell, J., Donner, G., & Wheeler, M. M. (2004). Outcomes of career planning and development program for registered nurses. *Nursing Economics, 22*(5), 231–238.

Meleis, A., Sawyer, L., Im, E., Messias, D., & Schumacher, K. (2000). Experiencing transitions: An emerging mid-range theory. *Advances in Nursing Science, 23*(1), 12–28.

Noyes, B. (2002). Midlevel management education. *Journal of Nursing Administration, 32*(1), 25–26.

Perry, B. (2008). Shine on: Achieving career satisfaction as a registered nurse. *The Journal of Continuing Education in Nursing, 39*(1), 17–25.

Porter-O'Grady, T., & Malloch, K. (2007). *Quantum leadership: A resource for health care innovation* (2nd ed., pp. 259–294). Mississauga, ON: Jones & Bartlett Canada.

Raup, G. H. (2008). Make transitional leadership work for you. *Nursing Management, 39*(1), 50–53.

Redman, R. (2006). Leadership succession planning: An evidence-based approach for managing the future. *Journal of Nursing Administration, 36*(6), 292–297.

Rodts, M. F., & Lamb, K. V. (2008). Transforming your professional self: Encouraging lifelong personal and professional growth. *Orthopaedic Nursing, 27*(2), 125–132.

Santucci, J. (2004). Facilitating the transition into nursing practice: Concepts and strategies for mentoring new graduates. *Journal for Nurses in Staff Development, 20*(6), 274–284.

Schoessler, M., & Waldo, M. (2006). The first 18 months in practice: A developmental transition model for newly graduated nurses. *Journal for Nurses in Staff Development, 22*(2), 47–52.

Scoble, K., & Russell, G. (2003). Vision 2020. *Journal of Nursing Administration, 33*(6), 324–330.

Sherman, R. O., & Bishop, M. (2007). The role of nurse educators in grooming future nurse leaders. *Journal of Nursing Education, 46*(7), 295–296.

Sherman, R. O., & Bishop, M., Eggenberger, T., & Karden, R. (2007). Development of a leadership competency model. *Journal of Nursing Administration 37*(2), 85–95.

Sullivan, J., Bretschneider, J., & McCausland, M. P. (2003). Designing a leadership development program for nurse managers: An evidence-driven approach. *Journal of Nursing Administration, 33*(10), 544–549.

Thomka, L. A. (2001). Graduate nurses' experiences of interactions with professional nursing staff during transition to the professional role. *The Journal of Continuing Education in Nursing, 32*(1), 15–19.

Tomey, A. M. (2009). *Guide to nursing management and leadership* (8th ed.). St. Louis, MO: Mosby.

Top Rhine, D., & Davis, J. A. (2007). Career development. In R. A. Patronis Jones (Ed.), *Nursing leadership and management: Theories, processes and practice.* Philadelphia: F. A. Davis.

Tourangeau, A. (2003). Building nurse leader capacity. *Journal of Nursing Administration, 33*(12), 624–626.

Twedell, D. M., & Jackson Gray, J. (2007). Role transition. In P. S. Yoder-Wise (Ed.), *Leading and managing in nursing* (4th ed., pp. 515–529). St. Louis, MO: Mosby.

Upenieks, V. (2003). Nurse leaders' perceptions of what compromises successful leadership in today's acute inpatient environment. *Nursing Administration Quarterly, 27*(2), 140–152.

Waddell, J. (2008). Career planning and development: Creating your path to the future. In P. Kelly & H. Crawford (Eds.), *Nursing leadership and management* (1st Canadian ed., pp. 385–400). Toronto, ON: Nelson Education.

CHAPTER 14

CURRENT ISSUES IN LEADERSHIP

urses are becoming leaders in the greening of health care worldwide. This is a natural development; because of their scientific education and communication skills, nurses are uniquely qualified to comprehend and interpret environmental issues as they relate to health for their clients and their co-workers.

—Lucille Auffrey, RN, MN
Chief Executive Officer, Canadian Nurses Association

Before joining Canadian Nurses Association in March 2001, Madame Lucille Auffrey was the executive director of the Nurses Association of New Brunswick/Association des infirmières et infirmiers du Nouveau-Brunswick. A leader in the nursing community, Madame Auffrey has served on a number of federal and provincial advisory committees as well as the boards of various health care organizations. She served as a member of the interim committee to establish the Canadian Patient Safety Institute. Madame Auffrey has been involved in a number of international projects. For example, she served as a consultant on a joint Canadian Nurses Association–Uganda Nurses Association project. She has represented Canadian nurses at meetings of the World Health Organization and World Health Assembly and was invited by World Health Organization to attend a seminar on community health care and evolving partnerships.

A native of Moncton, New Brunswick, Madame Auffrey holds a Baccalaureate in Nursing from the University of New Brunswick and a Master of Science in Nursing and Health Studies from the University of Edinburgh, Scotland (1993). Clinical nursing practice was her first professional commitment, reflecting, to this day, the values that guide her professional aspirations.

Overview

Nursing is a dynamic profession—continually changing as societal trends and multifaceted issues relevant to health care become increasingly more visible. Nurse leaders are expected to contribute their knowledge, beliefs, analysis, and resolution toward the ever-changing events that occur in health care over time. As well as collaborating with other health team members, nurse leaders are looked upon to play a variety of different political roles in major issues that stem from the societal trends of the time. It is important that nurse leaders unite as a group and that they take clearly stated positions on pertinent issues. Doing so is essential to enable nursing to exert its particular and unique influence on the future of the profession and at the same time maintain and advance the quality of health care to clients and their families.

Objectives

By critically reflecting upon and processing knowledge throughout this chapter, you will be able to respond effectively to the following objectives:

1. Examine population aging and its effect on nurse leaders.
2. Develop innovative strategies whereby society can develop more positive attitudes toward aging.
3. Prepare a report about the chronic conditions affecting the older adult.
4. Debate the concept of successful aging.
5. Summarize briefly the impact of the Human Genome Project on health.
6. Plan a critical path to implement genetic knowledge in the nursing curricula.
7. Evaluate the five recommendations to support genetic practice in Canada.
8. Design a questionnaire to assess a nurse leader's current knowledge regarding the environment in your practice setting.
9. Analyze research studies that examine the chronic conditions related to hazards in the environment.
10. Illustrate how the Canadian Nurses Association Code of Ethics (2008) can be used in your nursing practice to deal with environmental threats.
11. Discuss the findings of the Survey on Nurses Environmental Health (2008).
12. Compare and contrast ethical leadership with transformational leadership.
13. Develop a whistleblowing policy for use in your workplace.

Current Trends

Trends are best understood as the directions taken as a result of events and societal attitudes that have been observed over time. Examples of trends examined in this chapter include population aging in Canada, the influence of genetics, and attention to environmental health. Issues arise from trends, and these issues often create local challenges that require a response from individuals, such as nurse leaders, to initiate changes within the health care system.

Population Aging in Canada

In Canada today, the global phenomenon of population aging is probably one of the most frequently discussed and heatedly debated of current topics. McPherson and Wister (2008) state, "We live not only in an aging world where people live longer and older people are more visible, but in a society in which older citizens are healthier and more active" (p. 7). In Canada, life expectancy is increasing, and the results of aging carry a profound effect on health care, transportation, and housing, to name but a few. These life expectancy developments will have serious implications on the demands of health care professionals, especially nurses educated to work with older people (Baumbusch & Andrusyszyn, 2002; Williams, Anderson, & Day, 2007).

Gerontology, the discipline that systematically studies the aging process and aging individuals, discusses practices and policies designed to assist older adults (Novak & Campbell, 2006). These practices and policies are based on research studies conducted in a wide range of interdisciplinary fields. Gerontology is becoming so relevant and so important that nurses are seeking special qualifications through both undergraduate and graduate studies, as well as through certifications in the speciality.

> *reflective* **THINKING**   As the Canadian society ages, what are some of the more specific effects that aging exerts on the health care system and that particularly affect nurse leaders? What can the nurse leader do about such effects?

Demographic Profile

Relatively lower rates of birth, longer life expectancy, and the effects of the baby boom generation are among the factors contributing to the aging population. Between 1981 and 2005, the number of elderly in Canada increased from 2.4 to 4.2 million, and their share of the total population increased from 9.6% to 13.1% (Statistics Canada, 2007). As individuals from the Baby Boom years of 1946 to 1965 begin turning 65, the extent of the aging population will accelerate appreciably over the next three decades. That is, as individuals from the Baby Boom

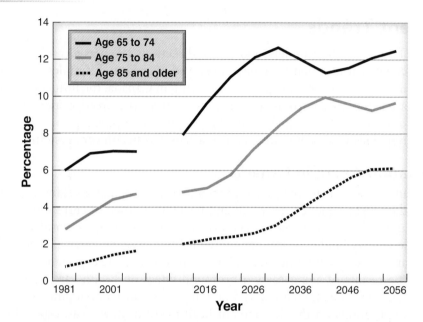

FIGURE 14.1 Percentage of total population comprised of seniors by group, Canada 1981 to 2005, projections from 2011 to 2056. (Adapted from Statistics Canada. [2007]. A Portrait of Seniors in Canada 2006 [p. 12]. Ottawa, ON: Author. Catalogue no. 89-519-XIE. Reproduced with permission.)

generation enter this age group, the number of 65- to 74-years-olds is projected to increase to 4.8 million by 2031, accounting for 12.4% of the total population at that time (Statistics Canada, 2007). A graphic illustration of the total population comprising Canadian seniors, by age group, from 1981 to 2005, with projections from 2011 to 2056, is seen in Figure 14.1. As the Baby Boomers age, the number of retired people will increase alarmingly (Wilson & Palha, 2007). In fact, with retirements lasting 10 years or more, a chief concern is the expected increased demand for health care (Rapoport, Jacobs, Bell, & Klarebach, 2004).

Attitudes Toward Aging

According to McPherson and Wister (2008), attitudes toward aging are influenced by a number of factors, including age, gender, ethnicity, level of education, and the socioeconomic status of individuals in society. Although a new trend urges society to view old age in a new light, ageism remains prevalent (Boissonnault, 2008).

Ageism is a socially constructed way of thinking about and behaving toward the elderly. It begins with negative attitudes and stereotypes about aging and older people and continues to express itself by focusing on the deterioration of the older adult. The effects of ageism lead steadily toward discrimination and the marginalization of elderly people (Lovell, 2006; McPherson & Wister, 2008). In Canada, a few developmental changes suggest that ageism will decrease over time. One such change is that individuals who now enter old age have more education and technological knowledge than did their age mates a generation earlier (Novak & Campbell, 2006). Another change is that older people tend to be perceived now as useful contributors to the labour force. Duchesne (2004) states that in Canada, 1 in 12 seniors age 65 and older were employed in 2001.

However, ageism and negative stereotypes persist. Older people tend to be devalued, and their human rights are frequently limited or denied (Lovell, 2006). Ageism affects the health care of older people by influencing the attitudes of health care professionals and policymakers regarding the care of the elderly. One example of such discrimination is that experienced by gay and lesbian seniors and their caregivers in Canada, who continue to face discrimination, particularly within the mainstream health and social service agencies. Brotman et al. (2007) conducted a study to explore the experiences of caregivers of gay and lesbian seniors living in the community and to identify issues that emerged from an examination of access to, and equity in, health care services for these populations. Based on the results, the researchers recommend expanding the definition of caregiver to be inclusive of gay and lesbian realities, advocating eliminating discrimination faced by these populations and developing specialized services to care for their needs.

> *reflective* **THINKING** What subpopulation other than the aging population might be experiencing discrimination within the health care system?

Another example of elder discrimination concerns sexuality and the older person. Sexuality has been described as one of the most natural and basic aspects of life that affects the individual's identity as a human being. Yet attitudes toward sexuality have generated devaluing reactions from society regarding older adults (Pangman & Seguire, 2000). Such reactions have relegated sexuality to invisibility. However, as the Baby Boom generation enters old age, sexuality may become more visible. Bauer, McAuliffe, and Nay (2007) state, "One factor that will act as a catalyst for this reconceptualization of sexuality in old age will be the impact of new drugs such as Viagra" (p. 65).

Older people are now being recognized as experiencing health-related sexual problems, and their concerns are being voiced. For example, diseases such as rheumatoid arthritis and other chronic illness can limit or impact on one's sexual activity. As well, it can adversely affect the relationship between partners (Hill, Bird, & Thorpe, 2003; Steinke, 2005). Many older people welcome the opportunity to discuss sexual issues. Nurses, however, are frequently either embarrassed or uncomfortable at either raising the topic or responding to the concerns of clients and their families (Reynolds & Magnan, 2005). In a study evaluating the attitudes of nursing staff toward love and intimacy in older people, the researcher found that the majority of rehabilitation nurses were sympathetic and supportive of the older person's expression of sexuality (Ali, 2004). Despite these results, there is a growing recognition that nurses need to change their attitudes toward sexuality and sexual health (Hordern & Currow, 2003).

Health Issues

Older adults live relatively healthy lives. In 2005, more than 74% of seniors assessed their health as either good, very good, or excellent, compared with 70% who rated their health 5 years earlier (National Advisory Council on Aging, Government of Canada, 2006). A longitudinal study conducted in Manitoba examined health status trends over a 14-year period. The researchers found noticeable improvements in health related to heart attack, stroke, cancer, and hip fractures. The prevalence of chronic illnesses, such as diabetes and dementia, however, increased significantly over that period (Menec, Lix, & MacWilliams, 2003).

Several Canadian researchers analyzed the Canadian National Population Health survey data (Denton, Prus, & Walters, 2004). The results indicated certain gender differences occur in health (measured by self-rated health, functional health, chronic illness, and distress). Women have lower rates of mortality, but they report higher rates of depression, arthritis, hypertension, and rheumatism than men (McDonough & Walters, 2001). Women, compared with men, also reported more falls (Fletcher & Hirdes, 2002). The fear of falling can lead to reduced activity and a higher risk of fatal falls (Cousins & Goodwin, 2002).

In Canada, chronic conditions, such as cancer, arthritis, chronic obstructive pulmonary disease, diabetes, heart disease, high blood pressure, and mood disorders, impact health and well-being of the population. These conditions represent a significant and growing burden on health care and the economy (Canadian Nurses Association [CNA], 2008a). Chronic illness detracts from the quality of life for individuals and will cost the health care system insurmountable amounts of money. One way to improve the quality of life of older persons and to reduce costs is to prevent the onset of these conditions and to ensure that health professionals manage the needs of these people so as to minimize avoidable exacerbations or complications (Broemeling, Watson, & Prebtani, 2008).

reflective **THINKING**   What approaches can be taken to prevent the onset of chronic conditions in the elderly?

Implications for Nurse Leaders

The impact of retiring Baby Boomers will influence every aspect of society, including health care. Because they are expected to be more demanding than current elderly people, Baby Boomers will challenge health care professionals, including nurses, when their health needs are not met (Villeneuve & MacDonald, 2006). Because of their interest in sports, nutrition, and their own health, they might profile a generation of healthier people who age successfully. In fact, this generation will remain engaged in life and community for years to come (Pascucci, 2008). However, as they grow older and are beset with chronic illnesses, an increased demand for health care, and for health services at all levels, will be needed both in the community and in the hospital (Rapoport, Jacobs, Bell, & Klarebach, 2004; Villeneuve & MacDonald, 2006).

The notion of successful aging was introduced by Rowe and Kahn (1987). Successful aging is characterized by older individuals who have the ability to maintain three distinct characteristics:

1. Low risk of disease and related disability
2. High mental and physical function
3. Active engagement with life (Rowe & Kahn, 1998).

These characteristics are important for nurse leaders to keep in mind as they develop programs and services for older people. Rowe and Kahn (1987) propose that despite the reality of chronic illnesses that plague older adults, most function well in the community. In fact, many acquire new knowledge and contribute significantly to society. To achieve the characteristics listed above, members of the health profession, including nurse leaders, must take political action to dispel ageism. In fact, enlightened nurse leaders can lead the way in facilitating this critical attitude shift (DiBartolo, 2008).

One of the principles in primary health care is health promotion, which is devoted to increasing the capacity of individuals to promote their own well-being (CNA, 2005a). Because health promotion is critical, two nurse researchers, one from Canada and the other from Brazil, found through databases 20 research-based articles that focus on health promotion immediately before or after retirement (Wilson & Palha, 2007). The articles were reviewed with qualitative content analysis methods, but the researchers found scant data on health promotion strategies at retirement that they believed to be of any considerable importance. Wilson and Palha (2007) recommend that political, social, and health leaders draft policies and promote programs to help improve health and wellness in older adults.

Nurse leaders need to be aware of the dynamics of this generation and plan policies to maintain and enhance health promotion strategies, such as regular exercise and social activities, for healthy and successful aging. The inclusion of exercise is probably the greatest weapon that can be used against the onset of

Reflections on Leadership Practice

You are a community health nurse in an inner-city health centre. You note that most of your clients are elderly and many are homeless. Most of them were successful when they retired, but due to several crises in their lives, they have been left without family or financial support. You believe that this population has numerous unidentified health needs. Beyond the basic requirements, they demonstrate mental deficiencies and substance abuse problems, and they seem to lack coping skills. This morning at a meeting, you were asked by administration to develop a health promotion program for this population.

1. In planning health promotion services for this special population, what facts are necessary for you to know?
2. What barriers must you overcome in planning health care?
3. Develop a 7-day program for this population. Present and discuss your innovative plan in class.
4. What steps are necessary to implement this program?
5. What resources do you need?

age-related disease and disability (Harman-Stein & Potkanowicz, 2003). Nurse educators can design and continue to develop innovative methods to integrate geriatric content in the curriculum (Williams, Anderson, & Day, 2007). Creative education approaches are important to foster positive attitudes and intergenerational relational skills. Nurse leaders can be highly instrumental in endeavours to foster research on their units to develop evidence-based guidelines for managing chronic illnesses and improving the quality of life of this population (DiBartolo, 2008; Harrington, Adams, & Titler, 2008).

Genetics

Shah (2003) indicates that the sequencing of the human genome, which is the complete set of molecular information that encodes the instruction for developing a human organism, is the beginning of a new paradigm in medicine as well as other health-related professions. The Human Genome Project has mapped the human genome and decoded some of the genetic sequences that may predispose individuals to certain disease (Government of Canada, 2006).

Human Genome Project

Current estimates indicate that approximately 5,000 human diseases have some type of genetic component. Some causes of congenital anomalies, such as Down syndrome, in which an extra copy of chromosome 21 prevails, are easy to identify. In other diseases, such as cancer, heart disease, and mental illness, which carry some genetic component, the causes are more difficult to identify because they involve multiple genes that are, in turn, controlled by environmental factors (Williams, 2000).

Presently, many of the related ethical, legal, and social issues are being considered with respect to the Human Genome Project. One such issue is genetic testing, which involves the examination of the individual's deoxyribonucleic acid for a variety of diseases (Wilson, 2002). Many individuals are struggling with the ethical and practical implications of the testing procedure (Williams, 2000). It is believed that over the next few years, as a result of the Human Genome Project, many other issues will surface. These issues will prevail upon society to cope with the even further areas of uncertainty regarding genetic disease and disability.

> *reflective* **THINKING**   Find out what types of prenatal genetic testing have been carried out in Canada. What is the role of the nurse leader regarding such testing?

Role of the Nurse in the Genomic Era

The development of genetics studies and genomics plays a strategic role in health care in the 21st century, and it has a special influence on nursing (Holtzclaw Williams, 2008). An urgent need exists in Canada for nurses in all settings to be informed about genomics (Bottorff et al., 2005b).

Nurses in the United States have been leaders in the development of genetic nursing. Jenkins and Calzone (2007) describe the development and process of consensus used to establish essential genetic and genomic nursing competencies relevant to the entire nursing profession in the United States, regardless of academic preparation, role, practice setting, or clinical speciality. In essence, this is the first step. The next step is to formulate a strategic action plan for the integration of genetic and genomic competency throughout education, practice, regulation, and quality control. Through conference calls and meetings, plans for implementation will be finalized. Jenkins and Calzone (2007) state that the progress of this particular effort has universal implications for all nurses worldwide. Partnering with nurses and other disciplines in other countries can lead to improved international nursing competency in genetics and genomics. In fact, integrating genetic and genomic competencies into nursing practice is directly focused on improving the quality and safety of care provided to clients and their families (Pestka, 2008).

International developments regarding nursing roles in the provision of genetic services are now being described (Feetham, 2004). Organizations such as the International Society of Nurses in Genetics, the American Nurses Association, and the Association of Genetic Nurses and Counsellors (in the United Kingdom) have developed standards of practice for basic and advanced nursing roles in genetic services (Bottorff et al., 2005b).

In Canada, only limited discussion has taken place on the nursing role in providing genetic services. Bottorff et al. (2005a) conducted a survey that included 975 nurses nationwide. The results indicate that nurses believe they play a critical role in providing genetic services for adult-onset hereditary disease. In fact, the nurses supported the notion of nursing roles in risk assessment and health teaching related to adult-onset hereditary disease and genetic testing. They also indicated support for providing counselling in addressing emotional reactions to perceived risk and in guiding individuals and families in implementing the management plans (Bottorff et al., 2005a). However, at this time, Canadian nursing organizations do not appear to have identified genetics as a priority within the scope of professional nursing practice. According to the CNA (2005b), no genetics educational program has yet been designed for nurses. Only a limited number of professional opportunities exist; most of them are geared to genetic counsellors and medical doctors.

> *reflective* **THINKING**   Form a study group and bring scholarly articles and reports of research studies in the field of genetics. How can you, as nurse leaders, develop competencies in genetics for nursing practice?

Implications for Nurse Leaders

In 2004, a planned Canadian forum began to identify opportunities, priorities, and strategies to support the incorporation of genetics and genomics into nursing practice (Bottorff et al., 2004). During the forum, nursing scholars and researchers shared the results of their studies and surveys regarding nursing and genetics. The findings were consistent and indicated that an urgent need exists for genetic education to support new and practicing nurses as they integrate genetics services into their nursing practice role. Nurses believe that they have important roles to play in providing genetic services to their clients and families (Bottorff et al., 2004).

Five recommendations were developed, accompanied by strong directive strategies to support genetic nursing practice in Canada, as outlined in Table 14.1. It is clear that nurse educators and nurse leaders need to come together to find ways to incorporate developed competencies in genetics into current nursing education programs and professional nursing practice. One way is for nurse leaders to design and conduct workshops that provide solid genetic theoretical and practical opportunities. In these workshops, nurses can explore ways to develop competencies in genetics. These nursing competencies will directly impact health care outcomes (Kirk, Tonkin, & Burke, 2008).

Another way is to develop the appropriate resources for an interdisciplinary team while the team is developing the knowledge, skills, and attitudes that are essential in practice roles (Calzone, Jenkins, & Rust, 2007). As more is learned about the contribution of genetics to health and wellness, nursing roles should be expected to expand appreciably in all clinical settings for the delivery of genetic health care (Burke, 2007). Figure 14.2 portrays the nurse educator and

TABLE 14.1	RECOMMENDATIONS AND STRATEGIES TO SUPPORT GENETIC NURSING PRACTICE IN CANADA
Recommendations	**Strategies**
Define genetic competencies to guide nursing practice and education.	Seek funding to support the involvement of a wide range of stakeholders in a broad consultation process. Consult with Canadian nurses who have pioneered roles in genetic nursing. Review nursing competencies in genetics developed in other countries. Develop a national competency framework to reflect different nursing roles and required levels of expertise in genetic nursing.
Increase awareness about the relevance of genetics to nursing.	Establish a network of nurses who are incorporating genetics into their practice and could champion key initiatives. Identify opportunities for the Canadian Nurses Association and other professional nursing groups to lobby for the inclusion of genetics as a priority for local, provincial, and national nursing organizations. Ensure the availability of educational resources to support awareness initiatives. Participate in multidisciplinary meetings related to genetics.
Make the integration of genetics into nursing education programs a national priority.	Identify where and how genetics is currently taught in nursing curricula. Introduce questions assessing genetics competencies into national registered nurse examinations. Support the involvement of Canadian nurses who have pioneered roles in genetic nursing in the development and implementation of genetics education and related resources. Develop summer institutes to train a cohort of nursing educators from across the country to be champions in the integration of genetics into nursing education. Conduct pilot projects to design and evaluate innovative approaches to enhance teaching of genetics in nursing programs (e.g., development of case studies, interactive Web-based strategies, and interdisciplinary courses/modules in genetics). Review existing genetics educational resources developed in the United States and United Kingdom and modify as necessary for Canadian context.

(table continues on page 366)

TABLE 14.1	RECOMMENDATIONS AND STRATEGIES TO SUPPORT GENETIC NURSING PRACTICE IN CANADA (continued)
Recommendations	**Strategies**
Increase the capacity of nurse researchers to focus on topics related to genetics.	Establish research units in several regions of the country using existing nursing research programs in genetics as a foundation. Capitalize on existing funding opportunities for research training to increase the number of nurses conducting research in genetics. Identify priorities for nursing research in genetics in Canada. Foster opportunities for nurse scientists to engage in interdisciplinary research in genetics. Develop innovative approaches to attract, train, and mentor nurse scientists whose research is not currently focused on genetics (e.g., summer institutes, co-mentorship).
Create a national strategy to support and lobby for the development of genetic nursing roles in Canada.	Create a database of Canadian nurses who have roles or interests in genetic nursing to facilitate networking and mentorship. Hold a national forum to engage stakeholders in a consultative process to set directions and goals for incorporating genetics into nursing. Form a national working group mandated to address priorities related to nursing genetics. Identify opportunities for nurses to influence policies that impact nursing roles in genetics. Lobby Canadian Nurses Association to develop a nonexamination route for specialty certification to provide an opportunity for credentialing nurses in genetics. Develop links with the International Society of Nurses in Genetics (United States) and the Association of Genetic Nurses and Counsellors (United Kingdom).

From Bottorff, J., McCullum, M., Balneaves, L., Esplen, M., Carroll, J., Kelly, M., et al. (2004). Nursing and genetics. *Canadian Nurse, 100*(8), 24, 28. Reproduced with the permission of Canadian Nurses Association. Copyright © 2008.

service leader walking the distance together to ensure that genetic competency for the nursing care of clients and their families is complete.

According to CNA (2005b), there are many ways nurse leaders can shape the delivery of health care to Canadians. By adding new knowledge and by developing competencies to reflect genetic practices, nurses can make an invaluable contribution to this emerging field.

Environmental Health

The care of the environment has been receiving considerable amounts of attention in both the private and public sectors for several years. The environmental

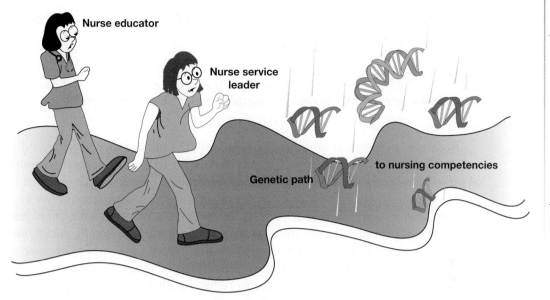

Nurse educator

Nurse service leader

Genetic path

to nursing competencies

FIGURE 14.2 Togetherness: Nursing practice competencies in genetics.

component has grown in its effect on the health status of individuals, families, vulnerable populations, and communities around the world (Jones, 2002). Increasingly, nurses are becoming the primary contact for clients and their families concerned about their health issues related to their environment (Larsson & Butterfield, 2002).

The CNA centennial environmental health initiative came at a prime time. CNA (2007) states that nurses will play critical roles in assessing and responding through the integration of environmental health strategies into their practice settings.

Environmental Issues Impacting Health

Today, the health of Earth and the health of its people are becoming inseparable. Because the environment is critically interdependent with health, the quality and sustainability of the environment impacts the health of Canadians every day (CNA, 2000). For example, the contamination of the public water supply in places like Walkerton, Ontario, and North Battleford, Saskatchewan, highlights the reality of environment-related health issues (CNA, 2005c). A retrospective study was conducted to review the available data on waterborne disease outbreaks in Canada from 1974 to 2001. The study set out to identify disease occurrences and to determine the contributing factors and implications for public health (Schuster et al., 2005). Based on their findings, these researchers recommended the development of a federal surveillance system for the consistent reporting of such outbreaks.

> _reflective_ **THINKING**   As a nurse leader, what strategies will you undertake to promote an environmentally responsible community?

Recently, a study was conducted to examine the environmental burden disease in Canada for respiratory and cardiovascular diseases, cancer, and congenital affliction (Boyd & Genuis, 2008). The researchers found that the burden of illness resulting from adverse environmental exposures is significant. They recommend that stronger efforts are warranted, including research, education, and regulation, to prevent adverse environmental exposures. The health, social, and economic impacts of global warming are likely to grow much worse because of the inevitable extent of climate change. The effects of these impacts are of special concern given the time it will take to reduce worldwide emissions of greenhouse gases (Lemmen & Warren, 2004).

Air pollution is most harmful to the very young, the very old, and individuals with respiratory and cardiac disease. According to Frank (2006), children are especially vulnerable to the health effects of air pollution for a number of reasons: they have a smaller body size, they generally spend more time being active outdoors than adults, and their lungs are still developing. It is important for health care professionals to note that evidence has increased significantly for the effects of air pollution on children. That is, evidence implicates pollution exposure in the environment with the development of chronic diseases such as asthma.

> _reflective_ **THINKING**   What steps can you recommend to reduce potential risk factors in health care facilities regarding the threat of an asthmatic attack?

Role of the Canadian Government

Health Canada is committed to making the population of Canada among the healthiest in the world. It works toward this by collaborating closely with other federal agencies, departments, and health stakeholders to reduce health and safety risks in Canada (Health Canada, 2007). Further, Health Canada is responsible for ensuring that human health is included as a component of environmental assessment. Environmental assessment is a planning tool that provides decision makers with the information they need to approve projects that are compatible with a healthy and sustainable environment (Western Economic Diversification Canada, 2008).

In 2004, the federal government of Canada realized the need for more reliable and clearly defined environmental indicators—measuring sticks that could track the results and be held accountable in striving for cleaner air, lower greenhouse gas emission, and cleaner water. The indicators are air quality, greenhouse gas emissions, and freshwater quality. These three Canadian environmental sustainability indicators provide important information—not only about Canada's environmental sustainability, but also about the health and well-being and economic growth and lifestyle choices of the people (Government of Canada, 2006).

reflective **THINKING** How can nurse leaders be certain of a clean water supply for clients in rural communities that use well water?

Definition of Environmental Health
The World Health Organization (2004) defines environmental health as comprising those aspects of human health that include quality of life as determined by physical, chemical, biological, social, and psychosocial factors present in the environment. It also refers to the theory and practice of assessing, correcting, controlling, and preventing those factors in the environment that can potentially affect adversely the health of current and future generations. In essence, these factors in the environment could include any aspect that is not genetic. However, it could be argued that even genes are influenced by the environment, either in the short or long run (Rutter, 2007).

Guidelines for Practice
CNA (2007) states that the World Health Organization's definition of environmental health is particularly useful in guiding nursing practice, research, education, and policy. One of the reasons is that it includes the determinants of health that nurses routinely address, such as biological, psychological, and social factors. Furthermore, it also provides specific guidance for areas of nursing intervention (assessing, correcting, controlling, and preventing), which are part of the theoretical frameworks used by nurses.

reflective **THINKING** On your unit, observe for the health condition of clients who have been diagnosed with, or who have been associated with, environmental health threats. How could these risks have been prevented? What health promotion strategies would you plan for these clients? An example of such a case may be a child with asthma.

Another guideline for practice is the *Code of Ethics for Registered Nurses* (CNA, 2008b). The code serves as a foundation for nurses' ethical practice. The first part of the code consists of nurses' primary values. The second part addresses ethical endeavours, which are broad aspects of social justice associated with health and well-being. These aspects relate to the need for change in systems and societal structures in order to create equity for all. Of the 13 statements entitled "ethical endeavours," three relate to the environment, as follows:

- VI: Supporting environmental preservation and restoration and advocating for initiatives that reduce environmentally harmful practices in order to promote health and well-being.
- XI: Maintaining awareness of broader global health concerns such as violation of human rights, war, world hunger, gender inequities, and environmental pollution. Nurses work individually and with others to bring about social change.
- XIII: Working collaboratively to develop a moral community. As part of the moral community, all nurses acknowledge their responsibility to contribute to positive, healthy work environments (CNA, 2008b).

By acting on these ethical endeavours, nurses should strive individually and collectively to advocate for, and work toward, eliminating social inequities in all settings locally, nationally, and globally.

For example, Canada has recognized that Aboriginal and northern communities in the country face unique challenges regarding climate change and its impact on health. Furgal and Seguin (2006) reviewed experiences from two projects that have identified and assessed the effects of a vulnerability to climate change and the impact of health in two Inuit regions of the Canadian Arctic. They conclude that the results argue for a multi-stakeholder, participatory framework to identify and assess risk, while advocating for and enhancing the capacity of local areas to respond to health issues that are a result of climate change. Nurses who work in such areas can certainly be part of the health team to respond to vulnerabilities and capabilities in Aboriginal and northern communities.

reflective **THINKING** If you are a nurse leader in one of the communities in the Canadian Arctic, what steps would you take with other members of an interdisciplinary team to create an assessment tool to identify health risk behaviours of the Inuit population due to climate change?

Implications for Nurse Leaders

Nurse leaders need to be aware of current environmental issues that affect not only the health of the client and family, but also professional health team members and staff. Providing a safe environment, both physically and psychologically, must be ongoing in the promotion of health and well-being. Gaudry and Skiehar (2007) state that nurses can take steps toward reducing, reusing, and recycling material.

Nurses can play an active and dynamic role through advocacy, education, and the implementation of strategies to reduce medical wastage and exposure to chemical toxins (Gaudry & Skiehar, 2007). Nurse leaders can lobby in the community for environmentally responsible health care practices by holding seminars about harmful toxins and proposing ways that individuals can eliminate these toxins from their home. In support of nursing practice regarding environmental health, the CNA has issued two position statements: *The Environment Is a Determinant of Health* (CNA, 2000) and *Joint CNA/CMA Position Statement on Environmentally Responsible Activity in the Health Sector* (CNA, 2005d). CNA has also issued the backgrounder *The Ecosystem, the Natural Environment, and Health and Nursing*. All of these documents are available on the CNA Website (see Websites at the end of this chapter).

reflective **THINKING** Examine the CNA Backgrounder (2005c) *The Ecosystem, the Natural Environment, and Health and Nursing.* What strategies would you advocate for "green" health care to make the health care team more environmentally responsible?

A survey of Canadian nurses was conducted by CNA in December 2007. This survey, as part of CNA's centennial project on environmental health, was conducted to identify the nurses':

- Awareness of environmental health issues.
- Education about environmental exposures.
- Use of teaching resources with client or patients.
- Perception of the sustainability of the health system in which they work (CNA, 2008c).

A synopsis of the results, discussion, and conclusions are outlined in Box 14.1. CNA (2008c) states that the findings will support the development of nursing educational modules to address gaps that nurses encounter. The first of these modules contains objectives, a reading list, and a PowerPoint presentation with notes; and they can be found on the home page of the CNA (see Websites at the end of this chapter). The three modules available at the time of writing are *Environmental Health Principles, Greening the Health System, and Climate Change.* Nurse leaders, both in the educational and service sectors, are encouraged to use these modules to enhance the knowledge of both student nurses and health team members to

(text continues on page 374)

BOX 14.1 NURSES AND ENVIRONMENTAL HEALTH: SURVEY RESULTS

Synopsis of Results

The CNA surveyed Canadian nurses to identify:

- Their awareness of environmental health issues.
- Their education about environmental exposures.
- Their use of teaching resources with patients or clients.
- Their perception of the sustainability of the health system in which they work.

Characteristics of sample:

- A total of 221 nurses responded.
- Education: Registered nurses, 91.4%; advanced practice nurses, 7.7%.
- Age: 75% were older than 40 years.
- Work setting: Hospitals, 53.8%; community or public health, 17.1%
- Previous education or training in environmental health: Had training, 41.4%; had no training, 39.2%.
- Location of respondents: Representation resulted from each of the provinces and territories, but significant proportions were from Ontario (44%), B.C. (29%), Alberta (18%), and Nova Scotia (17%); less than 2% worked in Quebec.

Indicated having an awareness of environmental hazards:

- Types of hazards: Indoor air quality, 79%; environmental tobacco smoke, 79%; mould, 68%; contaminated water, 53%; smog, 50%; organic solvents, 43%.
- Had been admitted to hospital due to environmental exposure: 31%
- Knew of the existence of Canadian legislation to protect health: 49%

Teaching experience with patients and clients about environmental health:

- Had discussed environmental exposures: 56%
- Had never discussed environmental exposures: 31%
- Teaching tools included fact sheet developed by health organization: 59%

Synopsis of Discussion

Characteristics:

- Participants were older and better educated than Canadian nurses generally.
- The high proportion of academics who responded to the survey made available on the Web might account for nursing schools' interest in increasing the coverage of environmental health in their curricula.

Environmental health:

- Environmental content did not seem available in either undergraduate or graduate level curricula.
- Nurses independently bolstered their environmental knowledge through various resources.

- Only half the sample reported routinely assessing exposure to environmental tobacco smoke during assessments.
- Half of the respondents were aware of legislation to protect Canadians from environmental hazards, but few felt they had the skills to engage in policy issues related to environmental health.

Sustainable health care system:

- Hospitals appear to be actively engaged in becoming more energy efficient.
- *Green Teams.* Several hospitals across Canada have established green teams with the goal of *reducing the institution's environmental footprint.* Team members include staff members from departments across the institution, and they focus on: *promoting energy efficiency, product longevity, use of less toxic products, and the attractiveness of the hospital environment.*
- Of the group of nurses who were sufficiently interested in environmental health to respond to the CNA survey, only 15% were aware of a green team at their place of work.

Conclusions
1. Nurses have an understanding of scientific methodologies, health conditions, and human behaviours, all of which could assist in transforming evidence-based information into policy-relevant initiatives and communication tools for environment health.
2. Nurses could play a more active role in reducing or preventing the health consequences of environmental hazards.
3. Training required to support nurses in this area could include:
   a. Focus on environmental health in both undergraduate and graduate nursing curricula.
   b. Educational opportunities for nurses in the workforce.
4. Strategies that can be used to disseminate information on environmental health issues outside of the formal educational system:
   a. Articles in nursing journals
   b. Presentation of information on the Internet
   c. Workshops and conferences
5. CNA is working with associate and provincial and territorial members to develop tools that can be used by schools of nursing, continuing education providers, and individual nurses across Canada to increase awareness of environmental health issues.

Adapted from Canadian Nurses Association (2008). *Nurses and Environmental Health: Survey Result.* Ottawa. ON: Author. Retrieved June 2008 from: http://www.cna-aiic.ca/CNA/documents/pdf/publications/Survey_Results_e.pdf

provide effective quality care to clients and their families who experience environmental health issues.

Nurse leaders, who have day-to-day contact with clients and families, must encourage and implement measures to achieve environmental responsibility in the settings where they practice, as well as in the health care system in general (CNA, 2005d). It will be of some interest to students to realize that nurse educators are urged to re-examine the curricula in their nursing faculties and initiate updates in course content to reflect the impact of environmental changes on health.

Leadership Issue

*P*roject yourself into the responsibilities of a nurse leader in a community setting within the next 5 years. You are thinking of replicating the survey on *Nurses and Environmental Health* in your own and surrounding communities and in several hospitals as well. After reflecting on the objectives provided in the survey conducted by CNA in December 2007, what objectives would you add to reflect your present environmental concerns?

List the set of objectives you would use.

What changes would you expect to find after 5 years?

Estimate how your findings may or may not change the practice of nursing.

Becoming an ethical nurse leader is important not only regarding environmental health but also with other issues that may arise. Ethical leadership is the demonstration of appropriate conduct through personal actions and interpersonal relationships to foster responsible decision making. Ethical leaders model to others appropriate behaviours such as honesty, trustworthiness, fairness, and care. Ethical leadership is an emerging area of leadership research, and to date, very little research has been conducted. However, one of the few studies indicates that ethical leadership was associated with more employee satisfaction, more willingness to devote extra effort on one's job, and more willingness to report problems to management (Johns & Saks, 2008). It is important that nurse leaders make ethics salient in the workplace and draw attention to it by setting ethical standards.

This type of leadership may advocate for team members who are concerned about the actions of another, especially if such actions might result in harm to clients, colleagues, or to the public. One such possible option is to "whistleblow" (Shah, 2005). The decision to whistleblow on a colleague, an associate, or an employer is never an easy one. Unless there is a legal obligation to report, it should be considered a step one takes when all else has failed (Ray, 2006). It is important that nurse leaders develop a whistleblowing policy that encourages nurses to raise genuine concerns about wrongdoing and that offers protection to those who initiate the action (Shah, 2005).

reflective **THINKING** | If someone had a concern that you were not being environmentally safe—specifically, smoking close to the entrance of the hospital—how would you want them to raise the issue?

Contemporary nursing is a complex and challenging practice that reflects influences arising from changing population demographics, exploding genetic knowledge, and the integration of environmental health in work settings. Figure 14.3 depicts the notion that it is time for nurse leaders to become more aware and more prepared for the enormous impact that climate change is expected to exert upon health. Examining and acting on these issues will assist the nurse to continue playing an important role in providing quality care to clients and families and to contributing even more emphatically to the health of society.

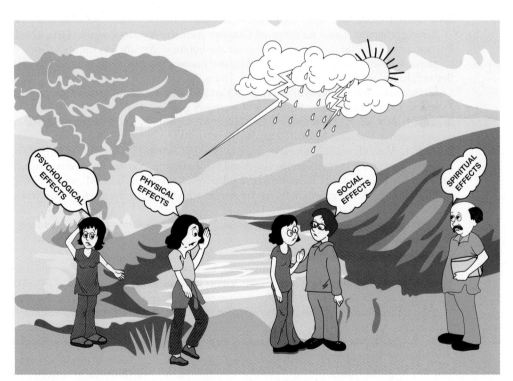

FIGURE 14.3 Effects of climate change on health: A Canadian priority.

WEBSITES

■ Canadian Nurses Association and Nursing and Environmental Health: Environmental Health Websites

http://www.cna-aiic.ca/CNA/issues/environment/websites/default_e.aspx#healthtutorials
Nurses need access to accurate information when reducing health risks from environmental hazards. These Websites provide information on a number of areas of environmental health. Under each section links are provided to both Canadian and international sites.

■ Seniors Canada

http://www.seniors.gc.ca/home.jsp?lang=en
The Seniors Canada site is Canada's premier information source for seniors, caregivers, families, and health care.

REFERENCES

Ali, K. M. (2004). Attitudes among rehabilitation nurses towards love and intimacy in older people. *Geriatrics Today: Journal of the Canadian Geriatrics Society, 7*(2), 46–48.

Bauer, M., McAuliffe, L., & Nay, R. (2007). Sexuality, health care and the older person: An overview of the literature. *International Journal of Older People Nursing,2*(1), 63–68.

Baumbusch, J. L., & Andrusyszyn, M.-A. (2002). Gerontological content in Canadian baccalaureate nursing programs: Cause for concern? *Canadian Journal of Nursing Research, 34*(1), 121–160.

Boissonnault, P. (2008). Look out! Here come the boomers: Ageism and the apocalyptic demographic. *Transformative Dialogues: Teaching and Learning Journal, 1*(3), 1–9.

Bottorff, J., Blaine, S., Carroll, J., Esplen, M., Evans, J., Nicolson Klimeck, M., et al. (2005a). The educational needs and professional roles of Canadian physicians and nurses regarding genetic testing and adult onset heredity disease. *Community Genetics, 100*(8), 24–28.

Bottorff, J., McCullum, M., Balneaves, L., Esplen, M., Carroll, J., Kelly, M., et al. (2004). Nursing and genetics. *Canadian Nurse, 100*(8), 24–28.

Bottorff, J., McCullum, M., Balneaves, L., Esplen, M., Carroll, J., Kelly, M., et al. (2005b). Canadian nursing in the genomic era: A call for leadership. *Nursing Leadership, 18*(2), 56–72.

Bottorff, J., McCullum, M., Balneaves, L., Esplen, M., Carroll, J., Kelly, M., et al. (2005c). Establishing roles in genetic nursing: Interviews with Canadian nurses. *Canadian Journal of Nursing Research, 37*(4), 96–115.

Broemeling, A.-M., Watson, D. E., & Prebtani, F. (2008). Population patterns of chronic health conditions, co-morbidity and healthcare use in Canada: Implications for policy and practice. *Healthcare Quarterly, 11*(3), 70–76.

Brotman, S., Ryan, B., Collins, S., Chamberland, L., Cormier, R., Julien, D., et al. (2007). Coming out to care: Caregivers of gay and lesbian seniors in Canada. *The Gerontologist, 47*(4), 490–503.

Boyd, D. R., & Genuis, S. J. (2008). The environmental burden of disease in Canada: Respiratory disease, cardiovascular disease, cancer, and congenital affliction. *Environmental Research 106*(2), 240–249.

Burke, B. (2007). Nurses play key role in translating genomic developments into health benefits. *Connecticut Nursing News, 80*(2), 12–13.

Calzone, K., Jenkins, J., & Rust, J. E. (2007). Establishing and implementing the essential nursing competencies and curricula guidelines for genetics and genomics. *Clinical Nurse Specialist, 21*(5), 265–266.

Canadian Nurses Association. (2000). *Position statement: The environment is a determinant of health.* Ottawa, ON: Author. PS-45.

Canadian Nurses Association. (2005a). *Backgrounder: Primary health care: A summary of the issues.* Ottawa, ON: Author. BG 007.

Canadian Nurses Association. (2005b). Nursing and genetics: Are you ready? *Nursing now: Issues and trends in Canadian Nursing, 20*(May).

Canadian Nurses Association. (2005c). *Backgrounder: The ecosystem, the natural environment, and health and nursing: A summary of the issues.* Ottawa, ON: Author. BG 004.

Canadian Nurses Association. (2005d). *Joint CNA/CMA position statement on environmentally responsible activity in the health sector.* Ottawa, ON: Author.

Canadian Nurses Association. (2007). *The environment and health: An introduction for nurses.* Ottawa, ON: Author.

Canadian Nurses Association. (2008a). CNA leads dialogue on healthy aging. *Canadian Nurse, 104*(6), 22.

Canadian Nurses Association (2008b). *Code of ethics for registered nurses: 2008 centennial edition.* Ottawa. ON: Author.

Canadian Nurses Association (2008c). *Nurses and Environmental Health: Survey Result.* Ottawa. ON: Author. Retrieved June 2008 from http://www.cna-aiic.ca/CNA/documents/pdf/publications/Survey_Results_e.pdf

Cousins, S. O., & Goodwin, D. (2002). Balance your life! The metaphors of falling. *Wellspring, 13*(3), 6–7.

Denton, M., Prus, S., & Walters, V. (2004). Gender differences in health: A Canadian study of the psychosocial, structural and behavioural determinants of health. *Social Science & Medicine, 58,* 2585–2600.

DiBartolo, M. C. (2008). The demographic tidal wave: Are we ready? *Journal of Gerontological Nursing, 34*(4), 3–4.

Duchesne, D. (2004). More seniors at work. *Perspectives on Labour and Income. 5*(2), 5–17. Statistics Canada Catalogue no. 75-001-XIE.

Feetham, S. E. (Ed.). (2004). *Genetics in nursing.* Geneva, Switzerland: International Council of Nurses.

Fletcher, P. C., & Hirdes, J. P. (2002). Risk factors for serious falls among community-based seniors: Results from the national population health survey. *Canadian Journal of Aging, 21*(1), 103–116.

Frank, J. (2006). CIHR research: Catching your breath: Research efforts to analyze the negative effects of air pollution on human health. *Healthcare Quarterly, 9*(4), 18–20.

Furgal, C., & Sequin, J. (2006). Climate change, health, and vulnerability in Canadian northern Aboriginal communities. *Environmental Health Perspectives, 114*(12), 1964–1970.

Gaudry, J., & Skiehar, K. (2007). Promoting environmentally responsible health care. *Canadian Nurse, 103*(1), 22–26.

Government of Canada. (2006). *BioBasics: Genetic testing.* Retrieved June 2008 from http://biobasics.gc.ca/english/View.asp?x=780

Harman-Stein, P. E., & Potkanowicz, M. A. (2003). Behavioral determinants of healthy aging: Good news for the baby boomer generation. *Online Journal of Issues in Nursing.* Retrieved June 2008 from http://www.nursingworld.org/mods/mod642/ceagfull.htm

Harrington, C. C., Adams, S., & Titler, M. G. (2008). Evidence-based guideline: Assessing heart failure in long-term care facilities. *Journal of Gerontological Nursing, 34*(2), 9–14.

Hill, J., Bird, H., & Thorpe, R. (2003). Effects of rheumatoid arthritis on sexual activity and relationships. *Rheumatology, 42,*280–286.

Holtzclaw Williams, P. S. (2008). Genetic and genomic public health strategies: Imperatives for neonatal nursing genetic competency. *Newborn and Infant Nursing Reviews, 8*(1), 43–50.

Hordern, A. J., & Currow, D. C. (2003). A patient-centred approach to sexuality in the face of life-limiting illness. *The Medical Journal of Australia, 179*(Supplement 6), S8–S11.

Jenkins, J., & Calzone, K. A. (2007). Establishing the essential nursing competencies for genetics and genomics. *Journal of Nursing Scholarship, 39*(1), 10–16.

Johns, G., & Saks, A. M. (2008). *Organizational behaviour: Understanding and managing life at work* (7th ed.). Toronto, ON: Pearson Education Canada.

Jones, S. L. (2002). Critical thinking and environmental health: Challenging the status quo. *Journal of Nursing Education, 4*(4), 143–144.

Kirk, M., Tonkin, E., & Burke, S. (2008). Engaging nurses in genetics: The strategic approach of the NHS national genetics education and development centre. *Journal of Genetic Counselling, 17*(2), 180–188.

Larsson, L. S., & Butterfield, P. (2002). Mapping the future of environmental health and nursing: Strategies for integrating national competencies into nursing practice. *Public Health Nursing, 19*(9), 301–308.

Lemmen, D. S., & Warren, F. J. (2004). *Climate change impacts and adaptation: A Canadian perspective.* Ottawa, ON: Government of Canada. Catalogue no. M174-2/2004E.

Lovell, M. (2006). Caring for the elderly: Changing perceptions and attitudes. *Journal of Vascular Nursing, 24*(1), 22–26.

McDonough, P., & Walters, V. (2001). Gender and health: Reassessing patterns and explanations. *Social Science & Medicine, 52*, 547–559.

McPherson, B. D., & Wister, A. (2008). *Aging as a social process: Canadian perspectives* (5th ed.). Don Mills, ON: Oxford University Press.

Menec, V. H., Lix, L., & MacWilliams, J. (2003, October). *Living longer, living healthier? Trends in the health status of older Manitobans.* Paper presented at the 32nd Annual Scientific and Educational Meeting of the Canadian Association of Gerontology, Toronto, ON.

National Advisory Council on Aging. (2006). *Seniors in Canada: 2006 report card.* Ottawa, ON: Government of Canada. Catalogue no. HP30-1/2006E.

Novak, M., & Campbell, L. (2006). *Aging and society: A Canadian perspective* (5th ed.). Toronto, ON: Nelson.

Pangman, V. C., & Seguire, M. (2000). Sexuality and the chronically ill older adult: A social justice issue. *Sexuality and Disability, 18*(1), 49–59.

Pascucci, M. A. (2008). A message to baby boomers: Take good care of yourselves! *Journal of Gerontological Nursing, 34*(3), 3.

Pestka, E. L. (2008). Are you including genomics in nursing practice? *Journal of American Psychiatric Nurses Association, 14*(1), 63–68.

Rapoport, R., Jacobs, P., Bell, N. R., & Klarenbach, S. (2004). Refining the measurement of the economic burden of chronic diseases in Canada. *Chronic Diseases in Canada, 25*(1). Retrieved June 2008 from http://www.phac-aspc.gc.ca/publicat/cdic-mcc/25-1/c_e.html

Ray, S. (2006). Whistleblowing and organizational ethics. *Nursing Ethics, 13*(4), 438–445.

Reynolds, K. E., & Magnan, M. A. (2005). Nursing attitudes and beliefs toward human sexuality: Collaborative research promoting evidence-based practice. *Clinical Nurse Specialist 19*(5), 255–259.

Rowe, J. W., & Kahn, R. N. (1987). Human aging: Usual and successful aging. *Science, 237*, 143–149.

Rowe, J. W., & Kahn, R. N. (1998). *Successful aging.* New York, NY: Pantheon Books.

Rutter, M. (2007). Gene-environment interdependence. *Developmental Science, 10*(1), 12–18.

Shah, C. P. (2003). *Public health and preventative medicine in Canada* (5th ed.). Toronto, ON: Elsevier Canada.

Shah, F. (2005). Whistleblowing: It's time to overcome the negative image. *British Journal of Community Nursing, 10*(6), 277–279.

Schuster, C. J., Ellis, A. G., Robertson, W. J., Charron, D. F., Aramini, J. J., Marshall, B. J., et al. (2005). Infectious diseases outbreaks related to drinking water in Canada, 1974–2001. *Canadian Journal of Public Health, 96*(4), 254–258.

Statistics Canada. (2007). A portrait of seniors in Canada 2006. Ottawa, ON: Author. Catalogue no. 89-519-XIE.

Steinke, E. E. (2005). Intimacy needs and chronic illness: Strategies for sexual counselling and self-management. *Journal of Gerontological Nursing, 31*(5), 40–50.

Villeneuve, M., & MacDonald, J. (2006). *Toward 2020: Visions for Nursing.* Ottawa, ON: Canadian Nurses Association.

Western Economic Diversification Canada. (2008). *Canadian environmental assessment act.* Retrieved July 2008 from http://www.wd.gc.ca/4767_ENG_ASP.asp

Williams, B., Anderson, M. C., & Day, R. (2007). Undergraduate nursing students' knowledge of the attitudes toward aging: Comparison of context-based learning and a traditional program. *Journal of Nursing Education, 46*(3), 115–120.

Williams, T. (2000). *The human genome project and its ethical, legal and social implications.* Ottawa, ON: Government of Canada, PRB 00-08E. Retrieved June 2008 from http://dsp-psd.tpsgc.gc.ca/Collection-R/LoPBdP/BP/prb0008-e.htm

Wilson, D. M., & Palha, P. (2007). A systematic review of published research articles on health promotion at retirement. *Journal of Nursing Scholarship, 39*(4), 330–337.

Wilson, R. D. (2002). Cystic fibrosis carrier testing in pregnancy in Canada. *Journal of Obstetrics and Gynaecology Canada, 24*(8), 644–647.

World Health Organization. (2004). *Improving the public's health through environmental health education and health promotion.* Retrieved June 2008 from http://www.who.int/phe/en/

NURSING LEADERSHIP: TOMORROW'S VISION

That robot running up the hall to fetch towels is freeing up time for the nurse on the unit to spend with patients. . . . We keep saying there are not enough of us, and we don't have enough time—and yet we're not using the technology that is there now, or could be there if we helped to design it. Every nurse should have a BlackBerry, a laptop computer, and/or other appropriate communications devices to connect instantly and more fully with needed information.

—**Michael Villeneuve, RN, BScN, MSc**
Scholar-in-Residence

From Canadian Nurses Association. (2007).
Toward 2020—Encouraging discussion on future directions.
Canadian Nurses. 103(2), 12.

Michael Villeneuve has more than 25 years of progressive experience in the Canadian health care system. He has held positions as a nursing attendant, staff nurse, instructor, lecturer, and clinical nurse specialist in neurosurgery and trauma. On the management side, Mr. Villeneuve has worked for Health Canada in charge of an outpost nursing station in Northern Manitoba and was Patient Care Manager of the Neurosurgical Intensive Care and Neuro/Trauma Units at Sunnybrook and Women's Health Sciences Centre in Toronto. For 4 years he held the position of Senior Consultant in the federal Office of Nursing Policy, and during that time, he represented Health Canada at the Organization for Economic Cooperation and Development. Mr. Villeneuve has published and presented widely on a variety of nursing and health policy topics. He maintains strong interests in diversity and social justice issues. Currently he is scholar-in-residence at the Canadian Nurses Association.

Overview

The dynamic changes that are occurring in our society, and specifically in the health care environment, present new and exciting challenges for the professional nurse. Nurses have always played an important role in providing care and contributing to the health of society. The call for reflection by nurse leaders is not new, but reflection becomes more critical as nurses struggle with the myriad of issues that require creative change through innovative problem solving by all members of the organization.

For example, the influences of exploding health information have shaped, and will continue to direct, the future of the nursing leadership. Personal and creative development must be allowed to flourish, and meaningful experiences must be validated to bring about organizational change so that quality nursing care can be effectively provided to all people. A need exists for nurse leaders to value the concept of spirituality. Spiritual leaders are those who incorporate all levels of interaction, have affection for risk taking, tolerate ambiguity, encourage curiosity and complexity, and share in the profession's adaptation and growth. Human capacity is the key for nurse leaders who seek to attain a paradigm shift toward the novel and endless possibilities to be found in tomorrow's challenges concerning nurse leadership.

Objectives

By critically reflecting upon and processing knowledge throughout this chapter, you will be able to respond effectively to the following objectives:

1. Summarize the various impacts of globalization.
2. Design a plan for nurse leaders to become politically involved in advocating for global health and equity.
3. Outline the responsibilities of a nurse in emergency and disaster response.
4. Critique the use of information and communication technology in health care.
5. Describe the nurse's role in telehealth.
6. Debate the importance of electronic health records to improve client safety.
7. Analyse the research findings regarding health disparities in Canada.
8. Justify nurses becoming involved in addressing the social determinants of health.
9. Critique the four core principles of change as proposed by Margaret J. Wheatley.
10. Examine the concept of spirituality in nursing practice.
11. Illustrate how nurse leaders can promote the concept of spirituality in the workplace.

Reflection

Reflection is an important and valuable process that allows nurse leaders to observe and ponder issues before extending their hand toward other health team members in the organization as they shape the future health care delivery system. Figure 15.1 depicts nurse leaders looking as far ahead as possible at visible issues on the horizon. Possibly, these nurse leaders are creating a vision of different models of practice, or they might be considering a vibrant new health care system that is aligned with the Canadian Nurses Association (CNA) (2008a) bold new *Vision for Change*. This vision entails an optimistic view of the future of health care, with registered nurses having a vital and an enhanced role.

Challenges and Changes

An examination of recent literature reveals that globalization, communication technology, and information management are now distinct concepts that continually raise relevant challenges, and these challenges have been addressed extensively among various disciplines, including nursing (Villeneuve & MacDonald, 2006). With the advent of a shrinking world, a number of predictable and unpredictable changes will occur. The impact of globalization and health informatics will certainly be felt within the continued restructuring of the health care system and increasing visibility of the profession of nursing in Canada.

Health disparities are a prime concern in Canada because the overall high standard of health is not shared by all people. One example is that those who are

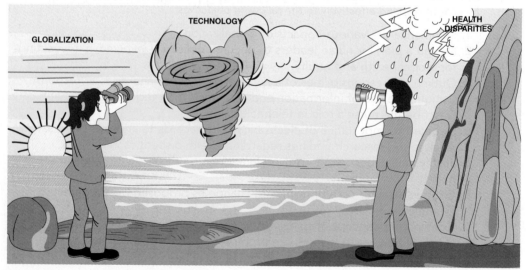

FIGURE 15.1 Tomorrow's vision.

better educated and have higher incomes can expect to have better health. Nurse leaders need to be aware of the social determinants of health, which are the social and economic conditions that influence the health of the Canadian people (CNA, 2005a).

Globalization

One impact of globalization is the mobility of nurses—moving to Canada or to other countries. Internationally educated nurses are coming to Canada and bringing with them a somewhat different set of skills and abilities, as well as individual personal experiences. As they seek licensure and registration to practice nursing, some find the procedure and adaptation easy, others find it difficult and frustrating (McGuire & Murphy, 2005; Ogilvie, Leung, Gushuliak, McGuire, & Burgess-Pinto, 2007). CNA (2005b) has developed a regulatory framework for the integration of international applicants. This framework identifies the infrastructure needed to assist internationally educated nurses to meet regulatory requirements and to make the transition into the Canadian health system. It is critical to note that CNA (2005b) recognizes the right of individual nurses to migrate, and it confirms the potential benefits of multicultural practice and learning opportunities supported by migration. However, the association also acknowledges the adverse effect that international migration can have on health care quality in countries seriously depleted of their nursing work force. Therefore, CNA (2005b) does not support the unethical recruitment of registered nurses from countries that are experiencing a nursing shortage either currently or in the future.

On the other hand, regarding mobility, many new graduates seek a career as a travel nurse, which is becoming a norm of Generation Y. The opportunity to live and practice nursing in Paris or Tuscany—or any other place in the world—is highly attractive (Yoder-Wise, 2007). The career path of nurses from Generation Y is not linear in nature. A linear route is distinguished by upward mobility favoured by the Baby Boomers. The career path of Generation Y is spiral in nature, with a mix of lateral and promotional movement more suitable to the expectations of their new work world (Boychuk Duchscher & Cowin, 2004).

Other alarming changes include the anticipation of a global disease, such as the feared Avian influenza, or the possibility of another terrorist attack (Landesman, 2001; Sheff, 2005). The current increased potential for an epidemic spread of disease and the occurrences of disasters are actually a reality in our global society (Stirling, 2004). In the World Health Organization Report (2007), the Director-General states that the disease situation is anything but stable. Population growth, the invasion of previously underpopulated areas, rapid urbanization, intensive farming practices, environmental degradation, and the misuse of microbial agents have disrupted the equilibrium of the microbial world. New diseases are emerging at the historically unprecedented rate of one per year. This rate is most alarming to those health professionals who must care for individuals who succumb to the disease.

In the second outbreak of SARS in Toronto, on May 23, 2003, a multidisciplinary approach was undertaken at the North York General Hospital to manage the impact of the disease. The successful approach was made possible because of the hard work and thoughtful effort of individuals, as well as through quick and effective collaborations of many people. In addition, active and open communication was maintained among all departments, employees, clients, and families. These actions proved to be essential during the outbreak (Loutfy et al., 2004). The question that arises is: Are nurses in Canada adequately prepared for disaster management (Langan & James, 2005)?

> ***reflective* THINKING**   What is your understanding of disaster management?

Many scholars argue that globalization has provided vast opportunities for women, lesbians and gay men, disabled individuals, and indigenous people, whereby they are able to mobilize their abilities and talents to a degree that was generally unavailable to them several years ago (Kickbusch, 2006). Unfortunately, the other dimension of globalization has exacerbated social inequality and social exclusion within both developed and developing countries (Herdman, 2004). Many humanitarian movements have been created to address global inequality and poverty, emphasizing that social justice and health are human rights (De Feyter, 2005). These actions suggest that a strong dialogue on global health is needed at the national level, whereby citizens and politicians become engaged in a unified global health agenda. One item on the agenda might be an exploration of new forms of financing that move beyond a charity model of foreign aid and at the same time, establish mechanisms of accountability among the many actors involved (Kickbusch, 2006).

> ***reflective* THINKING**   How can nurse leaders contribute to the dialogue on global health at the political level?

Implications of Globalization for Nurse Leaders

The CNA, in its Position Statement on Global Health and Equity (CNA, 2003), recounts the belief that global health—the optimal well-being of all humans from the individual and collective perspective—is a fundamental human right. CNA (2003) believes that governments have an obligation to promote the best interest of the public and urges the Canadian government to be a strong advocate for global health and equity on several fronts.

Advocacy and Partnership With Nursing Agencies

One of those fronts is for governments to improve factors that determine health in communities and countries at risk. Through funding from the Canadian International Development Agency, CNA has been creating partnerships with national nursing associations in developing countries for more than 30 years. The goal of the partnership is to increase the capacity of national nursing associations and consequently strengthen the nursing profession, including the quality of nursing and health services delivered to their populations (CNA, 2007a). Encouraging and establishing international health partnerships to advance global health and equity is part of CNA's commitment to social justice (CNA, 2005c). Figure 15.2 portrays a virtual meeting with Canadian and African nurse leaders

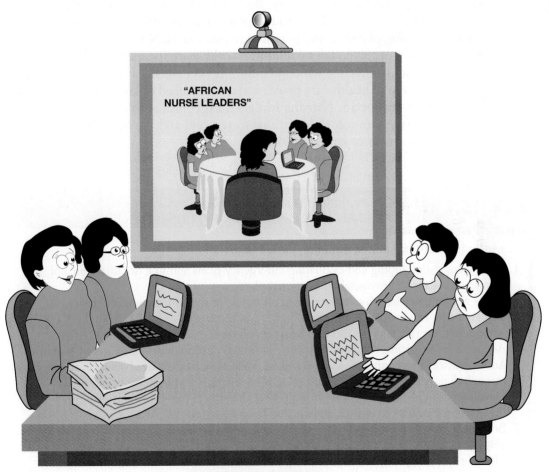

CANADIAN NURSE LEADERS

FIGURE 15.2 Nurse leaders collaborating on global issues.

who are trying to advance professional regulation for improved client safety and outcomes.

Disaster Preparedness

Regarding national disasters and emergencies in Canada, all levels of government are involved in preparing for, and responding to, an emergency or a disaster (Public Health Agency of Canada, 2005). Gebbie and Qureshi (2002) discuss core competencies for nurses after the terrorist attacks in the United States. They believe that an imperative need exists for nurses to know how to serve effectively as a member of an emergency and response team. The CNA has prepared a Position Statement on Emergency Preparedness and Response. CNA believes that the nursing profession plays an integral role in all aspects of emergencies, including mitigation, preparedness, response, and recovery. Box 15.1 outlines the responsibilities of the nurse in emergency preparedness and response with the underlying realization that extensive ongoing planning and practice are essential (CNA, 2007b).

Health care professionals around the world share increasing vulnerability to emergency and disaster for which planning is needed. Because nurses comprise the largest group of health care professionals, they need to know how to respond when tragic events occur. Nursing leaders must continue to support nurses who need additional education to learn how to respond and the best methods to use in response (Langan & James, 2005).

BOX 15.1 EMERGENCY PREPAREDNESS AND RESPONSE: THE CANADIAN NURSES ASSOCIATION POSITION

Canadian health professionals, including nurses, will:

1. Participate in developing and evaluating emergency plans and link organization and community plans to provincial and national plans.
2. Deliver emergency health care services at all points of the continuum: mitigation, preparedness, response, and recovery.
3. Articulate their role and the value of being involved in emergency planning.
4. Advocate for involving vulnerable groups and other stakeholders in emergency planning.
5. Address factors that contribute to emergencies, such as climate change, violence, and poverty, through their roles in clinical practice, education, research, administration, and policy.
6. Develop personal emergency plans that reflect the ethical values of their profession and recognize the needs of family members and pets.
7. Before an emergency, think through and discuss ethical issues and questions with colleagues, employers, union representatives, and others.
8. Maintain the competencies required to participate in emergency management.
9. Before an emergency, join registries of volunteer health care providers.

From Canadian Nurses Association. (2007). *Position Statement: Emergency Preparedness and Response.* Ottawa, ON: Author. PS–91.

Reflections on Leadership Practice

*Y*ou are a nurse unit manager in an emergency department of a large rural hospital. You have just been alerted to the fact that the ambulance is bringing in many people, children included, who were rescued from a forest fire that engulfed their communities.

1. What is the emergency plan in your department?

2. How will you mobilize your health care team to act in an ethical manner recognizing the immediate needs of the clients and their families?

3. What types of competencies are needed by nurses to cope with such an emergency?

Technology

The use of information and communication technology (ICT) is on the increase as an interactive means of transmitting health information (Côté, 2006). That is, the use of health informatics, including such innovations as virtual education, tele-health, decision-support systems, and workload measurement through electronic charting, is widespread in nursing practice (Hannah, 2007). It appears to be critical in meeting the challenges of accessibility and continuity of care and services faced by our present health care system (Côté, 2006). Information systems enable nurse leaders to capture effectively cost and quality indicators that are used to improve nursing practice, thereby improving efficiency and efficacy of health care (Vlasses & Smeltzer, 2007).

Nurse leaders will need to perform a range of activities in developing practice models to fit the coming age, when space and time will be more compressed, and the locus of control will shift from the provider to the user (Porter O'Grady & Malloch, 2007).

reflective **THINKING** What are your own thoughts and feelings regarding the use of ICT in health care?

According to Hannah (2007), the ". . .information revolution has been the driving force in the formation of the Canadian Institute for Health Information and a pan-Canadian electronic health record (EHR) through Canada Health Infoway" (p. 19). Infoway considers that the EHR will hold the "key health history" of Canadians, the scope of which currently includes information related to such aspects as past medical history and current diagnoses (Nagle, 2007). Although the health information is owned by the individual, the EHR will be accessible to any authorized health care provider from any point of care within a jurisdiction and from authorized providers outside the jurisdiction (Nagle, 2007).

EHRs and enhanced information exchange could improve health care quality. For example, one emerging focus is the design and deployment of "client portals." Using the Internet, these portals (windows or views of one's own personal health information) could empower individuals and families by providing access to diagnostic results, health information and education, and client support communities and forums as well (Nagle, 2007). These new monitoring approaches are revolutionizing the ways in which nurses organize their work, allowing nursing care to be available to a greater number of clients and their families. These advances in ICT will continue to change consumers' attitudes toward engaging in their own health care and their interface with the health care system (Dickerson & Brennan, 2002).

The use of eHealth tools, such as telehealth technologies, holds tremendous promise for supporting and enabling health behaviour change, for example, in the management of chronic diseases (Nguyen, Cuenco, Wolpin, Benditt, & Carrieri-Kohlman, 2007). CNA (2007c), in its position statement *Telehealth: The Role of the Nurse*, claims that nursing practice in telehealth is consistent with the philosophy and approach of primary health care. Telehealth should enhance existing health care services by improving their accessibility, appropriate use, and efficiency. However, a recent survey of the eHealth landscape found that despite progress in the field, significant evidence to support the effectiveness of these applications remains limited (Ahern, Kreslake, & Phalen, 2006). More research is warranted to analyze and interpret data that support these health care preferences.

reflective **THINKING** Design a research question to test the effectiveness of telehealth on a group of diabetic clients.

Even though the accelerated transformation of information and the rapid delivery of goods and services are both seen as increasingly normal today, a question remains. Will an increase in the radical changes in technology and information systems, consumer demand, and service structure create more chaos then currently experienced (Porter O'Grady & Malloch, 2007; Stanhope, Lancaster, Jessup-Falcioni, & Viverais-Dresler, 2008)? More importantly, are nurses sufficiently well prepared to meet the challenges and work systematically with decision makers on the principles, values, and intent of health actions?

Implications of Technology for Nurse Leaders

Improving the development and use of health information are high priorities for health care providers and governments around the world who focus on strengthening health care systems for a greater positive impact on the health of their citizens. In fact, CNA (2006) believes that information management and communications technology are integral to nursing practice. The association advocates for a client-centred, pan-Canadian EHR to improve client safety. In doing so, the EHR must meet the following criteria:

- Respect and protect the privacy of client information.
- Include the establishment and integration of unique identifiers for registered nurses.
- Include clinical care data from all disciplines.
- Design changes in collaboration with registered nurses to ensure that clinical data is captured in a standardized way to reflect the practice and impact of nursing care (CNA, 2006).

CNA (2006) believes that to implement the ICT while maintaining the data standards that the Canadian health system needs, registered nurses must be provided adequate support in making the transition to electronic health care systems.

As Canada seeks to maintain its leadership position in the health care field, while continuing to improve the effectiveness of the health care system, nurse leaders need to improve their competencies and their use of ICT in their own nursing practice. Then they need to go on to assist other health care team members to achieve the same results.

Health Disparities

Most Canadians enjoy a relatively high level of health (Public Health Agency Canada, 2002). However, Canada is a stratified society in which certain groups are more vulnerable to poverty than others as a result of the unequal distribution of both income and wealth. Most of these disadvantaged people are women, children, persons with disabilities, and Aboriginal people (Harman, 2000).

Research Findings Related to Health Disparities

A study conducted by Kosteniuk and Dickenson (2003), from the University of Saskatchewan, found that higher household income, being retired, and growing older are all significantly associated with lower stress levels. In another Canadian study, when the effects of low income on infant health were studied, the researchers concluded that less than sufficient household incomes were associated with poorer health and higher hospital admissions in the first 5 months of life (Seguin, Xu, Potvin, Zunzunegui, & Frohlick, 2003). After studying 6,748 women between ages 20 and 64 years, another group of Canadian researchers found that women in the lowest income group are about five times more likely to report poor or marginal health. Not surprisingly, those with higher incomes are more likely to report better health (Ing & Reutter, 2003).

Raphael (2002) states that the incidence of cardiovascular disease is particularly related to the incidence of poverty—a situation that applies to a number of diseases. No public consideration has been noted in Canada about the role societal factors, such as job loss, play in the incidence of cardiovascular disease, nor has there been mention of how recent changes in income distribution and social exclusion may be affecting the cardiovascular health of Canadians. Canadian researchers from all disciplines, including nursing, need to investigate more seriously the role of societal determinants of health such as income on the incidence of cardiovascular disease (Raphael, 2002).

> *reflective* **THINKING**   What other diseases may be particularly related to poverty? What may be other social determinants affecting disease?

Poverty Levels

In Canada, an uncomfortable number of children, adults, elderly people, homeless people, and new immigrants are poor. Further, chronically ill and disabled individuals and divorced women all may become poor. For example, child poverty rates are disproportionately high among vulnerable social groups. Such children are more likely to drop out of school and become unemployed. Lone mothers and their children continue to be one of the most economically vulnerable groups in Canada. One in eight children lives in poverty when income is measured after income taxes. Ontario, as the largest province, remains the child poverty capital of Canada, with 44% of Canada's low-income children living in that province (Campaign 2000, 2007).

An increasing body of research indicates that lone mothers and their children are at a higher than average risk for health problems (Curtis & Pennock, 2006). Based partly on the increase in the Aboriginal population, the plight of First Nations children in their communities as well as the conditions of urban Aboriginal children require sustained action to ensure that these children will thrive, not merely survive (Raphael, 2002). For example, infant mortality is higher among the poor in isolated communities and among Aboriginal peoples (Macionis & Gerber, 2008).

Implications of Disparities for Nurse Leaders

Nurse leaders should be aware that at a 2002 Toronto conference, a special group of social and health policy experts, community representatives, and health researchers considered the state of 10 key social determinants of health. A few of the social determinants identified as important and relevant to the health of Canadians were early childhood development, employment and working conditions, income, and equitable distribution of health care services. Because of the concern that the conditions surrounding the determinants were eroding, the Toronto Charter on the Social Determinants was developed to outline action for government at all levels, the media, public health, health agencies, and associations. The Toronto Charter on Social Determinants of Health is, and will continue to be, a valuable tool for promoting health and social justice (Raphael, Bryant, & Curry-Stevens, 2004).

Working in the health care system, nurses are able to observe the impact of the social determinants of health every day. They see individuals and groups of people who are more susceptible to illness, who experience more complications, or whose recovery process is much longer. During the assessment process, nurses often find links between these people and issues such as low income, high level of stress, job insecurity, poor housing, and social isolation. Nurses can play an important role in addressing social determinants of health by working in their individual practices, helping to reorient the health care system, and advocating for healthy public policies (CNA, 2005a). The CNA Code of Ethics argues that nursing ethics is concerned with how broad societal issues affect the health and well-being of individuals. This means that nurse leaders should undertake to address social inequities by becoming politically active and advocate for change (CNA, 2008b).

reflective **THINKING** What steps can you take as a nurse leader to advocate for change regarding several social inequities?

Human Capacity

Margaret J. Wheatley is one of the most innovative and influential organizational thinkers of our time. She has written about humanizing organizations and assisting people to work together more creatively, compassionately, and cooperatively. Her recent book *Finding our Way: Leadership for Uncertain Times* addresses this premise as a theme (Wheatley, 2007). Nurse leaders who find themselves in the midst of rapid change in organizations will find the insights and ideas provided by this author particularly motivating. Box 15.2 illustrates four core principles of change that seem especially relevant to all nurses and that can be enacted by nurse leaders.

BOX 15.2 FOUR CORE PRINCIPLES OF CHANGE

If it can be understood that an essential freedom to develop one's self exists in organizations, then behaviours can be interpreted in a more positive light, and thoughts can be directed toward ways to work with this great force (rather than deal with the consequences of ignoring its existence). Here are four very important principles for practice.

1. Participation is not a choice
   - We have no choice but to invite people to rethink, redesign, and restructure the organization.
   - We ignore people's need to participate at our own peril.
   - If they (people) are involved, they will create a future that has them in it, and they will work to make it happen.
   - People *only* support what they create.
   - Life insists on its freedom to participate and can never be coerced into accepting someone else's plans.
2. Life always reacts to directives. It never obeys them.
   - Regardless of how clear or visionary or important the message is, it can only elicit reactions, not straightforward compliance.
   - If we recognize that this principle is always at work, it changes expectations of what can be accomplished with any communication.
   - If we can offer our work as an invitation to others to engage with us, rather than as a plan or solution, we will develop good thinking relationships with colleagues.
3. We do not see "reality"; we each create our own interpretation of what's real.
   - No two people have exactly the same interpretation of what is going on. Yet at work and at home, we act as if others see what we see and assign the same meaning as we do to events.
   - If we stop and compare observations, we soon discover significant and useful differences in what we noticed and how we interpret the situation.
   - If we talk with colleagues to share perceptions, if we expect and even seek out the great diversity of interpretations that exist, we learn and change.
   - Entering a world of shared significance is achieved *only* by engaging in conversations with colleagues.
4. To create better health in a living system, connect it to more of itself.
   - When a system is troubled, it needs to start talking to itself, especially to those about whom the system has tended to overlook, such as clients and their families.
   - Without feedback, members of the organization are unaware of how or what to change.
   - Quality standards increase when clients and their families are connected to the system.

You are a nurse unit manager on a paediatric unit. After reviewing several policies with the members of the health care team, one policy needs to be clarified and reworked. It is the policy that deals with nurses providing care to clients in hospitals and then in clients' homes after discharge. You have thought deeply about the four principles and are drawn to the fourth principle, which reads, to *create better health in a living system: connect it more to itself.*

What steps will you take to enact the fourth principle through policy change?

What steps will you take to evaluate the effects of the policy change?

The four principles of change focus on connectedness with others. Perry (2008) claims that those relationships with clients and colleagues seem central for nurses' satisfaction. The heart and soul incentives are cherished, but nurses tend to become disillusioned when these humanitarian assets are not as highly valued as other skills in nursing (Peter, Macfarlane, & O'Brien-Pallas, 2004). These nursing scholars extended their observation, stating that salary, vacations, and sick leaves do not adequately compensate for the lack of sufficient opportunity to care for individuals in a deeply meaningful way.

reflective **THINKING** What can nurse leaders do to provide a milieu whereby the "heart and soul" incentives, which are so important to nurses, can flourish?

Spirituality

Heart and soul incentives and the caring for individuals in a meaningful way are inherent in the concept of spirituality. Delgado (2005) states, "Spirituality is characterized by faith, a search for meaning and purpose in life, a sense of connection with others, and a transcendence of self, resulting in a sense of inner peace and well-being" (p. 157). Yet Molzahn and Shields (2008) claim that spirituality is often overlooked and not addressed with clients or even among nurses (Molzahn & Shields, 2008). The question that arises is whether the care-related experiences of compassion, caring, listening, and helping clients and families to find meaning in their illness experience are being realized without nurses thinking that this actually is spiritual care. Nurses are privileged, in a way, to be in a position to work closely with others so that they can provide help to cope with many aspects of the human condition. When one reflects on spirituality and affirms that it warrants a prominent position in the profession of nursing, that is the moment when the nurse leader has begun to connect authentically with others (Molzahn & Shields, 2008).

reflective **THINKING**   What is your understanding of spirituality?

Implications of Meaningfulness for Nurse Leaders

Nurse leaders must be ready to become involved and assist with the development of health care organizations to make them creative and compassionate. This building process can be accomplished in large part through meaningful daily encounters with other nurses, members of the health care team, clients, and families. The main ingredient in the process is listening to and learning from each other. Wheatley (2007) reminds us that, realistically, the process of change cannot be challenged alone; the critical aspect is relying on others and helping them move into relationship with uncertainty and chaos. Spiritual teachers have been doing this for a very long time. Wheatley (2007) argues that to succeed as good leaders, the domain of spirituality needs to be entered and embraced. Researching and developing the methods that promote spiritual leadership and spiritual care have the potential to identify effective nursing care strategies that can foster a healthy workforce and milieu that improve the well-being of clients and their families (Burkhart, Solari-Twadell, & Haas, 2008).

Wheatley (2007) writes that leaders who embrace themselves and others in totality become the energizers for the total organization. Every change begins with the identification of issues that one finds meaningful. Leaders must allow those thoughts to flourish, and they must invite others to share their unique perspective. Wheatley (2007) again reminds us, "Life never stops teaching us about change" (p. 127). Creative nursing leaders embrace those words; they guide, as well as coach, individuals to discover their own experience with life's true nature. Creativity and commitment are the leader's greatest resources.

WEBSITES

■ Canada Health Infoway

http://www.infoway-inforoute.ca/

Canada Health Infoway is a federally funded, independent, not-for-profit organization whose members are Canada's 14 federal, provincial, and territorial Deputy Ministers of Health. *Infoway* is Canada's catalyst for collaborative change to accelerate the use of electronic health information systems and electronic health records across the country. *Infoway* invests in a common, pan-Canadian framework of electronic health record systems where best practices and successful projects in one region can be shared or replicated in another.

■ Bioterrorism and Emergency Preparedness

http://www.phac-aspc.gc.ca/ep-mu/bioem-eng.php

In Canada, all levels of government are involved in preparing for and responding to an emergency or disaster. Municipal governments respond to local emergencies. Provincial and territorial governments respond to emergencies within their borders, but may ask for federal government assistance if the emergency exceeds their resources. The responsibilities of the Public Health Agency of Canada regarding bioterrorism and emergency responses are outlined in this Website.

■ Campaign 2000: End Child Poverty in Canada

http://www.campaign2000.ca/

In 2007, Campaign 2000 released the 2007 Report Card on Child and Family Poverty, revealing that 18 years after the 1989 all-party resolution of the House of Commons, the child poverty rate is *exactly the same*, despite a growing economy, a soaring dollar, and low unemployment. See further details at this Website.

REFERENCES

Ahern, D. K., Kreslake, J. M., & Phalen, J. M. (2006). What is eHealth (6): Perspectives on the evolution of eHealth research. *Journal of Medical Internet Research, 8*(1), e4.

Boychuk Duchscher, J. E., & Cowin, L. (2004). Multigenerational nurses in the workplace. *Journal of Nursing Administration, 34*(11), 493–501.

Burkhart, L., Solari-Twadell, P. A., & Haas, S. (2008). Addressing spiritual leadership. *The Journal of Nursing Administration, 38*(1), 33–39.

Campaign 2000. (2007). *2007 report card on child and family poverty in Canada.* Toronto, ON: Family Service Association of Toronto. Retrieved July 2008 from http://www.campaign2000.ca/

Canadian Nurses Association. (2003). *Position statement: Global health and equity.* Ottawa, ON: Author. PS–69.

Canadian Nurses Association. (2005a). *Backgrounder: Social determinants of health and nursing: A summary of the issues.* Ottawa, ON: Author. BG 008.

Canadian Nurses Association. (2005b). *Position statement: Regulation and integration of international nurse applicants into the Canadian health system.* Ottawa, ON: Author. PS–79.

Canadian Nurses Association. (2005c). *Position statement: International health partnerships.* Ottawa, ON: Author. PS–82.

Canadian Nurses Association. (2006). *Position statement: Nursing information and knowledge management.* Ottawa, ON: Author. PS–87.

Canadian Nurses Association. (2007). *Position Statement: Emergency Preparedness and Response.* Ottawa: Author. PS–91.

Canadian Nurses Association. (2007a). *Knowing no boundaries: The Canadian nurses association and its international health partnerships 1976–2006.* Ottawa, ON: Author.

Canadian Nurses Association. (2007b). *Position Statement: Emergency Preparedness and Response.* Ottawa: Author. PS–91.

Canadian Nurses Association. (2007c). *Position statement: Telehealth: The role of the nurse.* Ottawa, ON: Author. PS–89.

Canadian Nurses Association. (2008a). A vibrant new health care system by 2020: CNA's bold vision. *Canadian Nurse, 104*(2), 13.

Canadian Nurses Association. (2008b). *Code of ethics for registered nurses* (2008 centennial edition). Ottawa, ON: Author.

Côté, J. (2006). Using interactive health communication technology in a renewed approach to nursing. *Canadian Journal of Nursing Research, 38*(4), 135–136.

Curtis, L. J., & Pennock, M. (2006). Social assistance, lone parents, and health: What do we know, where do we go? *Canadian Journal of Public Health, 97*(Supplement 3), S4–S10.

De Feyter, K. (2005). *Human rights—social justice in the age of the market.* London, UK: Zed Books.

Delgado, C. (2005). A discussion of the concept of spirituality. *Nursing Science Quarterly, 18*(2), 157–162.

Dickerson, S. S., & Brennan, P. F. (2002). The internet as a catalyst for shifting power in provider-patient relationships. *Nursing Outlook, 50*(5), 195–203.

Gebbie, K. M., & Qureshi, K. (2002). Emergency and disaster preparedness: Core competencies for nurses. *American Journal of Nursing, 102*(1), 46–51.

Hannah, K. J. (2007). The state of nursing informatics in Canada. *The Canadian Nurse, 103*(5), 18–19, 22.

Harman, L. D. (2000). Family poverty and economic struggles. In N. Mandell & A. Duffy (Eds.), *Canadian families: Diversity, conflict, and change* (3rd ed., pp. 241–275). Toronto, ON: Nelson.

Herdman, E. A. (2004). Globalization, internationalization and nursing. *Nursing and Health Sciences, 6*, 237–238.

Ing, J. D., & Reutter, L. (2003). Socioeconomic status, sense of coherence, and health in Canadian women. *Canadian Journal of Public Health, 94*(3), 224–228.

Kickbusch, I. (2006). Mapping the future of public health: Action on global health. *Canadian Journal of Public Health, 97*(1), 6–8.

Kosteniuk, J. G., & Dickinson, H. D. (2003). Tracing the social gradient in the health of Canadians: Primary and secondary determinants. *Social Science & Medicine, 57*(2), 263–276.

Landesman, L. Y. (2001). Essentials of disaster planning. In L. Y. Landesman (Ed.), *Public health management of disasters* (pp. 109–119). Washington, DC: American Public Health Association.

Langan, J. C., & James, D. C. (2005). *Preparing nurses for disaster management.* Upper Saddle River, NJ: Pearson Education.

Loutfy, M., Wallington, T., Rutledge, T., Mederski, B., Rose, K., Kwolek, S., et al. (2004). Hospital preparedness and SARS. *Emerging Infectious Diseases, 10*(5), 771–776.

Macionis, J., & Gerber, L. (2008). *Sociology* (6th Canadian ed.). Toronto, ON: Pearson Prentice Hall.

McGuire, M., & Murphy, S. (2005). The internationally educated nurse: Well-researched and sustainable programs are needed to introduce internationally educated nurses to the culture of nursing practice in Canada. *The Canadian Nurse, 101*(1), 25–29.

Molzahn, A., & Shields, L. (2008). Why is it so hard to talk about spirituality? *The Canadian Nurse, 104*(1), 25–30.

Nagle, L. M. (2007). Informatics: Emerging concepts and issues. *Nursing Leadership, 20*(1), 30–32.

Nguyen, H. Q., Cuenco, D., Wolpin, S., Benditt, J., & Carrieri-Kohlman, V. (2007). Methodological considerations in evaluating eHealth interventions. *Canadian Journal of Nursing Research. 39*(1), 116–134.

Ogilvie, L., Leung, B., Gushuliak, T., McGuire, M., & Burgess-Pinto, E. (2007). Licensure of internationally educated nurses seeking professional careers in the province of Alberta in Canada. *International Migration & Integration, 8*(2), 223–241.

Perry, B. (2008). Shine on: Achieving career satisfaction as a registered nurse. *The Journal of Continuing Education in Nursing, 38*(1), 17–25.

Peter, E., MacFarlane, A., & O'Brien-Pallas, L. (2004). Analysis of the moral habitability of the nursing work environment. *Journal of Advanced Nursing, 47*(4), 356–367.

Porter-O'Grady, T., & Malloch, K. (2007). *Quantum Leadership: A resource for health care innovation* (2nd ed.).Mississauga, ON: Jones & Bartlett Canada.

Public Health Agency Canada. (2002). *Population health, towards a Canadian understanding: Clarifying the core concepts of population health.* Ottawa, ON: Author. Retrieved July 2008 from http://www.phac-aspc.gc.ca/ph-sp/docs/common-commune/intro.html

Public Health Agency Canada. (2005). *Bioterrorism and emergency preparedness.* Ottawa, ON: Author. Retrieved July 2008 from http://www.phac-aspc.gc.ca/ep-mu/bioem-eng.php

Raphael, D. (2002). *Social justice is good for our hearts: Why societal factors – not lifestyles – are major causes of heart disease in Canada and elsewhere.* Toronto, ON: CSJ Foundation for Research and Education.

Raphael, D., Bryant, T., & Curry-Stevens, A. (2004). Toronto charter outlines future health policy directions for Canada and elsewhere. *Health Promotion International, 19*(2), 269–273.

Seguin, L., Xu, Q., Potvin, L., Zunzunegui, M.-V., & Frohlick, K. L. (2003). Effects of low income on infant health. *Canadian Medical Association Journal, 57*(2), 263–276.

Sheff, B. (2005). Avian influenza: Are you ready for a pandemic? *Nursing, 35*(9), 26–27.

Stanhope, M., Lancaster, J., Jessup-Falcioni, H., & Viverais-Dresler, G. A. (2008). *Community health nursing in Canada.* Toronto, ON: Elsevier Canada.

Stirling, B. (2004). Nurses and the control of infectious disease: Understanding epidemiology and disease transmission is vital to nursing care. *The Canadian Nurse, 100*(9), 16.

Vlasses, F. R., & Smeltzer, C. H. (2007). Toward a new future for healthcare and nursing practice. *Journal of Nursing Administration, 37*(9), 375–380.

Villeneuve, M., & MacDonald, J. (2006). *Toward 2020: Visions for Nursing.* Ottawa, ON: Canadian Nurses Association.

Wheatley, M. J. (2007). *Finding our way: Leadership for an uncertain time.* San Francisco, CA: Berrett-Koehler Publishers.

World Health Organization. (2007). *The world health report 2007, a safer future: global public health security in the 21st century.* Geneva, Switzerland: Author.

Yoder-Wise, P. S. (2007). Key forecasts shaping nursing's perfect storm. *Nursing Administration Quarterly, 31*(2), 115–119.

Index

In this index, *italic* page numbers designate figures; page numbers followed by the letter "t" designate tables; "b" indicates boxed material; *(see also)* cross-references designate related topics or more detailed subtopic breakdowns.

A

Aboriginal communities
  climate change and, 370
  diabetes and, 91–92
  nursing career encouragement in, 195
Aboriginal Head Start On-Reserve, 63
Aboriginal Health Transition Fund, 15
Aboriginal nurse leaders, influence of, 195
Aboriginal Nurses Association of Canada (ANAC), 195
Academy of Canadian Executive Nurses, 160
Accommodation, conflict resolution and, 292
Accountability
  in education/practice settings, 106
  as standard of practice, 203t
Achieving Health for All: A Framework for Health Promotion, 8, 38
Achieving Public Protection Through Collaborative Self-Regulation: Reflections for a New Paradigm (Conference Board of Canada), 202
Action Plan 2007–2010, of CPHI, 65
Adhocracy, 128
Adult population
  ageism and, 358–360
  elder discrimination and, 359–360
  health inequality, for homeless, 44
  health issues of, 360
  nursing and, 358–361
  program development for, 361
  successful aging of, 361
Advisory Committee on Health Delivery, 95
Advocacy. *See also* Political advocacy
  nurse leaders and, *385*, 385–386
    action taken by, 216
Ageism, 358–360
Aherne, M., 125
Aiken, L. H., 182
Akhavan, J., 186
Allen, M. N., 216
Almeida-Filho, N., 43
Almost, J., 290
American Philosophical Association Delphi Research Project, 255
ANAC. *See* Aboriginal Nurses Association of Canada
Anderson, D., 74
Anderson, Judy, 245

Appreciative inquiry
  four-D cycle of, 272–273
  leadership and, 273
  nurse leaders and, 272–273
Argyris, Chris, 118
Arnold, L., 337
Assess Use, Compliance and Efficacy Nursing Workload Measurement Tools (Hadley/Graham/Flannery), 185
Assessment
  of conflict resolution, 290, 291t
  for population health approach, 59–60, 62–70, 63t
    character/growth/size of groups, 62–65
    health status indicators, 65–66
  of team member, 234
  of team performance model, 241–242
Au, A., 121
Auffrey, Lucille, 355
Authority, centralized/decentralized, 129
Avoidance, conflict resolution and, 292

B

Baby Boomers, 286, 357
  Canada population and, 63–64
Baccalaureate degree, Canadian Association of Schools of Nursing/CNA on, 208
Bailey, S., 271
Baker, J. J., 175
Baker, R. W., 175
Barker, A. M., 122, 178
Barriers, to time management, 308–311
  perfectionism, 310
  personal/system, 311
  pessimism, 310–311
  procrastination, 308, 310
Bassendowski, S. L., 213
BATNA. *See* Best alternative to negotiated agreement
Bauer, M., 359
Beaton, M. R., 211
Berger-Wesley, M., 129
Best alternative to negotiated agreement (BATNA), 298
Bishop, M., 340
Black, J., 334
Bloom, Benjamin, 262